Bone Marrow
Structure and Function

Bone Marrow
Structure and Function

Mehdi Tavassoli, M.D., F.A.C.P.
Professor of Medicine
University of Mississippi School of Medicine
Chief, Hematology-Oncology
Director, Cell Biology Laboratory
Veterans Administration Medical Center
Jackson, Mississippi

Joseph Mendel Yoffey, D.Sc., M.D., F.R.C.S. (ENG.)
HON. LL. D. (Manchester)
Emeritus Professor of Anatomy
University of Bristol
Visiting Professor of Anatomy
The Hebrew University-Hadassah
Medical School, Jerusalem

Alan R. Liss, Inc., New York

Address all Inquiries to the Publisher
Alan R. Liss, Inc., 150 Fifth Avenue, New York, NY 10011

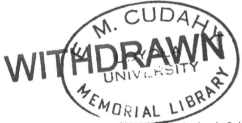

Library of Congress Cataloging in Publication Data

Tavassoli, Mehdi, 1933–
  Bone marrow, structure and function.

  Bibliography: p.
  Includes index.
  1. Bone marrow. I. Yoffey, Joseph Mendel. II. Title.
[DNLM: 1. Bone marrow—Anatomy and histology.
2. Bone marrow—Physiology. WH 380 B7118]
QM569.Y63 1983   612'.491   83-14888
ISBN 0-8451-0226-5

To Marie and Betty

About the Authors

Mehdi Tavassoli is Professor of Medicine at the University of Mississippi Medical Center. He was trained as a hematologist at Tufts University in Boston where he subsequently began a research career in hemopoiesis. For a decade he was affiliated with Scripps Clinic and Research Foundation in LaJolla, California. His research interest centers around the bone marrow and its hemopoietic function, a subject about which he has published extensive original work. He was among the first to demonstrate the microenvironmental requirements for hemopoiesis and to study their nature, and interactions with hemopoietic cells. He has received numerous awards for his original research and has trained a number of investigators who have subsequently done, in their own right, meritorious research in hemopoiesis.

A pioneer investigator and acknowledged world authority on the lymphoid tissues and bone marrow, **Joseph Mendel Yoffey** has pursued an illustrious and influential career devoted to the service of anatomy. In the 1940s he became especially interested in the lymphocytes and related cells in mammalian bone marrow. He developed the concept, which has since stimulated extensive research, that the bone marrow and lymphoid tissues constitute a single system, "The Lymphomyeloid Complex," unified by a continuous interchange of cells. The bone marrow is the central organ of the complex, and provides its main cellular driving force.

After reaching the conventional retirement age he went as a Visiting Professor to the Australian National University to produce a final edition of his major book. Since 1967 he has resided in Jerusalem and held an active Professorship in the Department of Anatomy, Hebrew University-Hadassah Medical School.

Contents

Foreword

Science in our time is incredibly fashion-oriented. Certain subjects and areas may now ride the crest of popularity only to be buried in the well of oblivion before long. They may be reincarnated again. The reasons for this periodicity in the popularity of scientific subjects are not clear, but the tendency has been increasingly amplified as science has become a mass profession and therefore heavily dependent on public funds. The nefarious influence of mass media may be another factor.

A deleterious effect of this fashion orientation is the neglect that non-fashionable areas may suffer. Certain disciplines may entirely be submerged and never recover. Others may move with some regularity from the top to the bottom and vice versa. And yet others may not be totally neglected but the angle of study may become fixed, thus providing a channelized rather than comprehensive view.

Studies of the bone marrow have suffered this last distortion. An observer sitting through one of the frequent meetings and symposia on this subject may come out with the impression that the bone marrow grows in culture dishes and not inside the bone. Undoubtedly, the application of tissue culture techniques, and particularly the clonal analysis of hemopoietic progenitor cells, has given a great impetus in furthering our understanding of hemopoiesis. It has opened new vistas in this field and brought to the surface many new questions for resolution. By simplifying the system, the application of tissue culture permits the analysis of different steps in hemopoiesis. Yet, the marrow is clearly a complex tissue which can also synthesize and integrate all these different steps in such a way that it can respond, in an orderly fashion, to physiological regulatory stimuli. The present volume is an attempt to present a different view of the bone marrow: a view that has been considerably neglected in recent years; a view that considers the marrow as the organ which it actually is. In this attempt the book intends to rectify, to a certain extent, the channelization of views on this subject.

Because we intend to treat only certain neglected aspects of bone marrow studies, the book has been designed as a collection of essays on particular aspects of this subject and not as a complete treatise on bone marrow as a whole. Some of the material has previously appeared in a different form and has been revised and updated in this volume. Because much of the data, collected in this volume, are scattered throughout the literature, this book can be of some reference use as well. Chapters I, II, III, IV, VI, and XI were written by M. Tavassoli and chapters V, VIII, IX, X, XII, XIII, XIV are the work of J.M. Yoffey. Chapter VII is a collaborative effort. J.M. Yoffey would particularly like to place on record his thanks to the following for their kind permission to draw freely on previously published material: (1) Messrs. Edward Arnold, publishers of "Bone Marrow Reactions" in 1966, (2) The Charles C. Thomas Co., publishers of "Bone Marrow in Hypoxia and Rebound" in 1974, and (3) The Academic Press. For permission to use previously published materials in chapters I and XI, M. Tavassoli is grateful to McGraw-Hill and Grune & Stratton, and adds his thanks to Academic. We are also grateful to Mrs. Jackie Davis whose highly organized administrative assistance was indispensable to the completion of this volume.

I.

Historical Perspective

INTRODUCTION

The marrow of our bones is the seedbed of our blood. Like blood, it is essential to life. It is, after the blood itself, the largest and most widely dispersed organ in our body. We harbor more than 1 trillion cells in our marrow at any one time. Every day more than 200 billion red cells, 10 billion white cells, and 400 billion platelets are produced in the marrow. Here is where all lymphocytes and scavenger monocytes originate. A variety of other functions are attributed to the marrow. Birds carry air in their marrow not only to aid in levitation but apparently to serve a respiratory function as well [Meyer and Meltzer, 1916]. There is an interesting cyclic change in pigeons: Before ovulation, the marrow cavity is almost entirely obliterated by bone, which is then resorbed during ovulation and the bone minerals are used to form the egg shell [Bloom et al, 1941].

As one might surmise, a production center of this magnitude is highly vulnerable to malfunction or to the deleterious effects of various factors such as anticancer drugs. In fact, the marrow is currently the single most important limiting factor in cancer treatment. The reason that the treatment of cancer is often not definitive is because the marrow cannot tolerate it. However, the marrow is endowed with considerable potential for self-renewal, which mitigates the impact of its exquisite sensitivity. In this regard its wide dispersion is a distinct advantage.

We have not known all this for very long. For centuries, poets, healers, and philosophers saw and described the close link between blood and life. Not so the marrow. Its role as the seedbed of blood lay hidden, like a seed in the soil. It began to sprout hardly more than a hundred years ago when Ernst Neumann (Fig. I.1) and Giulio Bizzozero (Fig. I.2) established the link between blood and marrow. Ever since, marrow research has been a fertile field, fruitful not only to medicine but to the fundamental understanding of life itself. Scientists have used the marrow as a model for the elucidation of basic questions in biology. In some instances, new fields of biomedical

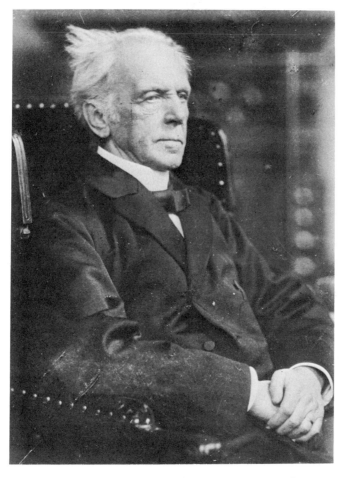

Fig. I-1.   Ernst Neumann (1834–1918).

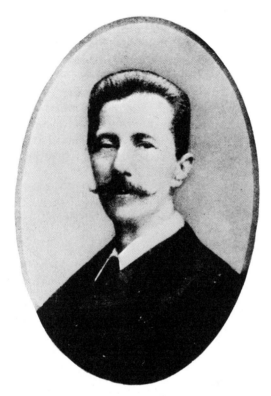

Fig. 1-2. Giulio Bizzozero (1846–1901).

research have emerged from studies of the marrow—eg, radiobiology, cell kinetics, and transplantation.

A TRACE IN THE REALM OF IDEAS

In most languages, marrow denotes the inmost of the central part. Metaphorically, it connotes the essence, the substance, the vital part, or the "goodness." Thus, in the prologue of Gargantua, Rabelais invites us to "break the bone and to suck the substantive marrow." And in Hamlet, we are told:

> It takes
> From our achievement through perform'd a height
> The pith and marrow of our attribute.

From the ancient days, the marrow of animals was used for food and was considered to be rich and nutritious. During the 12th century, marrow was considered a "dainty," and cookbooks gave recipes for preparing it. In 1539, Sir Thomas Elyot thought, "Marrowe is more dilectable than the brayne."

In modern times, as everything came to have a scientific aroma, the nutritious effect of marrow was tested by physicians. In the 1890s, first Brown-Sequard [Brown-Sequard and d'Arsonval, 1891, 1892] and then others fed marrow to patients with blood dyscrasias, but to no avail. The matter was then laid to rest only to be revived in the 1920s. Whipple's study of the effects of different foods on hemoglobin production stimulated further interest. Isolated, anecdotal case reports claimed that patients recovered from blood dyscrasias after eating marrow. By 1929, however, it was clear that the only nutritious effect of marrow was due to its iron content. These experiments were the forerunners of marrow transplantation, as some physicians naively hoped that they could transfer living cells by feeding the marrow [Pegg, 1966].

During the 16th and 17th centuries, the marrow was considered a source of warmth, energy, and inner heat: "Thy bone is marrowless, thy blood is cold," said Shakespeare. "Love" was said to burn, or to "melt the marrow." Perhaps in this connotation, the marrow was also considered the seat of vitality and strength: "Marrowy and vigorous manhood," said Oliver Wendell Holmes. "Spending his manlie marrow in her armes," said Shakespeare. Prior to the discovery of its blood-forming function, the marrow was believed to be the source of bone nutrition. Identification of large bones with physical strength and manhood might have led to the designation of the marrow as a source of strength. In 1926, Mechanik, who was measuring the volume of the marrow, found that "under comparable conditions, man has more marrow than woman, a highly noteworthy characteristic of the normal sex differences in man until now unknown." The major product of the marrow, red cell mass, also is known to be lower in the female sex than the male.

THE PATH OF A DISCOVERY

Historic events do not take place in a vacuum. The course of history is a continuum wherein every event relates to a preceding one and leads to the next. Neumann's revelation that the marrow is the seedbed of blood was the culmination of a search for the origin of red cells that had begun much earlier.

Red cells were first described in the 17th century, but it was not until the 19th century that a search for their origin could begin. The intervening period, the entire 18th century, was spent in a seemingly endless squabble, which achieved little more than establishing the identity of the red cell. In fact, for biology as a whole, this was a century of indolence, torpor, and inaction. Nothing positive could be achieved without the synthesis of a conceptual frame that could serve as a *point de depart* for future work; this came in 1838 with the formulation of the cell theory.

The formulation of a cell theory, the conceptualization of the cell (the "little room") as the fundamental unit of life, was the dawn of a new era in biology. It was conceived in 1838 by Mathias Schleiden [Schleiden, 1838] and Theodor Schwann [Schwann, 1847]. From then on, biology moved rapidly. The rest of the 19th century was the *aurea aetas*, when the foundations of many disciplines were laid—bacteriology and immunology, pathology and histochemistry, modern biochemistry and genetics, and antisepsis and modern surgery. This was the century that provided great workers in biology. The essence of this period is well reflected in two quotations from Claude Bernard. In 1855, when he was appointed professor of experimental medicine, the opening sentence of his inauguration lecture was, "Experimental medicine which I am supposed to teach you, does not exist." Some 15 years later, as the president of the Paris Academy of Sciences, he amended this statement: "The dawn of experimental medicine is now visible on the scientific horizon."

It was within this scientific ambience that the search for the origin of red cells began and for several decades was focused on embryonic life. This was only natural: Scholars of this period did not know that blood formation is a continuous process, and takes place throughout life. The finite life-span of red cells, and therefore the necessity for their continuous replenishment, was not recognized. As late as 1923, Peyton Rous wrote, "So subtly is normal blood destruction conducted and the remains of the cells disposed of, that, were it not for indirect evidence, one might suppose the life of most red corpuscles to endure with that of the body" [Rous, 1923]. As late as 1905, Jolly found remnants of the nucleus in some red cells and none in others. He postulated two cell lineages and wrote, "In search of their origin, I have naturally searched the blood of mammalian embryos" [Jolly, 1905]. Evidently, the assumption was that blood cells, once formed in the embryo, remain in the body throughout life.

Neumann is rightly credited with the recognition of the marrow as the seat of blood formation. However, it is generally unrecognized that, conceptually, his most fundamental contribution was his recognition that blood formation is a continuous process, occurring during postnatal life. It was this concept that formed the frame of reference for much of the work that followed. His first brief communication of 1868 does not reflect this, suggesting that he attained this conceptual view gradually. But, the opening paragraph of his 1869 note [Neumann, 1869a] reads:

> The present work intends to demonstrate the physiologic importance of the bone marrow and that it is an important organ for blood formation which has not been recognized. It operates continually in a *de novo* formation of red blood cells.

To reach this conclusion, Neumann used deductive logic based on a premise that later proved incorrect. For a different reason, however, the conclusion remains valid: Neumann thought that proliferation of marrow cells occurred inside the blood vessels of the bone marrow, and reasoned that these continuously proliferating cells must also continuously move out into the general circulation; otherwise the blood circulation in the marrow would stop. We now know that red cell proliferation does not take place inside the blood vessels, but Neumann's conclusion remains valid because all blood formation takes place within a fixed volume inside a rigid frame of bone, where for every cell that is born, within or outside the blood vessels, one must leave to maintain the fixed volume.

Here, a corrective note is necessary. Most historical introductions on the marrow suggest that a substantive contribution was made by Claude Bernard [Michels, 1931; Ness and Stengle, 1974]. These all refer to Volume 68 of *Comptes Rendues* of the Paris Academy of Sciences. Examination of the original document [Neumann, 1869a] indicates that in this particular year, Claude Bernard, in his capacity as a member of the Academy, introduced a paper by Neumann, who was not a member. The title reads, "The Function of Bone Marrow in the Formation of Blood. Note by Mr. Neumann, presented by Mr. Claude Bernard."

Opposition to Neumann's discovery was most intense in Paris, where almost every eminent histologist had a theory on red cell production (vide infra). Bernard recognized Neumann's depth of vision and strongly supported his views. But there is nowhere, in this or other volumes of *Comptes Rendues*, an indication that Claude Bernard himself made a substantive contribution to this subject.

A VISIONARY DUO

Neumann's discovery was announced in the form of a preliminary report, which appeared as the lead article in the issue of 10 October 1868 of the

Centralblatt fur die medizinischen Wissenshaften [Neumann, 1868]. Here is a translation of "About the Significance of Bone Marrow for Blood Formation, Preliminary Communication by Prof. E. Neumann":

> In the so-called red bone marrow of man as well as the rabbit, one can regularly find, in addition to the well-known marrow cell, certain other elements which have not been mentioned until now; namely nucleated red blood cells, in every respect corresponding to embryonic stages of the red blood cells.
>
> Also in the marrow rich in fat, the same cells are present but in lower quantity and their number decreases parallel to the decrease in the number of marrow cells and the increase in the number of fat cells.
>
> It is possible to trace the origin of these elements to the marrow cells. The high content of colorless elements in the blood of the marrow makes it likely that there is a migration of contractile marrow cells into the vessels.
>
> A thorough description of my observations will be published.

The promised thorough description appeared the next year in an extensive article in *Archiv der Heilkunde* [Neumann, 1869b]. In the interim, however, two communications appeared in Italian and were soon translated in the *Centralblatt* [Bizzozero, 1868, 1869]. They were both by Bizzozero, confirming the observation that nonnucleated red blood cells are formed from nucleated red cells in the marrow. Bizzozero extended the blood-forming function of the marrow to include the formation of white cells.

A careful reading of these interesting communications leaves one with the impression that perhaps Bizzozero might have come to this conclusion even before Neumann, but that he was unsure of the reception he might receive if his findings were announced. The rapidity with which Bizzozero's announcement appeared following publication of Neumann's announcement supports this speculation. It is worth mentioning that Neumann was a well-established professor in the European tradition [Askanazy, 1918], whereas Bizzozero was but a 22-year-old recent graduate facing considerable opposition in his hometown of Pavia. His appointment to the faculty of medicine was pushed through, thanks to the recommendation of his mentor, Mantegazza, in the face of opposition by other faculty members, who cited his youth [Ghisalberti, 1960]. It should also be noted that in some areas, the views of Neumann and Bizzozero were not exactly identical. Retrospectively, in all these instances, Bizzozero proved to be correct.

Of the two, however, Neumann was a more persistent student of the subject. He continued his work on the marrow, and toward the end of the century produced other classic contributions. Among his "firsts" was the identification of leukemia [Neumann, 1870] as a disease of the marrow. He coined the term "myelogenous leukemia" [Neumann, 1878].

Like Immanuel Kant, Neumann preferred to remain a lifelong citizen of Konigsberg, where he taught and worked almost all his life on blood production and blood pigments. His superb literary taste, reflected in his masterful German writings, provides the profile of a German scholar in the classical sense. Bizzozero, by contrast, led a very unsettled life. Born in Varese, he studied in Milan and completed his medical studies in Pavia. He subsequently trained with Virchow in Berlin and, for a brief period, settled in Torino. He then moved to Rome where he became a senator. The scope of his scientific interest was also varied. His early interest in the vascular system was soon replaced by interest in the marrow, but after a decade, he focused on the coagulation mechanism and recognized and coined the term "platelet." Toward the end of his life, he developed choroiditis, which interfered with the microscopic work. His interest then turned to issues affecting public health. He died at the turn of the century, rather prematurely, at the age of 55.

Even before Neumann and Bizzozero, the transition of the nucleated to nonnucleated red cell had been seen in the liver by Kolliker [1846], a German scholar. The French anatomist Charles Robin [1849] had also come close to this discovery, but he did not recognize the kinship of red cells to marrow cells. He coined the term "marrow cells" (*medullocelles*), which apparently is what Neumann referred to as *bekannten Markzellen* [Neumann, 1868]—the well-known marrow cells.

This frontier of knowledge was thus being explored intensively. Had not Neumann made his discovery known, it would surely have been made by others. It is the curious nature of science that, in Bergsonian terms, it has its own *elan vital*, its own momentum. With some exceptions, humanity is but an instrument of this momentum to expand the boundary of knowledge: "It is not the men that make science; it is science that makes the men [Chargaff, 1968]".[*]

---

[*]Variations on this theme also appear in Paul Valery's *Mauvaises pensées ou autres* [1941, Paris, Corti], wherein he concludes, "Ce qui fait un ouvrage n'est past celui qui y met son nom. Ce qui fair un ouvrage n'a pas de nom." (The one who does a piece of work has no name.) Bertolt Brecht's *Galileo* is even more emphatic on this note: "There is no scientific work that one man alone can write" (Collected Plays, 1972, New York, Vintage.).

THE MAZE OF THEORIES

The findings of Neumann and Bizzozero had two components. One related to the cellular origin of the red cell; it stated that nonnucleated red cells in the blood are derived from nucleated precursors. The second related to the tissue origin, and stated that this process takes places in the marrow.

The first component stood in contrast to a great number of divergent theories of that time [Michels, 1931; Jolly, 1907; Malassez, 1882], perhaps reflecting the intensity of search for the origin of the red cell. A number of investigators supported the nuclear origin of the red cell. Erb [1865] maintained that red cells are products of disintegration of white cell nuclei. Wharton-Jones [1846] believed that the nuclei of precursor cells swelled by acquiring hemoglobin and became red cells. Pouchet [1878] maintained that red cells might be derived from white cells by hemoglobinic degeneration, similar to fatty degeneration. Weber [1846], on the other hand, thought that red cells were made from fat globules in the liver. Several scholars played different notes on the tune that red cells are protoplasmic offsprings of a precursor cell which is in a state of continuous expansion and budding. To this group belonged Rindfleisch [1880], Rollet [1870], and Malassez [1882]. Generation of hemoglobin in the cytoplasm of vasoformative cells (scavenger cells) was the theory of Ranvier [1874], who maintained that from these cells, red cells are released, plasmidlike, into the circulation. Hayem [1889] thought red cells were made by platelets. Arndt [1881] believed that any protoplasmic fragment could absorb hemoglobin and turn into a red cell. Apparently, in drawing a parallel with nucleated red cells in birds, several investigators, including Boettcher [1866], Lowit [1891], and Stricker [1868], were of the opinion that mammalian red cells also had a nucleus (Innenkorper), albeit not as well defined as that of their avian counterparts.

Some of these theories may now appear strange and even naive, but it should be remembered that during this period, the viable nature of red cells had not yet been established. More than a quarter of a century later, Jolly [1907] observed that "these theories diverted the researchers in a direction completely inconsistent with the viable nature of the red cell." It was against this background that the observations of Neumann and Bizzozero appeared. To see straight through this cloud of confusion, vision was needed; that is what Neumann and Bizzozero offered. They belonged to a generation of scientists who could expand the range of possibilities.

Despite the intensity of the search, Neumann's observations did not catch on easily. His ideas were received with the same skepticism with which Immanuel Kant's *Critique of Pure Reason* had been greeted almost a century before. Neumann was supported by Bizzozero and by Claude Bernard, but there were also Pouchet and Hayem to repudiate him and Robin to accuse him of adding to the confusion by postulating yet another theory. Georges Hayem wrote an entire book in repudiation of Bizzozero! The preface of this book [Hayem, 1889], despite a haughty tone, is but a lamentoso for plausible theories that were about to sink. Later, in reference to Hayem, Jolly [1907] deplored the "unfortunate" influence that did not permit Neumann's theory to be accepted universally for about 20 years.

To understand this skepticism, we may remember that during this period all students of the subject had their pet theories, which they defended vehemently. Moreover, in their initial presentations, Neumann and Bizzozero could not provide compelling evidence to override the maze of theories. They saw nucleated red cells in the marrow and concluded that they are the source of nonnucleated red cells. Naturally, this was received as "yet another theory." At any rate, "compelling evidence" in those days consisted of demonstrating the transition forms between the two cells: *post hoc ergo propter hoc.*

The confusion may not have been all that unjustified. During this period, histologists were working at the limits of their methodological potential. Without further developments in fixation and staining techniques, little substantive information could be gained. Charles Robin is an example. He studied the marrow in 1849 using acetic acid in his preparations. Consequently, the hemoglobin was leached out of nucleated red cells, and he was unable to recognize their kinship to their nonnucleated products [Robin, 1849]. Apparently, with reference to Robin and mindful of his mistake, both Neumann and Bizzozero repeatedly emphasized the necessity of using a neutral fixative or no fixative at all.

Despite all the opposition, however, within two decades, Neumann's discovery was a scientific axiom! The brilliance of truth may first be blinding, but ultimately it supersedes all artificial illuminators.

BEYOND THE MARROW

The observations of Neumann and Bizzozero related not only to the cellular origin but also to the tissue origin of the red cell. They stated that the marrow is the major production center of red cells. On this issue, the scientific ambience was less opinionated and this concept should have fared better. Actually, it did not. Scholars of that period, being deeply entangled in the theories of the cellular origin of the red cell, were oblivious to the tissue in which the search should be made. Most searched in the blood; few found it necessary to look in other tissues. The epitome of this attitude is shown by the work of Georges Pouchet [1878]. In 1878, he reported on the regeneration of red cells in a dog that had been bled. He examined the blood but not the marrow. He found no nucleated red cells and concluded that nucleated cells could not be the origin of red cells, for, were it so, "it would be difficult to admit that none of these elements could find their way into the circulation." He then observed an increased number of platelets, now a well-recognized occurrence after blood loss, and concluded that platelets were the source of red cells. "In the field of experimentation, chance favors only the prepared mind," said Louis Pasteur, who, during the same period, was engaged in a battle with another Pouchet, Felix. The latter, believing in the spontaneous generation of microbes, repudiated Pasteur's germ theory [Dubos, 1950].

We may remember, however, that during this time, researchers were studying various species from frog to bat to human. Nucleated red cells had been seen in many other tissues, and even after the function of the marrow in blood formation had been generally accepted, there was no reason that this site should exclude other sites. Thus, in defense of their view, Neumann and Bizzozero began a systematic study of various tissues in a variety of species. Their studies lasted nearly two decades and showed that in adult humans, red cell production is limited to the marrow [Bizzozero and Torre, 1884; Neumann, 1890]. The only dissent came from Harvey Jordan, who, some 30 years later, maintained that lymph nodes also could produce red cells [Jordan, 1926]. He argued that plasma cells were but aborted red cells. This is the more interesting because during this period, Jordan [1927] raised another dissenting voice, this time against, to quote Florence Sabin [1928], the "majority opinion" that red cells originate from the vascular wall. The minority of one, Jordan, proved to be correct in his dissent, and proved once again that truth is not achieved by consensus. Indeed, science is not a democratic domain.

THE FAVORABLE ENVIRONMENT

The "majority opinion" to which Sabin refers had evolved as a corollary to Neumann's discovery. Once the marrow was established as the site of blood cell formation, it was natural to search in the marrow not only for the immediate parent cells but also for their ancestors. This led to the assumption that the ancestor cells of blood cells originate in the marrow. The assumption was based on plausibility, not logic. The bone marrow is certainly a production center for blood cells, but no logical dictum requires that the ancestor cells originate there. Simply because a product comes out of a factory, we do not assume that its basic constituents also originate there.

Yet, this assumption provided the frame of reference for students of the marrow during the first quarter of our century, and formed the basis of the "majority opinion" that the ancestor cell of the red cell is derived from the vascular wall [Maximow, 1924]. It was the advent of more appropriate methodology, radiobiologic methods and the transplantation technique, that placed the question in perspective: The marrow is a production center whose environment is favorable to the proliferation and growth of blood cells. The ancestor of these cells, the common stem cell, however, might circulate. In its course, it may pass through many organs, but, upon arrival in the marrow, it "homes" and begins to proliferate and produce blood cells like a seed in a fertile soil [Tavassoli, 1975a]. In our age of acronyms, this concept has become known as HIM, for "hematopoietic inductive microenvironment" [Trentin, 1970].

The foundation for this thinking was evident as early as the first decade of this century in the writings of such scholars as Max Askanazy [1911], a pupil of Neumann. Danchakoff [1909], who subscribed to the "majority opinion," remarked that in birds, red cells were produced inside the blood vessels; not so the white cells—they arose on the outside and wandered in. She was of the opinion that the vascular wall gave rise to both red and white cells, and, thus concluded that the environment on the two sides of the wall must be different and must determine which cell type is produced. A few years later, in 1916, in a lecture before the College of Physicians and Surgeons of Columbia University, she was arguing the case for the existence of a common stem cell [Danchakoff, 1916]. She drew an analogy to a heap of tree seeds. In a moderate climate the seeds will grow into tall trees, but in Arctic lands they will develop into trees no higher than our moss:

> How would it be possible to know if there were differences in the seeds? The only possibility of solving this problem would consist of sowing the seeds of arctic lands, the seeds of the different products of development will have been shown to have been identical.
> Similar experiments may be carried out with haematopoietic tissue.

Her prophecy was realized some 50 years later, thanks to the advent of transplantation techniques, which proves that in the absence of appropriate methods, the most brilliant concepts may lead nowhere but to oblivion or stagnation.

RED AND YELLOW MARROW

In the course of evolution, the bone marrow is a latecomer in the task of blood production, but it probably has achieved a high plateau of efficiency.

There are two types of marrow: blood-producing marrow, which is red because of its hemoglobin content; and yellow marrow, containing mostly fat, which imparts a yellowish color. It was Xavier Bichat [1802] who first, at the end of the 18th century, recognized the two types of marrow and coined the terms "red" and "fatty" marrow. He thought that the red marrow was seen in the fetus and the yellow or "true" marrow, in the adult. He recognized that the marrow fat is distinct from the usual variety of fat. Bichat could not yet know of the link between the blood and the marrow; nor could he discuss the changes from red to fatty marrow. The presence of red marrow in the adult was to be recognized later, including even the transitory state between the two, the gelatinous marrow [Gosselin and Regnauld, 1849].

Again, it was Neumann who provided us with the classic statement. In 1882, he enunciated the rule governing the development of yellow marrow. In effect, he recognized a phenomenon that is sometimes referred to as Neumann's law [Neumann 1882b]. It states that at birth, all bones that contain marrow contain red marrow. With age, the blood-producing activity contracts toward the center of the body, leaving the more peripheral bones with only fatty marrow.

For about 50 years, students of the marrow did not know what to make of this phenomenon. The mechanism underlying the development of yellow marrow after birth was not studied until 1936, when Charles Huggins and his co-workers [Huggins and Blocksom, 1936] observed a parallel phenomenon: At birth, the temperature of the marrow is comparable in all bones, but, soon after birth, cooling takes place in the bones of the extremities. This observation immediately suggested a relationship: The thermal environment in the bones of the extremities after birth is not optimal for blood production; consequently, the sites for blood production contract and are confined to the warmer bones in the central part of the body. To test this hypothesis, they looped the rat tail, which contains yellow marrow, and placed it within the warmer environment of the abdomen. Soon, the part located inside the abdomen became red. Here, one is faced with two separate elements of the scientific finding—the contraction of red marrow and the concomitant cooling of the bones; their discoveries were separated by a period of 50 years. Both discoveries, however, were necessary before a logical synthesis could be formulated and tested.

Huggins' explanation has now proved to be an oversimplification. Genetic, functional, and developmental influences may be even more important for the development of yellow marrow [Tavassoli and Crosby, 1970].

OF THE BONE AND ITS MARROW

The most ancient views about the function of the marrow are related to its strange case, the bone. Hippocrates maintained that the marrow is the source of the nutrient supply to the bone, an opinion also held by Galen. Aristotle took the opposite view—viz, the marrow is a waste product of the bone: excrementum ossium [Robin, 1875].

Impressed by the extensive vascularity of the marrow, anatomists of the 18th century expounded on the Hippocratic view and maintained that the marrow is but the vascular component of the bone and is located in the inner part for protection. Considerable interest centered around an ill-defined membrane, the "medullary membrane," which was believed to be an elaborate barrier controlling the nutrition of bone [Robin, 1875]. In 1700, the French anatomist Duverney [1700] argued that many bones, like those of the middle ear, do not have marrow; thus, the marrow could not be all that essential to the nutrition of bone. In the 19th century, Charles Robin [1875] noted that in the course of development, the marrow is formed after the bone and therefore cannot be the source of bone nutrition any more than it can be the origin of its development.

This was an era in science when mechanomorphic views were beginning to become popular. Robin postulated a purely mechanical function for the marrow in relation to the bone. He argued that of two cylinders of similar weights and substance, the one with an empty core—ie, with a larger diameter—is the stronger. Thus, the presence of a marrow cavity in the long bones strengthens them without adding to their weight and, in addition, creates more surface area for the insertion of muscles and ligaments than otherwise would be possible, a postulate hardly testable or contestable.

Experimental medicine, which was then beginning to thrive, provided an opportunity for exploring the relation between the bone and its marrow. Several researchers separated the two tissues by removing bits of the marrow out of the bone and grafting them elsewhere, usually in the abdomen. Some of the first such experiments were done by the French experimentalist Goujon [1866, 1869] and, later, by Bailkow [1870], who noted a somewhat surprising phenomenon: The grafted marrow may disappear entirely, but if it survives, it transforms into a piece of bone that has neither the volume nor the shape of the grafted tissue.

These were the first observations made on the bone-forming potential of the marrow. No marrow could be obtained from the grafted marrow in these experiments. Indeed, it was not until the present century that marrow was obtained after implantation of the marrow, and this marrow was still within a shell of bone [Tavassoli and Crosby, 1968]. Thus, the Hippocratic postulate was reversed: The bone must somehow be essential for the function of the marrow. This was the frame of reference for the marrow researchers of the 1920s. Sabin [1928] sets the tone by pointing out that bone provides a nonexpansile frame for the marrow, and "when there is any increase of cells in marrow, something has to pass out to make room." For lack of suitable methods, the question remains unsolved.

MARROW VESSELS

In a general way, one may say that marrow blood vessels, more than any of its components, have intrigued researchers. They also exemplify how the advance of knowledge depends on appropriate methods.

In ancient times, when the marrow was believed to be a source of nutrient supply to the bone, it was perceived as a mass of vessels interspersed with fat. During the 18th century, when the medullary membrane theory was fashionable, Duverney [1700] and, later, Bichat [1802], thought of it essentially as a vascular membrane. Duverney drew an analogy with the spinal cord. Both the marrow and the spinal cord are protected within a rigid frame of bone, and both are very soft tissues with a high fat content. Since the spinal cord has a vascular membrane, the arachnoid, so must the marrow. During the 19th century, Miescher exaggerated these views and considered the entire marrow cavity as a single, enormously enlarged vascular channel [Robin, 1875].

By the mid-19th century, however, methodologic developments permitted a more realistic view of the marrow vasculature, and by the turn of the century the problem had been reduced to two related questions. One question concerned the nature of the circulation in the marrow and asked whether it is a closed system or open to the extravascular space. This question involved enigmatic vascular structures for which the term "sinusoids" was soon to be coined by Minot [1901]. The second question related to the site of blood production and whether it is inside or outside the vessels. Thus, the lines were drawn for a battle which was to last for about half a century.

In 1892, Van der Stricht [1892] recognized that the sites of red cell formation differ in birds and mammmals. In birds, he maintained that the circulation is a closed system and that red cell formation takes place within the vessels, an opinion that was later confirmed. In mammals, however, he thought the circulation is wide open, with maturing red cells wandering about and entering the circulation only when fully mature. During the 1920s, a concerted effort by many students of the marrow led to the formulation of a coherent view, if not a complete answer [Jordan and Baker, 1927]. It was only after the advent of new microscopic techniques that a picture began to emerge, according to which, in mammals red cells are formed outside the vessels and delivered to the circulation through the "sinusoid" barrier. Now other questions puzzle us: the nature of the sinusoid wall, the mode of cellular migration across the wall, and the regulation of this phenomenon.

There is no final answer for a scientific question—only metamorphosis.

II.

Phylogeny

INTRODUCTION

In the course of evolution, the appearance of the bone marrow as the seat of hemopoiesis is a late event. The entire kingdom of invertebrates lack any bone and, therefore, the bone marrow. Even the pisces, inhabiting the vast expanse of oceans and lakes which cover three fourths of our planet surface, have no bone marrow [Siegel, 1970; Warren, 1965]. The first appearance of hemopoietic bone marrow is in amphibians in whom the blood-forming activity of the marrow is transitional and seasonal. The marrow takes on a more dominant hemopoietic role in reptiles, and, finally, it is in birds that the marrow becomes the major site of blood formation. In mammals, the marrow retains this preeminent role, and in primates the marrow is the sole site of hemopoiesis.

Hence, the bone marrow, although a latecomer to the function of hemopoiesis, reaches a summit of efficiency supplanting all other tissues that in the course of evolution are endowed by hemopoietic function.

It is a curious and unappreciated fact that, phylogenetically, the bone marrow's acquisition of the hemopoietic function coincides with the exit of vertebrates from the water when the bone begins to serve a weight-bearing function; yet it is also curious that in man, hemopoietic marrow evades the weight-bearing bones and its distribution is limited to the bones of the torso. Whatever functional significance there may be in these observations is not clear.

PHYLOGENY OF HEMOPOIESIS IN INVERTEBRATES

The scope of this volume is limited to the bone marrow. But to set the stage for the understanding of marrow phylogeny, the origin and evolution of blood cells and hemopoiesis will briefly be sketched. Providing such a sketch, however, is not an easy task. A major difficulty is the absence of adequate data that could provide a coherent picture. Moreover, the available data are usually discontinuous. Some species have been studied extensively; others not at all. Thus, the biological thread running through the course of evolution cannot be perceived; it must be surmised. Among invertebrates, insects are perhaps the most extensively studied [Wigglesworth, 1959; Jones, 1962]. Yet in 1970, Jones, a major contributor to our understanding of insect hematology, wrote:

> When it is realized that there are approximately one million species of insect that have been described, that at least one million remain to be discovered and described, that our present knowledge concerning insect hemocytes is based on probably not more than 200 insects and that detailed quantitative information exists on less than 25 species, an appreciation of the magnitude of our ignorance becomes quite evident.

And the picture has not really changed since then.

Another difficulty is the lack of a definition of the entities under study. Blood cells, of course, undergo evolutionary changes. What may be considered a "lymphocyte" in man is not the same as a lymphocyte in worms. Moreover, in some species blood cells may change their characters during the various phases of their life cycle, being disfigured beyond recognition. Compounding this difficulty is the fact that almost all conclusions in this area rely on purely morphologic observations. Data on invertebrates are based on crudely prepared specimens. For instance, living insects are immersed in hot water bath, 60°C, and preparations are made from these heat-fixed creatures. More modern techniques of observations have not been adopted for application, and may not be easily applicable to invertebrates. Nonetheless a few general impressions are possible.

The Origin of Blood and the Vascular System

In the course of evolution, the appearance of white cells (or what may be considered their equivalent) far precedes the appearance of red cells. Even the earliest metazoans, such as sponges, are endowed with motile and phagocytic cells. Thus, phagocytes antedate even the evolution of body cavities. These cells subserve digestive and excretory functions and are also involved in clotting [Beard, 1950], and therefore may be considered as the ancestors of thrombocytes. They are mesenchyme-derived and in view of their multiple function may be considered hemocytes. Their morphology changes during different phases of the organism's life. Their evolution is associated with the division of labor and the appearance of more specialized cells, leukocytes and thrombocytes.

In contrast to this primitive origin of leukocytes, erythrocytes do not exist in invertebrates.* The respiratory pigment in these organisms is in solution within the blood or celomic fluid. The respiratory pigment is generally hemoglobin, one of the most primitive proteins. It is only in vertebrates that packaging of the respiratory pigment comes about. Even in those species in which intracellular respiratory pigment is seen, it cannot be considered as a form of "packaging." Rather, it is an intermediate stage between synthesis of the pigment and its subsequent release into the hemolymph. Thus, horseshoe crab and certain other species have "cyanocytes" which synthetize hemocyanin and liberate it in the hemolymph [Fahrenback, 1970].

The absence of packaging may be due to the absence of an adequately advanced blood vascular system. Diffusion, through the celom and celomic

---

*Exceptions, of course, exist: At least in two genera of worms, *Thalassema* and *Magelona*, not only the genuine discoid hemoglobin-containing erythrocyte exists but they even become enucleated (erythroplastids) [Jordan, 1938]. Enucleation of erythrocyte is limited to mammals, and even in amphibian and avian species where hemoglobin packaging is the rule, the cells are still nucleated [Tavassoli, 1978c]. The presence of enucleated erythroplastids in worms is therefore quite intriguing, as if in the course of evolution nature toyed with an idea, shelved it, and took it up again when it was deemed useful. This may be an example of convergent evolution [Gould, 1980].

fluid, rather than circulation, is responsible for the oxygen transport by the hemoglobin. Celom, a cavity of mesodermal origin, develops as a space around the gut and subsequently assumes many functions. It contains celomic fluid and cells of different types including phagocytes [Dales and Dixen, 1981]. Celom may open to the outside [Dales and Dixon, 1981].

Development of the blood vascular system, however, is independent of that of hemocytes and celom [Dales and Dixon, 1981]. The simplest blood vascular system is in worms and insects, where a tube extends dorsally and ventrally from the abdomen to the head with occasional branching. The vessels surrounding the gut may enlarge into a sinus. The wall consists of a discontinuous endothelium and a collagenous connective tissue layer [Dales and Dixon, 1981]. In some species there may even be an accessory pulsatile structure [Jones, 1970] which may be considered as a primitive heart. In this manner, the circulatory fluid, known as hemolymph, bathes the internal organ. Hemocytes, which are primarily celomic (celomocytes) can now migrate into the circulatory channels, and there is a free exchange between the celomic and circulatory fluids. Thus the circulation, lacking a complex system of vessels and being in state of free exchange, is essentially an open system, primarily used to expedite the movement of celomic fluid and cells. This system, which gradually becomes more complex, is the origin of the circulatory system.

Origin of Hemopoiesis

The least developed invertebrates do not have hemopoiesis as commonly understood. Hemocytes are apparently produced in the hemocele during the embryonic life from a mesodermal origin [Dorn, 1978; Cowden, 1968]. They probably remain with the organism throughout its life-span. Celomocytes may be derived from the epithelial lining of the celomic cavity [Cooper and Stein, 1981], and may transform into hemocytes. In somewhat more developed invertebrates, such as worms and insects, these cells may undergo divisions [Siminia, 1974], usually in the primitive circulatory system. But even these divisions are in the form of amitosis in which the nucleus incorporates triated thymidine and divides without the cytoplasmic division's being consummated. In more developed invertebrates, however, division of hemocytes within the circulatory system may take place and be considered the most primitive form of hemopoiesis, if only a very diffuse one [Siminia, 1972, 1974; Lie et al, 1975]. Whether the proliferation is through the division of preexisting hemocytes or a pool of stem cell is present [Kinoti, 1971; Lie et al, 1975] is not known.

As concerns hemopoiesis, segmented worms provide a cornerstone in the course of evolution. In less developed invertebrates, the formation of blood cells is a migratory phenomenon. While in segmented worms migratory hemopoiesis is still a dominant form, dense accumulations of cells resembling hemocytes (blood islands or lymphogenous organs) occurs and is associated with the lateral vascular channels. The cells may or may not be sessile. These blood islands may be considered the most primitive form of *settlement* for hemopoiesis, to distinguish it from *migratory* hemopoiesis. Variations on this theme provide the "leukocytopoietic" or "lymphogenous" organs of the higher invertebrates.

One of the first *settlements* of hemopoiesis is seen in cephalopod mollusks. It is also a very unusual settlement and has attracted considerable attention [Bolognari, 1949, 1951; Cowden, 1968; Cowden and Curtis, 1973, 1981]. In these mollusks, the hemopoietic tissues are called white bodies because they impart a white color. They are located behind the eye in the orbital pit. This is a compact tissue which resists mechanical disruption. It is encapsulated with the capsule sending trabeculae inside the tissue. The trabeculae carry blood vessels inside the tissue. Within the tissue, blood-forming cells are interspersed with venous sinuses. This is reminiscent of a similar hemopoietic organ in some insects [Akai and Sato, 1971; Hoffman, 1972; Monpeyssin and Beaulaton, 1978]. From the description in the literature, it is not known if the hemopoiesis is extravascular or not; but if this is so, it is comparable to that in higher vertebrates, demonstrating a well-developed settlement of hemopoiesis in a fairly undeveloped invertebrate. In fact, the structure of some of these nodules [Wright, 1981] is reminiscent of erythroblastic islands in the mammalian bone marrow [Bessis 1973; Shaklai and Tavassoli, 1979].

In arthropods the hemocytopoietic organs are still diffuse, but they have taken more definitive and variegated form [Jones, 1970; Hoffman, 1972, 1973; Nutting, 1975; Zachary and Hoffman, 1973; Brehelin, 1973; Akai and Sato, 1971; Monpeyssin and Beaulaton, 1978]: stomachal glands in decapods, gland of Blanchard in scorpion, and spleens of Kowalevsky in myriopods. The latter structures are diffuse, multiple, and segmentally distributed. Spleens of Kowalevsky are indeed another cornerstone in the evolution of hemopoiesis. These dispersed and scattered islands of hemopoiesis are the most primitive form of the spleen which, in pisces, become quite compact, attaining the definitive shape of spleen.

The first settlements of hemopoiesis occur in the wall of gastrointestinal tract and particularly in the submucosa [Charmantier, 1972]. Here is where the first blood islands originate and evolve into such organs as the gland of Blanchard and spleens of Kowalevsky and, in more developed species, into the spleen. A factor that may render this site suitable to the task of hemopoiesis is probably its proximity to the absorptive surfaces where necessary nutrients can readily be obtained. Another factor may be the vascularity of this region. The common denominator of all hemopoietic tissues is the presence of an extensive vascular system providing a very slow rate of flow (sinusoidal microcirculation). The presence of this system may be essential for optimal hemopoietic function.

Settlement of Hemopoiesis

Even when migratory blood cell formation is evolved into a more "settled" hemopoiesis, intravascular division of blood cells does not cease to exist [Lavallard and Campiglia, 1975; Debaisieux, 1952, 1953; Shapiro, 1968]. The two phenomena may coexist. The intravascular proliferation of blood cell may show a circadian rhythm [Ravindranth, 1977] and, in certain species, may account entirely for the maintenance of hemocytes in certain insects [Jones and Lin, 1968, 1969]. Circulatory space continues to serve as a site of hemopoiesis in all piscine and even amphibian species, although the magnitude of its contribution to hemopoiesis is gradually reduced. In fact, even in the settlement sites of hemopoiesis (hemopoietic organs), much of blood formation is intravascular. Blood cells are formed *within* the lumen of large venous sinuses. As the cells mature, they become detached and move into the circulation. This pattern, seen even in birds [Campbell, 1967], is a continuation of the pattern that is first seen in segmented worm with accumulation of cells in the blood islands within the lateral vascular channels.

Leukocytes are the first cell types that are produced extravascularly and this occurs in the least developed pisces studied, the hagfish. In this regard, too, they take precedence over erythrocytes. In almost all piscine, amphibian, and avian systems, the extracellular leukopoiesis and intravascular erythropoiesis is the rule. Ultimately, however, erythropoiesis also moves to the extracellular site and the pattern of mammalian hemopoiesis is achieved.

Sites of Hemopoiesis

In pisces and amphibia the hemopoiesis is settled in several discrete sites. The relative contribution of these sites to blood formation varies with the species and depends on the cell type. In addition to the circulatory space, these sites include the spleen and the central lymphoid organ, intertubular stroma of kidney, intestinal submucosa, and to a lesser degree the liver and the gonads. The spleen is the product of the compaction of "blood islands" and, in invertebrates, spleens of Kowalevsky are predominantly erythropoietic. The central lymphoid organ is in fact a region of spleen that is primarily lymphocytopoietic. This organ, too, is the product of the compaction of the lymphogenous organs in invertebrates. It is the combination of these two functions (and organs) that, in vertebrates, gives rise to the dual structure of spleen with its red and white pulps.

Hemopoiesis in the intestinal submucosa may be considered a vestigial variation of splenic hemopoiesis. When blood islands undergo compaction to form the spleen, a few islands may escape this compaction and appear as separate hemopoietic foci in the intestinal submucosa. When kidney, gonads, or liver partake in the function of hemopoiesis, they are predominantly leukocytopoietic.

HEMOPOIESIS IN PISCES

Table II.1 summarizes the sites of hemopoiesis in several major piscine and amphibian species with the cell lineages produced. The following is a brief description of hemopoiesis in these species.

Hagfish

The major hemopoietic site is in the spleen. Here the spleen is quite dispersed, consisting of scattered islands of hemopoiesis in the submucosa of intestine. It represents a very early stage in the evolution of spleen. It produces erythrocytes, granulocytes, thrombocytes, and lymphocytes. Some of these cells, particularly erythrocytes and thrombocytes, can also divide within the circulatory space.

Lamprey

The spleen is here more compact but still in association with the submucosa of the intestine. Again it produces all four cell lines (erythrocytes, granulocytes, thrombocytes, and lymphocytes). In addition, some erythrocytes and granulocytes are produced in the intestinal submucosa independent of the spleen. Again, erythrocytes and thrombocytes are also produced within the circulatory space by division of preexisting cells.

Lungfish

In this fish, not only is the spleen more discrete but the formation of the dual structure of spleen (the white and red pulps) is quite evident. The organ consists of a central core of lymphoid mass surrounded by a pulp of cords and sinuses, very similar to the mammalian spleen. Also similar to the mammalian system is the primitive type of splenic circulation whereby the blood flows around the lymphoid tissue and receives developing blood

TABLE II.1. Sites of Hemopoiesis in Pisces and Amphibia

	Sites of hemopoiesis	Cell lineages produced[a]
Pisces		
Hagfish (cyclostome)	Spleen (diffuse)[b]	E, T, G, L
	Circulatory space (by division)	E, T
Lamprey (cyclostome)	Spleen (compact)[b]	E, T, G, L
	Intestinal submucosa	E, G
	Circulatory space	E, T
Lungfish (Dipnoi)	Spleen	E, T, L
	Intestinal submucosa	E, G, L
	Kidney	G, L
	Circulatory space	E
Ganoid fish	Spleen (discrete)	E, T, L
	Kidney (intertubular) stroma	G, L
	Intestinal submucosa	G, L
	Gonads (subcapsular area)	G
	Circulatory space	E, T
	Meninges and bone marrow	See text
Dogfish	Spleen	E, T, G, L
(Elasmobranch)	Gonads[b]	G
	Kidney	E, T, G, L
	Liver	E, T
	Pancreas (periportal space)	G
	Intestinal submucosa	G, T
	Circulatory space	E, T
Trout (Teleost)	Kidney[b]	E, T, G, L
	Spleen	E, T, L
	Pancreas (periportal space)	G
	Intestinal submucosa	T, G, L
	Circulatory space	T
Amphibia		
Salamander	Spleen	E, T, L
(urodeles)	Intestinal submucosa	G, L
	Liver (subcapsular)	G, L
Frog (Anurans)	Bone marrow	See text
	Spleen	E, L
	Kidney	G
	Intestinal submucosa	G
	Circulatory space	T

[a]E: erythrocyte, G: granulocyte, T: thrombocyte, L: lymphocyte.
[b]Clearly dominant in hemopoietic function.

cells from it [Yoffey, 1929]. Here again, the spleen is involved in the production of all four cell lines, which are also produced in the intestinal submucosa. In addition, erythrocytes divide in the circulatory space.

Ganoids

These fishes provide a transition in the evolution of spleen. The spleen here is a discrete organ completely separated from the intestinal wall, although close to the stomach. In all higher forms, the spleen has migrated a variable distance from the intestinal tube and is attached to the mesentery. The spleen produces erythrocytes, lymphocytes, and thrombocytes; the granulocytes are produced in the intestinal submucosa, kidney, and the subcapsular area of gonads. Again, division within the circulatory space provides a number of additional erythrocytes and granulocytes.

Cartilaginous Fishes

A representative of this group is the dogfish shark. Here, the hemopoiesis is somewhat more diffuse. Although the spleen appears to be a major site of production of all four cell lines [Yoffey, 1929], substantial contribution to the granulopoiesis is made by gonads. Other granulopoietic areas include the kidney, intestinal mucosa, pancreas, and the portal canal of the liver. In addition, the liver and the kidney as well as the circulatory space can produce a large number of erythrocytes and thrombocytes.

Bony Fishes

Kidney rather than spleen is the major hemopoietic organ in this group. Although considerable variation may exist, trout can be considered a representative species [Weinrel, 1958, 1963]. In trout the kidney is the predominant hemopoietic organ, producing all four cell lines. Spleen is also very active, particularly in lymphopoiesis, erythropoiesis, and thrombocy-topoiesis. Thrombocytes, granulocytes, and lymphocytes are also produced in the intestinal submucosa. Granulopoiesis may also occur in the periportal pancreatic tissue. Again, erythrocytes divide within the circulation.

AMPHIBIAN HEMOPOIESIS

Relatively more information exists on amphibian hemopoiesis than on invertebrates and pisces. This is in part because of the considerably less methodologic difficulties encountered in the study of hemopoietic tissues and the expanded possibilities for experimentation.

Furthermore, amphibians provide a cornerstone in the evolution of hemopoiesis. It is in amphibians that the bone marrow is initiated, although transiently, into the function of hemopoiesis. In this order, salamander (representing *urodeles*) and the frog (representing *anurans*) are most extensively studied.

Salamander

As in the dogfish shark, there is a dichotomy in the salamander with regard to the sites of hemopoiesis. Erythropoiesis is primarily in the spleen, which produces some thrombocytes and lymphocytes as well. Granulocytes, however, are formed primarily in the subcapsular area of the liver and to a lesser extent the intestinal submucosa. In salamander bone marrow is not yet a hemopoietic organ.

Interestingly, surgical removal of each of these organs is not associated with a compensatory function in the other. Splenectomy only shifts the erythropoiesis and granulopoiesis to the circulatory space but not to the liver [Ohuye, 1932] or other lymphogranulopoietic tissues [Jordan and Speidel, 1930]. Total hepatectomy is, of course, associated with death; partial hepatectomy shifts the granulopoiesis to the liver remnant, but not to the spleen [Jordan and Beam, 1930]. Thus, the microenvironments of theses two organs differ and do not support the hemopoietic function other than what they normally support.

Frog

In the frog, erythropoiesis is virtually restricted to the spleen, except when it occurs transiently in the bone marrow. In contrast to that of the salamander, spleen can also have some granulopoietic function but this is very limited. Granulopoiesis takes place largely in the kidney and intestinal submucosa, particularly in the cecal region.

The transiently hemopoietic marrow is both erythropoietic and granulopoietic. Hemopoietic marrow is evident immediately after metamorphosis and hibernation, but also in experimental postsplenectomy states when the marrow compensate for the splenic erythropoiesis [Jordan and Speidel, 1923, 1925]. Thus the bone marrow, in contrast to other hemopoietic organs, has an early potential to compensate for the hemopoietic function of other organs.

THE FIRST BONE MARROW

It is generally agreed that in the course of evolution, hemopoietic bone marrow first appears in the frog. Lower vertebrates have no hemopoietic bone marrow. However, Scharrer [1944] has demonstrated the presence of hemopoietic bone marrow in the ganoid fishes. In this piscine species the mininges overlying the fourth ventricle are greatly thickened, forming a large mass of tissue. Ths mass of tissue was always considered glandular in nature until Scharrer demonstrated that it is hemopoietic. Its general structure is highly reminiscent of that of the mammalian bone marrow—the most mature form of bone marrow. It consists of an elaborate reticular network and a sinusoidal system of circulation. Erythropoietic, granulopoietic, and lymphocytic cells are present in distinct foci or islands. Both erythropoiesis and granulopoiesis are extravascular, and mature cells must traverse the sinusoidal wall to enter the circulation. Even in the marginal part of this tissue, adipose cells are interspersed with the hemopoietic tissue, an association generally seen in the phylogenetically most advanced forms of the bone marrow. Although this mass is not located within the bone, it extends into little cavities inside the cartilaginous skull. The photomicrograph provided by Scharrer is almost indistinguishable from the hemopoietic marrow located within the cancellous bone of the most advanced mammalian species. Thus, in the strict sense of the term, this mass may be considered as "bone marrow." Scharrer recognized that this sort of hemopoiesis occurred only in ganoids, and not other fishes. This demonstration by Scharrer is instructive in several respects.

Firstly, it suggests that the marrow and the bone are no more than two strange bedfellows. Phylogenetically, the hemopoietic marrow does not *originate* in the bone. It originates outside the bone and, perhaps by evolutionary pressure, extends into the bone cavities, where the microenvironment may be more optimal for the hemopoietic function. Perhaps this should provide a frame of reference for investigating the relation between the marrow and bone, a totally neglected area. Moreover, the invasion of solid bone by the marrow is associated with the development of an extensive specialized vascular system (sinusoidal system) that appears to be essential for hemopoiesis. It is the common denominator of all hemopoietic organs. A similar vascular invasion is also noted during the ontogeny of the bone marrow when endochondral osteogenesis takes place.

Second, the structure of this most primitive marrow is comparable to that of the developmentally most advanced species—mammals. The shifting of erythropoiesis to the extravascular space and the development of a marrow-blood barrier are characteristics of the mammalian bone marrow and are absent in premammalian species. The degree of sophistication in this first experiment of nature in marrow hemopoiesis questions the validity of the concept that the evolution is in the direction of producing organisms of *higher* order, a concept based on value judgment.

Third, the meningeal origin of the bone marrow is intriguing. Before the hemopoietic function of the marrow was recognized, Duverney (see Chapter I) described the marrow of the bones as essentially a vascular membrane similar to the meninges. He drew a parallel between the nervous system and the marrow: Both are protected within the rigid frame of bone, and both are very soft tissues with high fat content. Duverney was, of course, unaware of the meningeal origin of the marrow in ganoids.

Finally, the presence of bone marrow in ganoid fishes is an anomaly in the course of evolution. No other species in the vast kingdom of pisces have marrow. Here again it appears that nature toyed with an idea, shelved it, and took it up again when it was deemed useful. This may yet be another example of convergent evolution [Gould, 1980], of which an example is seen in the presence of nonnucleated erythrocytes in worms (vide supra).

BONE MARROW HEMOPOIESIS

If in the frog the bone marrow is only initiated to the function of hemopoiesis, in reptiles it effectively competes with other hemopoietic organs. Moreover, with the advent of hemopoietic bone marrow in reptiles, the competition becomes restricted to the spleen. Such other organs as the kidney and the intestinal wall appear to be effectively out of the competition.

Three reptilian species—toads, turtles, and lizards—provide a line of evidence to indicate how the bone marrow's successful competition comes about (Table II.2). In the horned toad, the spleen is the dominant site of hemopoiesis, producing large numbers of erythrocytes and thrombocytes although it is less active in granulopoiesis. Hemopoietic activity of the bone marrow is decidedly less than that of spleen and is mostly granulopoietic. Liver and kidney are not hemopoietic, nor could they be so induced by splenectomy [Jordan and Speidel, 1930]. In the turtle, spleen and bone marrow equally share the burden of hemopoiesis. In lizards the bone

TABLE II.2. Sites of Hemopoiesis in Reptiles and Birds

	Sites of hemopoiesis
Reptiles	
Horned toad	Spleen dominant
Turtle	Spleen equal to marrow
Lizard	Marrow dominant
Birds	Restricted to marrow

marrow dominates, being active in the production of all blood cells. Some hemopoiesis also takes place in the spleen and liver as well as within the circulatory space. Reptiles in general present an evolutionary intermediate between amphibians and birds.

In birds hemopoiesis is restricted to the bone marrow, where erythropoiesis is still intravascular but granulopoiesis is extravascular. Here the spleen retains only its lymphocytopoietic function. Thus, in birds the lymphocytopoiesis and hemocytopoiesis begin to segregate, B lymphocytes are produced in the bursa of Fabricius, and, moreover, the presence of lymph nodes in water birds (the only birds having lymph nodes) heralds the appearance of this organ in mammals.

Although avian spleen is not erythropoietic, total splenectomy causes an immediate fall in the hemoglobin level, which returns to normal after a few days [Ohuye, 1932]. This, however, may be related to the function of spleen as a blood reservoir.

With the evolution of mammalia, the marrow retains the function of hemopoiesis to the exclusion of other sites. In lower mammals, the spleen still has a limited hemopoietic function; but in man and other primates, extramedullary hemopoiesis must be considered pathologic.

III.

Ontogeny

INTRODUCTION

Ontogeny of hemopoiesis was the focus of attention even before the postnatal hemopoiesis in the marrow had been recognized. "This was only natural: Scholars of this period did not know that blood formation is a continuous process and takes place throughout life. The finite life span of red cell and therefore the necessity for their continuous replenishment was not recognized" (see Chapter I). The assumption was that, like such cells as neurones, blood cells once formed in embryo remain in the body throughout life. The search for the origin of blood cells therefore began in the embryo. Studies on ontogeny of the hemopoiesis was fashionable for the half-century that spanned the last two decades of the 19th centry and the first three decades of the 20th. This period is characterized by much controversy, contradictory statements, and irreconcilable dogmas caused by the use of static histological methods which did not permit the dynamic observations needed to reach valid conclusions on such a dynamic developmental system. Nonetheless this period managed to provide us with most of our basic knowledge in this area. During the past two decades more information has become available, and most controversies have now subsided through the application of such new techniques as tracer methods (radioactive labeling, autoradiography, chromosome markers, etc) or functional assays (in vitro and in vivo clonal analysis of stem cells).

GENERAL CONSIDERATIONS

Hemopoiesis is a migratory phenomenon during the embryonic and fetal life. It begins in the *extraembryonic* mesoblastic tissue [Bloom and Bartelmez,

1940], particularly the yolk sac, and then moves to the *intraembyronic* sites, liver and spleen, to settle finally in the bone marrow. In mammals, this migration continues in postnatal life by centripetal regression of hemopoiesis so that in adult life, in many species including man, hemopoiesis is limited to the bones of torso. The limb bones are devoid of hemopoiesis.

This migration pattern is in some ways reminiscent of the evolutionary aspects of hemopoiesis, and it is often said that the ontogeny of hemopoiesis recapitulates its phylogeny [Metcalf and Moore, 1971]. This recapitulation is not exact. The two migration patterns differ in many respects, but they may be said to coincide in their essential features.

Parallel, but not necessarily coincident to this migration pattern, there is a switch in the type of hemoglobin synthesized, from embryonic to fetal to adult type. The regulatory mechanism for this switch is still unknown but probably is not related to the site of hemopoiesis, and will not be treated here. Extensive reviews are available on this subject, which has fascinated molecular biologists [Stamatoyannopoulos and Nienhuis, 1978, 1981].

Embryogenesis of hemopoiesis is fundamentally comparable in all mammals. Thus, apart from the temporal frame, some generalization can be permitted. In all species, hemopoiesis begins in extraembryonic mesoblastic tissue and then migrates to intraembryonic tissues, where it is again closely associated with the mesenchyme. It appears that all tissues of mesenchymal origin may be potentially hemopoietic under appropriate conditions, although these conditions are not always met and, thus, the potential is not always realized.

Ontogeny of hemopoiesis has best been studied in mice, perhaps because of the methodological applications. Thus, in the following treatment the baseline data are derived mostly from the mouse.

YOLK SAC HEMOPOIESIS

Hemopoiesis in the yolk sac occurs in distinct foci known as blood islands (Fig. III.1). In most species, including man and mouse, only erythropoiesis is expressed, as the environment of the yolk sac is restrictive in its inductive potential. In some species, particularly during the later stages, granulocyte precursors and megakaryocytes have been reported but not confirmed [Maximow, 1924; Knoll and Pingle, 1949; Playfair et al, 1963]. The precursor cells responsible for the formation of these islands and capable of differentiating into erythroid cells are known as hemangioblasts. They migrate from the primitive streak region of early blastoderm into the developing area opaca vasculosa [Murray, 1932; Rudnick, 1938]. They are organized in a

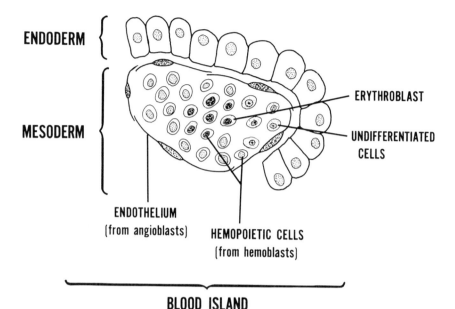

ENDODERM {

MESODERM {

ERYTHROBLAST

UNDIFFERENTIATED CELLS

ENDOTHELIUM
(from angioblasts)

HEMOPOIETIC CELLS
(from hemoblasts)

BLOOD ISLAND

Fig. III.1. Diagrammatic representation of a blood island in the yolk sac. The island is adjacent to the endoderm, which is required for the development of the island. The island itself consists of the peripheral cells which are flattened to form the capillary endothelium (angioblasts), and the central cells which are hemopoietic (hemoblasts). The latter cells are undifferentiated at the periphery, but they differentiate toward the center and become recognizable as erythroblasts.

horseshoe-shaped region surrounding the posterior and posteriolateral region of area pellucida [Settle, 1954; Metcalf and Moore, 1971]. ³H-thymidine-labeling studies have indicated that the cells destined to form blood islands invaginate through the primitive streak and then migrate laterally to produce the mesodermal layer [Rosenquist, 1966]. These cells can differentiate in two directions (Fig. III.1). The peripheral cells flatten to form capillary endothelial cells, and are known as angioblasts whereas the central cells round up, develop intense basophilia, and become detached from peripheral cells. These cells are hemopoietic precursor cells and are true hemoblasts. These two lines of differentiation may occur together, but they are not necessarily associated: Capillary endothelium can develop in the absence of hemopoiesis, and hemopoietic foci can be seen in the absence of endothelium. The current consensus maintains that the endothelium does not contribute to the differentiation of blood cells in the yolk sac [Edmunds, 1964, 1966] as was once thought to be the case [Jordan, 1916; Hauser et al,

1969]. The adjacent endoderm (Fig. III.1), however, is required for the development of these islands [Wilt, 1965; Miura and Wilt, 1969, 1970]. In fact, the formation of blood islands in the mesoderm is the result of interaction of mesoderm and endoderm. The culture of experimentally separated mesoectoderm does not lead to the formation of many blood islands unless it is coincubated with the endoderm. This dependence of yolk sac hemopoiesis on endoderm and other morphological observations in human fetuses [Thomas and Yoffey, 1962, 1964; Yoffey et al, 1961; Yoffey and Thomas, 1964; Yoffey, 1971] has led some investigators to question the origin of blood cells from primitive mesenchyme, as ardently advocated by Maximow [1907, 1909].

Blood islands (Fig. III.1) initially appear as thickening regions in the inner (mesodermal) layer of yolk sac, which is in contact with the extraembryonic endoderm. The undifferentiated hemangioblasts develop into an outer layer (in contact with the endoderm) of morphologically undifferentiated blast cells. The more centrally located cells soon become recognizable as erythroblasts (Fig. III.1), which then undergo further maturation into nucleated red cells filled with embryonic hemoglobin and devoid of organelles. The nucleus, however, is not extruded, and the cells circulate in nucleated form [Marks and Rifkind, 1972]. Maturation may not be exactly synchronous, but apparently only a cohort of cells develop in the yolk sac [Fantoni et al, 1968; De la Chapelle et al, 1969], and therefore the yolk sac hemopoiesis is relatively homogeneous. In vitro studies suggest that the yolk sac erythropoiesis cannot be stimulated by erythropoietin (EP) [Cole and Paule, 1966]. This could mean either that the yolk erythropoiesis is EP-independent or, less likely, that it is already maximally stimulated. With maturation, blood islands appear as large sinusoids filled with erythroid cells. These sinusoids then communicate with the circulation, and, in fact, later stages of maturation take place within the circulation. In the mouse, whose gestation period is 21 days, the yolk sac hemopoiesis begins at approximately the eighth day and the proliferation proceeds from the eighth day to the tenth (Table III.1), and by the ninth day cells begin to enter the circulation, where they proliferate further. Mitosis may be observed through day 13 of gestation [Marks and Rifkind, 1972]. In man, the yolk sac hemopoiesis continues for the first 6 weeks of gestation and then begins to decrease, and by the tenth week it is undetectable [Bloom and Bartelmez, 1940; Hesseldahl and Larsen, 1971].

Primitive and Definitive Hemopoiesis

Primitive hemopoiesis differs from definitive hemopoiesis in that its product is restricted to embryo and not seen after birth. This difference is most easily distinguished in the case of the erythroid tissue. Two characteristics make the primitive erythropoiesis different from the definitive types: The end cell is nucleated, and the synthesized hemoglobin is of embryonic types. None of these is characteristic of postnatal erythropoiesis. Moreover, the life-span of the primitive erythroblasts appears to be shorter than that of definitive cells [Bloom and Bartlemaz, 1940; Knoll and Pingle, 1949; Maximow, 1924]. By contrast, the red cells produced by definitive erythropoiesis undergo nuclear expulsion, similar to the red cells produced after birth. They can also synthesize hemoglobins that can be produced in postnatal life (hemoglobins F, A, and A2 [Clarke et al, 1979]). Post–yolk sac hemopoiesis is generally of definitive type. In most vertebrates, yolk sac hemopoiesis can embrace both primitive and definitive hemopoiesis. The mouse is an exception in which yolk sac hemopoiesis is highly restricted to primitive erythropoiesis [Marks and Rifkind, 1972]. The primitive type of hemopoiesis in the yolk sac does not depend on the presence of normal embryo. This is evident from experiments using whole mouse embryos. In these cultures, the embryo can be induced to undergo degeneration while the yolk sac continues to grow and develops blood islands [Chen and Hsu, 1979]. Thus, primitive hemopoiesis is strictly an extraembryonic phenomenon. By contrast, definitive hemopoiesis depends on the presence of normal embryo. Recent evidence indicates that humoral factors, appearing in the embryo, act on the hemopoietic stem cells to induce the onset of definitive hemopoiesis [Cudennec et al, 1981].

The relationship between these two types of hemopoiesis has been the subject of some debate [Marks and Rifkind, 1972]. Are the primitive erythroid cells the precursors of definitive erythroid cells, or are they both derived from a common precursor? Do the stem cells from the yolk sac migrate to seed the fetal liver, or does the embryogenesis of stem cells proceed in the two tissues independently? There is no evidence that the primitive erythroid cells of the yolk sac actually seed the fetal liver and become involved in definitive erythropoiesis [Baker et al, 1969]. But there is good evidence that both types of erythropoiesis may be the products of a common stem cells. If the same stem cell can migrate between two compartments and differentiate to give rise to two different end products, one must assume that the two compartments provide different directives for the stem cell. In fact, there is some evidence to indicate that the environment of yolk sac and liver control the differentiation of the stem cell.

Metcalf and Moore [1971] have advanced a line of evidence to indicate that the yolk sac is the precursor of all stem cell populations, both myeloid and lymphoid, that develop subsequently in the embryo and adult animal.

According to this hypothesis, the mesenchymal cells, which differentiate into the hemopoietic stem cell, migrate from one hemopoietic tissue to another, and the directive milieu of the hemopoietic tissue determines its subsequent path of development and consequently its end product. Although the migration of hemopoietic stem cells has been questioned [Rifkind et al, 1969], this hypothesis is based on the following experimental data:

1. During the period when it is erythropoietic, the yolk sac also contains a number of CFU-S (pluripotential stem cells) capable of forming erythroid, megakaryocytic, granulocytic, and mixed colonies in the spleen of lethally irradiated mouse. Moreover, they can give rise to definitive adult erythrocytes [Beaupain et al, 1979] whereas in the yolk sac they produce primitive erythrocytes. Similarly, yolk sac cells from chick embryo can repopulate the hemopoietic system of sublethally irradiated chick embryo [Moore and Owen, 1967]. In both the mouse and the chick [Metcalf and Moore, 1971], chromosome tracer studies indicate that these colonies are of yolk sac and not of endogenous origin. Moreover, the yolk sac contains a number of CFU-GM (progenitors of granulocytes-macrophages) capable of forming granulocytic colonies in vitro. The environment of the yolk sac, however, is restricted for the differentiation of erythroid cells and other lines of differentiation are not expressed. Both CFU-S and CFU-GM concentrations in the yolk sac are parallel in magnitude to erythropoietic activity and are reduced to zero when the yolk sac ceases to be erythropoietic.

2. Similarly, the yok sac cells can repopulate the thymus and secondary lymphoid tissues of lethally irradiated mice and sublethally irradiated chick embryo system [Tyan, 1968; Tyan and Herzenberg, 1968; Tyan et al, 1969; Moore and Metcalf, 1970], indicating that the lymphoid cells have their origin in the yolk sac as well. Again chromosome tracer studies indicate the donor origin of these repopulating cells.

3. Studies in lower vertebrates support the concept of the migration of stem cells between different hemopoietic compartments. Removal of blood islands from the embryo of *Rana fusca* at the beginning of the tail bud stage can result in the development of larvae devoid of erythrocytes [Federici, 1926]. Similarly, the removal of yolk sac blood islands, when well localized, resulted in complete suppression of hemopoiesis in the subsequent hemopoietic sites [Goss, 1928]. At somewhat later stage, this experimental manipulation reduced but did not completely suppress hemopoiesis in the subsequent sites.

4. With the establishment of circulation in the mouse embryo, both CFU-S and CFU-GM, as well as more differentiated cells, can readily be

detected in a very high concentration in the circulation (Figs. III.2, 3) [Barnes et al, 1964; Moore and Metcalf, 1970]. Similarly, circulating stem cells can be detected in the chick embryo [Moore and Owen, 1967]. The concentration of these cells may be reduced when the liver becomes hemopoietic. These findings are consistent with the hypothesis that the hemopoietic stem cells migrate through the circulation between the two hemopoietic sites.

5. Seven-day mouse embryos can be cultured in vitro on the surface of Millipore filters for 48 hours [Moore and Metcalf, 1970]. These embryos proceed with normal development of yolk sac hemopoiesis, actively beating heart and a circulation containing primitive erythrocytes as well as a large number of CFU-GM. If, however, they are cultured after the removal of the yolk sac, they again proceed with the development of actively beating heart but without evidence of hemopoiesis in the circulation or in the region of the developing liver, neither in the form of developing erythroid cells nor in the form of CFU-GM. Addition of a source of colony-stimulat-

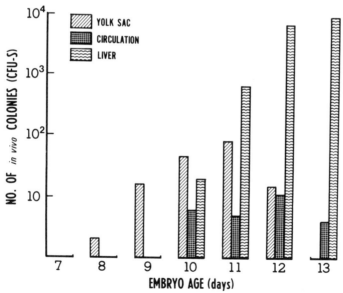

Fig. III.2. Histogram showing the concentration of hemopoietic stem cells as assayed in vivo by splenic colony technique (CFU-S) in the yolk sac, circulation, and liver. As the concentration decreases in the yolk sac, it increases in the circulation and then the liver, suggesting mobilization of stem cells from the yolk sac into the liver, via the circulation [from Moore and Metcalf, 1970].

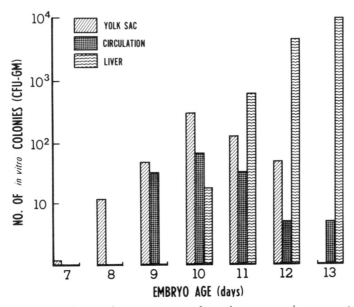

Fig. III.3. Histogram showing the concentration of granulocyte-macrophage progenitor cells assayed in vitro (CFU-GM). The concentration increases in the liver as it decreases in the yolk sac. During this period, CFU-GM also appear transiently in the circulation, suggesting mobilization of these progenitor cells from the yolk sac into the liver via the circulation [from Moore and Metcalf, 1970].

ing activity (CSA) has no effect in initiating the CFU-GM activity, but recombination with the addition of yolk sac to these cultures leads to the appearance of CFU-GM. This indicates that the progenitor cells, and not the colony-stimulating factor, is the missing factor when the yolk sac is absent from these cultures. Moreover, the addition of the yolk sac to the culture is ineffectual when it is separated from the embryo by a cell-impermeable filter. Thus, a direct cellular migration from the yolk sac leading to intraembryonic hemopoiesis is strongly suggested.

However, more recent experiments using chick-quail chimeras have demonstrated that the stem cells can also arise intraembryonically [Dieterlen-Lievre, 1975; Martin et al, 1980]. By grafting cytogenetically labeled tissue anlagen in frogs, Turpen et al [1981, 1982] have recently demonstrated that the blood islands of the ventral mesoderm contribute to embryonic erythropoiesis which then declines. On the other hand, dorsal anterior mesoderm contributes to a population of stem cells that can give rise to different lineages of hemopoietic cells. Thus, in addition to the extraembyronic yolk sac stem cells, a population of embryonic cells may also be capable of colonizing hemopoietic tissues.

LIVER HEMOPOIESIS

With the development of liver and when the formation of hepatic cords is in its definitive stages, hemopoiesis is transferred from the extraembryonic site to the liver within the embryo. In the mouse this occurs at day 10 of gestation, when the yolk sac erythropoiesis is at its peak. After hemopoiesis is settled in the new site, the yolk sac loses its hemopoietic capacity and, by day 13 in the mouse, no longer contains hemopoietic cells. In man hemopoiesis is detectable in the liver at approximately 6 weeks of gestation [Knoll and Pingle, 1949].

Hepatic hemopoiesis is initiated by the appearance of undifferentiated blast cells scattered in the liver cords [Karrer, 1961; Grasso et al, 1962; Thomas and Yoffey, 1964]. This is followed by the appearance of erythroid cells and then megakaryocytes and granulocytic cells [Mrsevic et al, 1970], although erythropoiesis remains the dominant process with an erythroid-granulocytic ratio of 5:1. As discussed above, the origin of the precursors of these cells is probably extraembryonic, from the yolk sac, reaching the liver through a hematogenous route. Granulopoiesis and megakaryopoiesis indicate that the environment of liver, unlike that of the yolk sac, is not restricted to the expression of erythropoiesis.

Liver hemopoiesis expands exponentially for the few days (doubling time 8 hours) and then stabilizes with a doubling time of 2 days [Paul et al, 1969]. Liver remains hemopoietic during the entire fetal period and even during the first postnatal week [Borghese, 1959], although the magnitude of its hemopoietic activity is considerably reduced during the latter part of this period. Thus, hepatic hemopoiesis in mammals may represent a true "settlement" of hemopoiesis.

The extravascular hepatic erythropoiesis is reflected in the fact that its product is nonnucleated red cells of 8 μ, somewhat larger than adult red cells (6 μ) [Russell and Bernstein, 1966]. The endothelial barrier which the nucleated cell must pass to enter the circulation can remove the nucleus [Tavassoli and Crosby, 1973; Tavassoli, 1978c, 1979b]. The liver CFU-GM is also larger than those in the marrow and homogeneous in volume [Symann et al, 1976], indicating a single noncycling population.

Simultaneous with the appearance of hemopoiesis, CFU-S becomes detectable in the liver. For a few days, this compartment enlarges to establish a CFU-S pool. Although the size of this pool remains stable throughout the fetal life, the subsequent enlargement in the size of hemopoietic pool results in dilution and a relative fall in concentration of the liver CFU-GM which remains fairly stable during the fetal life [Silini et al, 1976; Baker et al, 1969; Duplan, 1968; Moore et al, 1970; Moore and Metcalf, 1970]. There is a slight increase in this concentration immediately before birth and the concentration approaches zero within a week after birth, at which time the liver loses its hemopoietic function. A similar pattern is seen for CFU-GM except that the initial growth of the pool and the subsequent fall in CFU-GM concentration are much more prominent and rapid [Moore et al, 1970; Moore and Metcalf, 1970]. At least in the mouse, liver CFU-GM displays the same differentiating capacity and dependence on colony-stimulating activity as in adult bone marrow, and this seems to be somewhat different from the situation with the erythroid progenitor cells (vide infra).

There are differences, however between both CFU-S and CFU-GM in embryonic liver and adult bone marrow [Moore et al, 1970; Moore and Metcalf, 1970]. In embryonic liver, the CFU-GM is of relatively low and homogeneous density. As the course of embryogenesis proceeds, the density of CFU-GM increases progressively and the cells become more heterogeneous. A similar pattern can be seen for CFU-S [Haskill et al, 1970]. Thus, in adult bone marrow both CFU-S and CFU-GM are heterogeneous with regard to cell density and cell volume [Worton et al, 1969].

Because the light-density CFU-S and CFU-GM give rise to higher-density cells upon transplantation to irradiated host [Haskill and Moore, 1970; Metcalf and Moore, 1971], it is postulated that the homogeneous population of extremely light density cells are the stem cells with highest capacity to migrate and colonize other tissues. They migrate from the yolk sac to the liver and spleen and eventually to the marrow. By contrast, the more "settled" stem cells (with low capacity for migration) are of higher density, and their proportion increases as the embryogenesis of hemopoiesis proceeds and becomes mature.

Other differences exist between embryonic liver and adult marrow stem cells [Metcalf and Moore, 1971]. The former are more rapidly proliferating [Becker et al, 1965] than the latter, the majority of which are in a Go state. This may explain why embryonic liver stem cells are somewhat larger than adult marrow stem cells [Symann et al, 1976]: The size difference may be related to cycle status. This may also explain the higher radiosensitivity of fetal liver CFU-S [Siminovitch, 1965] as cells in S phase are more radioresistant than in Go phase [Boggs, 1973].

Moreover, passaging experiments have suggested that embryonic stem cells can undergo 20–80 more doubling time than adult stem cells. Liver

CFU-S has a shorter doubling time [Schofield, 1970], and a more rapid growth in diffusion chamber [Symann et al, 1976], and is more efficient than adult marrow CFU-S in preventing the lethal effects of radiation [Duplan, 1968]. All these differences suggest that there is a modulation of stem cell in the course of embryogenesis depending on the environmental conditions. It is possible but unlikely that different populations of stem cells may be responsible for these differences.

Regulatory mechanisms in fetal and embryonic erythropoiesis, and in particular their responses to erythropoietin (EP), are unclear. Inconsistent results have been reported [Bateman and Cole, 1971; Krantz and Jacobson, 1970; Cole et al, 1968; Rifkind et al, 1969; Rich and Kubranek, 1976, 1980].

A difference in EP sensitivity of erythroid progenitor cells (CFU-E) has been documented between fetal liver and adult marrow and spleen [Rich and Kubranek, 1976, 1980]. Undoubtedly, erythropoietin is present in the fetus that appears not to be dependent on the mother to produce it [Jacobson et al, 1959]. But its appearance is rather late in man, during week 32 of gestation [Halvorsen and Finne, 1968]. Its site of production appears to be not the kidney [Zanjani et al, 1974a] but the liver [Zanjani et al, 1977]. It is likely that during this late intrauterine life EP has a regulatory function in erythropoiesis [Krantz and Jacobson, 1970], as the intensity of erythropoiesis can be modulated by the use of anti-EP [Schooley et al, 1968; Zanjani et al, 1974b]. In earlier stages of liver erythropoiesis (as early as day 11 of gestation in the mouse), a response to EP can also be elicited in vitro [Cole and Paul, 1966; Gallien-Lartigue, 1966, 1967]. Yet the kinetics of stimulation suggest that the embryonic liver stem cell population may contain a component that is less dependent on erythropoietin than adult stem cells. Thus, erythroid colony formation in spleen by adult cells is almost entirely eliminated in polycythemic mice, whereas it is reduced only by about 50% for embryonic stem cells [Bleiberg and Feldman, 1969]. It is possible that the erythroid precursor cells acquire EP dependence gradually in the course of fetal life. In yolk sac, they are EP-independent; in liver, they are EP-sensitive and either this sensitivity gradually increases to total dependence on EP or, alternatively, a subpopulation of EP-sensitive cells appear and become dominant so that late in the course of intrauterine life, erythropoiesis is entirely EP-dependent.

SPLENIC HEMOPOIESIS

Embryologically, spleen originates from the thickening of mesenchymal tissue in the dorsal mesogastrium [Bloom, 1938; Klemperer, 1938]. Development of spleen occurs in two distinct phases. In the first phase, the condensation of mesenchymal cells is interspersed with vascular spaces where the circulating blood comes into direct contact with mesenchymal cells. This corresponds to the primordial red pulp of spleen. The tissue is then "seeded" by hemopoietic cells to form hemopoietc areas. In the second phase the white pulp develops through the formation of numerous circumscribed reticulum sheaths surrounding arterioles. These sheaths are then seeded by lymphocytes to form distinct demarcated nodules. The development of the white pulp and the lymphocyte repopulation of spleen are generally associated with a decline in its hemopoietic activity. The pattern of development is similar to the regenerative pattern of ectopic splenic implants during the postnatal life. The latter recapitulates splenic embryogenesis [Tavassoli et al, 1973b]. There is now good evidence based on cross transplantation or experiments with parabiotic animals that in both systems the spleen is repopulated with hemopoietic cells or lymphocytes from the circulation [Metcalf and Moore, 1971, Tavassoli et al, 1973a; Levy et al, 1976; Tavassoli and Khademi, 1980]. Temporal appearance of hemopoiesis in spleen is subsequent to that in the liver. For instance, in the mouse embryo, liver hemopoiesis appears on day 10 whereas splenic hemopoiesis begins by day 15 (Fig. III.4; Table III.1). A similar sequence is true for the loss of hemopoietic potential. Liver hemopoiesis regresses almost within 2 weeks after birth, whereas splenic hemopoiesis continues for a longer period and does not totally regress. In man splenic hemopoiesis is detectable at

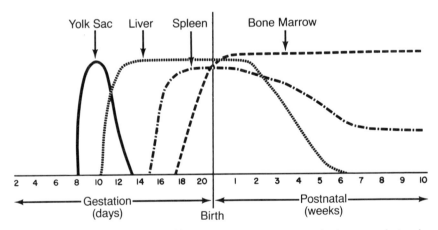

Fig. III.4. Temporal appearance of hemopoiesis in various organs in the mouse during the course of ontogeny. Gestation period is 21 days. The figure has been constructed from data in Table III.1.

TABLE III.1. Migration of Hemopoiesis in the Mouse Embryo (Days of Gestation, Gestation Period 21 Days)

	Initiation	Termination	Disappearance
Yolk sac	8	10	13
Liver	10	15 (postnatal)	Gradually
Spleen	15	Gradual, postnatal	Never
Bone marrow	17–18	No	No

approximately 12 weeks of gestation. As in the case of liver, initiation of hemopoiesis is associated with the appearance of CFU-S and CFU-GM. However, the rate of expansion of stem cell compartments is not as rapid as in liver (doubling time of 7–8 hours in liver vs 24 hours in spleen), but more rapid than in bone marrow. Receding of hemopoiesis in spleen after birth is not associated with a proportional reduction in the size of CFU-S compartment. Thus, in adult there is a discrepancy between the size of CFU-S pool and the hemopoietic activity of spleen [Metcalf and Moore, 1971]. It is of interest that the embryonic spleen in the mouse does not incorporate significant amount of ^{59}Fe into the heme even after exposure to erythropoietin [Cole and Paul, 1966; Cole et al, 1968]. In contrast to adult mouse spleen which has considerable erythropoietic potential [Fruhman, 1970], in embryonic spleen granulopoiesis predominates. The origin of CFU-S populating the mouse spleen is probably the liver, since at the time of splenic development, liver is the only tissue containing a pool of CFU-S. On the other hand, in chick embryo, the yolk sac is the only tissue with the potential for populating the developing spleen [Moore and Owen, 1967].

BONE MARROW HEMOPOIESIS

Bone marrow is the last site of hemopoiesis during the prenatal period. Development of marrow is generally thought to be the result of penetration of perichondrial mesenchymal cells and their associated blood vessels into the calcified zone of cartilage, which, in the tubular bones, is located in the central region of the shaft. This vascular mesenchyme then forms the reticular meshwork which, in hemopoietic marrow, constitutes the frame upon which hemopoietic cells proliferate. The invasion from outside the calcified cartilage by the mesenchyme, although not uniformly observed [Yoffey and Thomas, 1964], is highly reminiscent of the development of bone marrow in ganoid fish described by Scharrer [1944] (see Chapter II).

In both situations, one is dealing with the association of two distinctly separate tissues rather than the derivation of one from the other. It is the invasion of vascular mesenchyme that leads to the resorption of the cartilage matrix and the establishment of the marrow's structural framework. Nonetheless, organ culture studies indicate that there is a mutual interdependence between the vascular mesenchyme and the calcified cartilage or rudimentary bone. The vascular mesenchyme is not hemopoietic before the invasion into the bone. (This is in contrast to the development of marrow in ganoid fish.) On the other hand, the mesenchyme is necessary for the development of the rudimentary bone in organ culture. When the mesenchyme of the femoral rudiment is removed and the invasion of the bone and medullary cavity formation does not occur, the femoral rudiment degenerates [Petrakis et al, 1969]. However, when these two elements, the rudimentary bone and the vascular mesenchyme, are cocultured, the femur develops a marrow cavity which can be induced by the addition of erythropoietin or thyroxin to become hemopoietic [Petrakis et al, 1969].

In the mouse, marrow hemopoiesis appears by 17–18 days of gestation (Fig. III.4; Table III.1). In man this is quite apparent at approximately 20 weeks [Knoll and Pingle, 1949], but Yoffey and Thomas [1964] have observed some marrow as early as 12 weeks and Yoffey et al [1961] have illustrated a transitional cell spectrum in femoral marrow as early as 15 weeks. Hemopoiesis is then intiatiated by the appearance of large numbers of undifferentiated basophilic cells within the dilated marrrow sinuses. These are presumably hemopoietic stem cells which are populating the newly developed stromal meshwork. In the mouse embryo, marrow hemopoiesis is limited to granulopoiesis, and erythropoiesis does not appear until after birth. Granulopoiesis is entirely exravascular. Other mammals, such as rats, may share this pattern [Lucarelli et al, 1967] but in human, embryonic marrow is erythropoietic as well. In the chick embryo, however, marrow undertakes both erythropoietic and granulopoietic function, erythropoiesis being intravascular whereas granulopoiesis, as is the case with the mouse, is extravascular. The thin layer of marrow sinus endothelium separates these foci. This compartmentalization has been demonstrated after the injection of tritiated thymidine-labeled hemopoietic cells, which leads to the segregation of erythroid and granulocytic cells, respectively, to the intravascular and extravascular compartments [Metcalf and Moore, 1971]. This compartmentalized pattern (intravascular erythropoiesis, extravascular granulopoiesis) in birds continues after hatching. By contrast, in mammals, when the marrow becomes erythropoietic after birth, erythropoiesis switches to the extravascular. The product of intravascular erythropoiesis in birds is nucleated red cells characteristic of the avian system; the product of extra-vascular erythropoiesis in mammals is anucleated red cells characteristic of the mammalian system. This relationship has been one of the bases of the formulation of the concept of bone marrow–blood barrier which is treated elsewhere in this volume (see Chapter VI).

Evidence that the stromal meshwork is "seeded" by circulating hemo-poietic stem cell is derived from sex chromosome studies in parabiosed chick embryos of opposite sex, demonstrating high reciprocal chimerism ap-proaching 50% equilibrium level [Metcalf and Moore, 1971].

In the mouse marrow both CFU-S and CFU-GM can be detected by day 17 of the gestation and their number progressively increases. Their doubling time is about 34 hours—considerably longer than those of both the yolk sac and liver. Marrow hemopoiesis expands as the liver and spleen hemopoiesis declines during the first postnatal week, at which time 50–60% of the total body CFU-S and 65–70% of CFU-GM are localized to the marrow. Splenic hemopoiesis also begins to decline by the end of the third postnatal week. After the first postnatal week the incidence of CFU-GM increases 3- to 5-fold whereas the incidence of CFU-S remains stable. CFU-S, and possibly CFU-GM, appear to seed the newly developing marrow stroma through the circulating blood. The origin of the stem cells seeding the marrow is proba-bly the fetal spleen, and perhaps yolk sac in the chick embryo. In the mouse, fetal liver is thought to be the origin of the developing marrow stem cells. In fact the rapid decline in the liver hemopoiesis is thought to be caused by mass migration of stem cells into the marrow [Baker et al, 1969], but this view has not been confirmed [Metcalf and Moore, 1971].

IV.

Marrow Structure

INTRODUCTION

Within the confines of bones, the marrow exists as a richly cellular and highly vascular loose connective tissue. Two components may be recognized in the marrow: the hemopoietic cells that comprise the majority of the cellular elements, and a highly organized stromal component that supports the proliferation of hemopoietic cells [Weiss, 1976; Shaklai and Tavassoli, 1979]. Hemopoietic cells are transient in the marrow. Upon maturation they move into blood stream. The stroma, however, remains and serves as a scaffolding upon which the hemopoietic cells can differentiate and mature. Effective hemopoiesis is the product of the interplay between these two components.

ORGANIZATIONAL LAYOUT

The organization of marrow can best be approached by following its vascular layout [Branemark, 1959; DeBruyn et al, 1970]. In a tubular bone (Fig. IV.1), the nutrient artery enters the marrow cavity and runs parallel to the long axis in the central part of the cavity. It branches out toward the bone and these branches lead to specialized vascular structures known as sinuses or sinusoids. Few branches may lead directly to the venous system. Sinuses are the first efferent elements of the marrow vasculature, and several of them may combine to form collecting sinuses which lead to the central

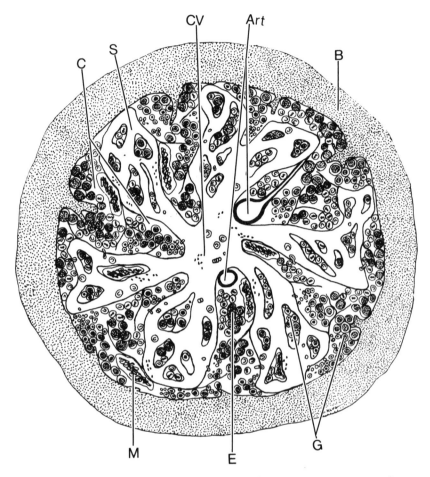

Fig. IV.1. A diagram of the organizational layout of bone marrow, as seen in the cross section of a tubular bone. The surrounding bone is identified (B). The central artery (Art) and vein (CV) run at the center parallel to the long axis of the bone. The artery gives out branches which run toward the periphery, leading to marrow sinuses (S). Sinuses are the first efferent elements of marrow vasculature, and lead to the central vein. Interspersed with sinuses is the hemopoietic space or cord (C), where developing erythroid (E) and granulocytic (G) cells appear in distinctive foci. Megakaryocytes (M) mature subjacent to the endothelium of marrow sinuses.

sinus or central vein. The latter vessel runs side by side with the nutrient artery and parallel to the long axis of the bone. The structural features of marrow vessels are discussed elsewhere in this volume (Chapter V).

As is evident from this general layout, within the marrow cavity the direction of blood flow is from the center of the cavity toward the bone and back again toward the center. This pattern yields an unusually high number of small vessels and, particuarly, sinuses in the periphery, in the vicinity of the bone. Because most exchanges occur through the wall of these small vessels and sinuses, the intensity of hemopoiesis is maximal at the periphery, leaving the central part of the bone with relatively little hemopoietic activity [Tavassoli, 1976b]. This is most evident in those bones that form a transition between red and yellow marrow (see Chapter VII and Fig. VII.2). In such bones, there is a gradient of increasing hemopoiesis from the central part of the cavity toward the bone. A gradient in the opposite direction is seen for adipocytes. Moreover, the spatial distribution of hematopoietic stem cells (CFU-S) and other progenitor cells (CFU-C, BFU-E, and CFU-E) shows a definite concentration gradient with relation to the bone. CFU-S and immature BFU-E have their highest concentrations near the bone with a decreasing gradient toward the center. More mature CFU-C and CFU-E concentration also demonstrates specific spatial distribution in relation to the bone [Frassoni et al, 1982; Lord et al, 1975; Lord and Hendry, 1972]. A similar pattern may also be present, although less appreciable, for cancellous bones where, in humans, most hemopoiesis takes place.

Within the hemopoietic areas of the marrow, hemopoiesis is highly compartmentalized. The two major compartments are vascular and hemopoietic compartments (Fig. IV.2). In mammals all hemopoietic cells proliferate extravascularly in the hemopoietic compartment, also known as hemopoietic cords. Upon maturation, they traverse the wall of specialized vascular sinuses to enter the blood stream [Tavassoli, 1978c; 1979b]. The walls of these vessels control the traffic of cells and molecules between the vascular and hemopoietic compartments. This traffic is the subject of a separate chapter in this volume (Chapter VI). Even in the hemopoietic cords, hemopoiesis is compartmentalized. Erythropoiesis takes place in distinct anatomical units, surrounding a central macrophage and known as erythroblastic islands [Shaklai and Tavassoli, 1979; Bessis, 1958]. Granulopoiesis also takes place in foci that, although less appreciable morphologically, are in association with a distinct reticular cell and thus recognizable as an entity [Westen and Bainton, 1979; LaPushin and Trentin, 1977]. Megakaryopoiesis occurs subjacent to the sinus endothelium, where the small cytoplasmic processes of the megakaryocyte penetrate the wall thereby anchoring the cell to the wall [Tavassoli, 1979a; Tavassoli and Aoki, 1981].

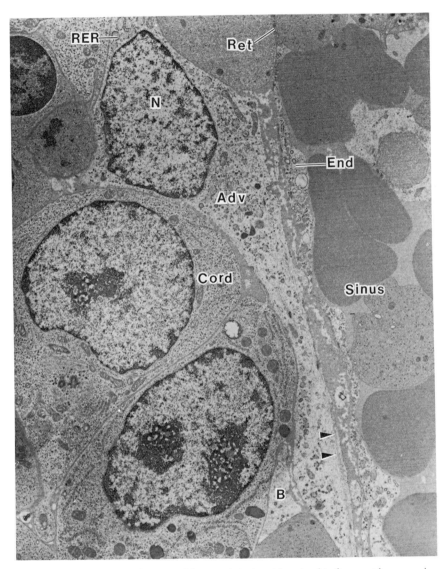

Fig. IV.2. Compartmentalization of hemopoiesis is evident in this figure with a vascular sinus on the right containing numerous red cells and newly released reticulocytes. Hemopoietic cord is on the left and contains parts of several developing cells, but is dominated by two developing granulocytic cells. The two compartments are separated by a wall consisting of a thin endothelial (End) and an adventitial (Adv) layer. The adventitial cell, the nucleus of which is identified (N), contains some fibers (arrowheads) and can thus be recognized as an adventitial reticular cell. The cell also contains profiles of rough endoplasmic reticulum (RER), suggestive of its protein synthetic activity. The cell and its branches (B) are in close association with the developing granulocyte. At the top, a fully mature reticulocyte (Ret) is attempting to move out into the sinus. It has elevated the adventitial cell and penetrated the endothelium. (× 9,000.)

Hemopoietic Cords

The hemopoietic cord is based on a meshwork of long, slender, and highly anastomosing branches of stromal cells. Two major types can be recognized: reticular cells and macrophages. Reticular cells are associated with fibers that can be visualized by light microscopy and after silver staining. The silver-staining fibers associated with reticular cells are known as reticulin fibers. By electron microscopy the seldom seen nuclear region of these cells may be located on the abluminal surface of the sinus endothelium, with the main body of the cytoplasm applied to the endothelium and forming a layer of the sinus wall. This makes the cells recognizable as "adventitial reticular cells" (Fig. IV.2). Slender cytoplasmic branches, however, penetrate deep into the hemopoietic cords, making frequent anastomoses with similar branches of other cells and thereby forming a scaffolding. The nuclear region can also be seen deep within the hemopoietic cords. In the latter situation, the cell is usually associated with granulopoietic foci.

Irrespective of the location of the main cell body and the nuclear region, this cell appears to be a single entity with distinct cytologic features. Its cytoplasm is often highly rarified, such that without the use of the tracer methods its branches may be confused with the extracellular space [Shaklai and Tavassoli, 1979; Tavassoli and Shaklai, 1979]. The salient feature of the cytoplasm is the presence of large numbers of ribosomes and rough endoplasmic reticulum (RER), usually in the perinuclear area. This feature suggests that the cell is highly active in protein synthesis. In addition the cell contains many filamentous structures, 6–9 nm in diameter, and it is possible that these fibers are the product of the protein synthetic activity in the cell (Fig. IV.2). The relation of these fibers to the reticulin fibers seen in light microscopy is not known. These fibers can be scattered in the cytoplasm, but they can also form bands—particularly in submembranous area. When the body's demand for blood cells is experimentally enhanced, the frequency of these submembranous bands increases. This observation has led to the suggestion that these bands are inserted into the membrane, causing retraction of the cell's cytoplasmic processes from the vicinity of the sinus wall and leading to an enhanced cell traffic across the wall [Tavassoli, 1977a].

Cytochemically, these cells are noted for their alkaline phosphatase positivity [Westen and Bainton, 1979], and in this regard they resemble osteoblasts that are also alkaline phosphatase–positive. Osteoblasts bear other similarities to these cells. They, too, have dominant features of protein synthesis and are associated with fibrous structures—eg, collagen. The association of this reticular cell with granulopoiesis is reported not only in the marrow but also in the spleen during the CFU-S formation [LaPushin and

Trentin, 1977], an observation suggesting the dependence of granulopoiesis on this stromal element.

A second cell type commonly seen in the hemopoietic cords is the macrophage. At least two subpopulations can be recognized; perisinal [Tavassoli, 1974d, 1977b] and central macrophages [Shaklai and Tavassoli, 1979; Bessis, 1958; Berman, 1967, Ben-Ishay and Yoffey, 1971a,b, 1972]. Perisinal macrophages are located in the vicinity of marrow sinuses, and their function in relation to the bone marrow–blood barrier is discussed in Chapter VI. Central macrophages (Fig. III.3) are surrounded by developing erythroid cells, and these formations are usually referred to as erythroblastic islands. In these islands, there is a spectrum of maturation in erythroid cells with the least mature cells located in the center and the most mature cells toward the periphery. This suggests that the cell maturation is associated with a displacement toward the periphery. This stratification, however, has been debated [Ben-Ishay and Yoffee, 1971a,b, 1972]. The main body and the nuclear region of the macrophage are located in the center, sending, octopuslike, long, slender cytoplasmic process to embrace the developing erythroid cells (Figs. IV.3, 4). The association of these processes with the developing erythroid cells is close, intimate, and extensive. It can best be appreciated with the use of freeze-fracture or tracer methods (Fig. IV.4) or when membrane-enhancing agents such as tannic acid are used (Fig. IV.3). Nearly two-thirds of the surface of every erythroid cell is covered by these processes. There is evidence that considerable exchange may take place between the two cells.

The salient morphologic feature of the central macrophage is the presence of large numbers of lysosomes and phagosomes, the latter consisting of extruded erythroid cell nuclei and occasionally an entire cell. Cytochemically, this cell is known for its acid phosphatase positivity, thus bearing a kinship to osteoclasts, which are also a form of macrophage. Acid phosphatase activity varies and seems to be proportional to the erythropoietic activity [Yoffey and Yaffe, 1980a]. When erythropoiesis is stimulated, the macrophage takes up an increased number of extruded nuclei, which must be subjected to digestion by lysosomes. The activity of lysosomal enzymes such as acid phosphatase then appears to be increased. Increased phagocytic activity of the central macrophage is necessary for recycling of the building blocks for the formation of new red cells. In addition to the DNA precursors present in the extruded nuclei, a small rim of hemoglobinized cytoplasm is also present around these nuclei which contains the iron needed for the formation of new cells. A most remarkable feature of the central macrophages is that, no matter how active erythropoiesis, they do not seem to be

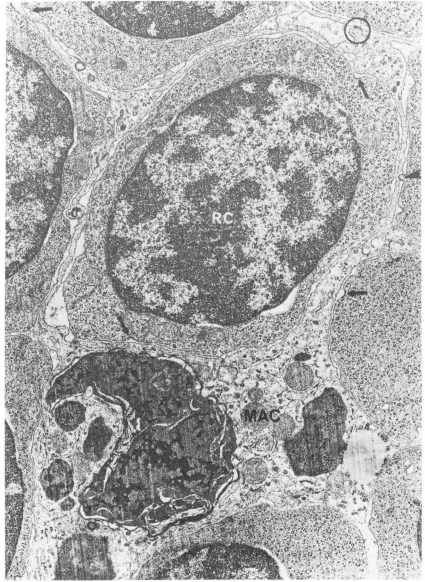

Fig. IV.3. Thin section of an erythroblastic island. To enhance the membrane contrast, the section has been treated with tannic acid. The central macrophage (MAC) contains some cellular debris including remnants of some nuclei. Note that the small, thin cytoplasmic processes of this cell run between erythroid cells and *completely embrace* one of them (RC), giving the false impression that the erythroid cell is actually located within the macrophage. Note numerous endocytic vesicles (arrows). In one area (arrowhead), an endocytic vesicle of the macrophage appears to "pinch off" another of the erythroid cell. A junctional density (circled) is also seen. [From Shaklai and Tavassoli, 1979. Courtesy of Academic Press.] (× 14,000.)

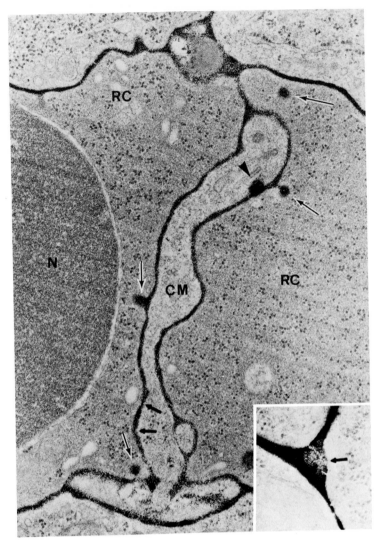

Fig. IV.4. Thin-section micrograph of a lanthanum-impregnated erythroblastic island. Lanthanum serves as an extracellular tracer and identifies slender, light cytoplasmic processes that may otherwise go unrecognized as cellular processes. In this figure, the light cytoplasmic processes of a central macrophage (CM) run between two erythroid cells (RC); the nucleus of one is identified (N). Lanthanum has also identified many endocytic vesicles in erythroid cells (arrows) and one within the CM (arrowhead). Note the thinning of the intercellular space (at the two black arrows toward the bottom), which may represent small adhering junctions. The inset shows a higher magnification of a small adhering junction delineated by lanthanum. [From Shaklai and Tavassoli, 1979. Courtesy of Academic Press.] (× 37,000; inset × 75,000.)

overloaded. On the other hand, when the demand for red cell formation is reduced by hypertransfusion, these macrophages are destroyed and do not readily regenerate [Brookoff and Weiss, 1982].

Association of macrophages with erythroid cells is also noted in spleen during CFU-S development [LaPushin and Trentin, 1977] and even in vitro in the course of BFU-E development [Parmley et al, 1978]. These observations suggest the dependence of erythropoiesis on this stromal element of the hemopoietic cord.

Other cell types have been described in the hemopoietic cord. A stromal cell is present that is recognizable only by its preferential uptake of lanthanum [Tavassoli et al, 1980], but these cell types may be the result of modulation of the two essential cell types.

Packed upon the scaffolding of these stromal cells are developing hemopoietic cells that are normally in close apposition, leaving little or no extracellular space.

The noncellular (extracellular) components of the hemopoietic cord have not been adequately studied. The presence of collagen fibers in developing marrow is well substantiated [Tavassoli and Weiss, 1971]. They may be produced by osteoblasts and thus related to bone formation, which is an integral part of the development of bone marrow.

In well-developed marrow, collagen-related silver-staining reticulin fibers are present in association with branching reticular cells which display numerous profiles of RER and appear to be involved in protein synthesis. These cells may bear a kinship to fibroblasts and osteoblasts. The chemical nature of the fibers remains to be better defined. The ground substance of the bone marrow probably consists of mucopolysaccharides (MPS), which can be neutral or acidic. There is some evidence that the ratio of these two types may influence the microenvironment of hemopoiesis, with the neutral MPS being favorable to this process [McCuskey et al, 1972; Tavassoli et al, 1976]. It has been postulated that some of the factors influencing hemopoiesis may do so by changing the nature of the MPS.

THE STROMA IN VITRO

There now exist methods to maintain the stromal elements of the marrow in culture. As is the case in vivo, these cultures can then support the proliferation and differentiation of hemopoietic cells [Dexter et al, 1977; Dexter and Testa, 1978; Greenberger, 1978, 1979, 1980; Sakakeeny and Greenberger, 1982].

In vitro, the stroma may also consist of several cell types. There exist some species variations [Wilson et al, 1981]. Stromal cells have the common characteristics of adherence to the substratum in vitro. The major component is a fibroblastic cell [Tavassoli and Takahashi, 1982] capable of producing collagen types I and III as well as fibronectin [Bentley, 1982]. This cell may be related to the in vivo reticular cells which are associated with reticulin fibers and may thus bear also a kinship to osteoblasts. As is the case in vitro, this cell is AP-positive [Tavassoli, 1982b]. In fact, AP positivity is a common denominator of this fibroblast, marrow reticular cells, and osteoblasts. However, marrow fibroblasts manifest species-specific differences. In human and hamster most of the fibroblast colonies are strongly AP-positive. This is also true of nearly half the colonies in mouse culture, whereas in rabbit and guinea pig cultures all the fibroblast colonies show a low AP activity. In continuous marrow cultures, this cell spreads widely over the surface of the culture dish, providing a "blanketing floor mat" upon which other cells can interact [Tavassoli and Takahashi, 1982].

It is now possible to grow these cells in the form of fibroblastic colonies (CFU-F) which can be quantitatively analyzed. When the initial explanation density of marrow cells does not exceed 10^4 cells per square centimeter, the nascent fibroblast colonies are clones, as proved by chromosome markers and by time-lapse cinematography [Friedenstein, 1976]. The fibroblasts in these colonies are distinguishable from the macrophages and endothelial cells by the following features: They synthesize type I and III collagen, but not type IV; they lack factor VIII and the F_c and complement receptors; their nonspecific esterase activity is low [Friedenstein, 1976; Friedenstein et al, 1982]. In addition to fibroblasts, colonies may also include macrophages and hemopoietic cells that adhere to fibroblasts, particularly in murine cultures.

CFU-F are highly adherent. In marrow they are nonproliferating, but after explantation they appear in their first S phase within 18–60 hours; on subsequent days they proliferate intensively, dividing every 20 hours. CFU-F concentration in mechanically dissociated guinea pig or mouse marrow is about 2×10^{-5}; in hamsters and humans the figures are 0.8×10^{-5} and 4×10^{-5}, respectively. In suspensions prepared by trypsinization, the CFU-F concentration increases 15-fold for mice and guinea pigs, and 20-fold for hamsters, remaining practically unchanged for rabbits and humans [Friedenstein, 1976; Friedenstein et al, 1982]. Hence, bone marrow stroma includes CFU-F of different adhesive capacity. However, these dissimilarities seem to be expressed differently in different species. In mice, the more adhesive CFU-F possess osteogenic properties and the ability to transfer the marrow microenvironment. It should be emphasized that the interpopulational hierarchy of the stromal cells, including the CFU-F, has not yet been established. Stromal fibroblasts of marrow and spleen in rabbits show no morphological or histochemical differences. However, in vivo reverse transplantation of these cells generates hemopoietic territories with different microenvironments: Fibroblasts from red marrow form red marrow ossicles; those of yellow marrow form yellow marrow ossicle [Patt et al, 1982]; yet spleen fibroblasts form lymphoid organs [Friedenstein et al, 1974]. Thus, stromal fibroblasts are capable of transferring the specific features of the microenvironment characteristic of the initial organ.

In the mouse, macrophages also constitute a major component of hemopoietic stroma in vitro [Wilson et al, 1981]. These are acid phosphatase-positive cells [Tavassoli, 1982b], bearing a kinship to in vivo marrow macrophages. They may also be related to osteoclasts that are also acid phosphatase–positive. In the mouse, in vitro macrophages differ from those in vivo by lacking characteristic crystalloid structures [Berman, 1967; Shaklai and Tavassoli, 1977] containing hemoglobin, but this may be the result of variations in the strains of mice studied. Adipocytes have also been described in continuous marrow culture [Dexter and Testa, 1978; Dexter et al, 1977; Greenberger, 1978], but this is probably not a distinct cell type: Both macrophages and epithelioid cells can accumulate fat under these culture conditions, and therefore the fat-containing cell must be considered a culture epiphenomenon [Tavassoli and Takahashi, 1982]. The presence of endothelial cells in continuous culture has been debated [Bentley, 1982], but recently good evidence of its presence has been provided by the demonstration of factor VIII antigen and other endothelial by-products such as collagen type IV and laminin [Zuckerman and Wicha, 1983].

STROMA AND HEMOPOIETIC MICROENVIRONMENT

Effective hemopoiesis is a multistep phenomenon. It consists of "lodging" of HSC, their proliferation and self-maintenance, their differentiation into various compartments of committed stem cells, their orderly maturation into functional cells that are then released into the circulation in an orderly fashion in response to the body's demand. Although in vitro experimental systems exist for many of these functions separately, it is only in the hemopoietic tissues and particularly in the bone marrow that these functions are integrated, and the integrated phenomenon is finely tuned to the body's demand. This integration is the function of the marrow stromal organization.

There is now considerable evidence that the marrow stroma provides a favorable microenvironment for sustained and controlled proliferation of hemopoietic cells [Trentin, 1971; Tavassoli, 1975a; Wolf, 1979; Tavassoli and Friedenstein, in press]. In man and other primates this microenvironment is unique, for in these species, during adult life, hemopoiesis is limited to the bone marrow, and extramedullary hemopoiesis is a pathologic phenomenon. Evidence for the role of stroma in regulation of hemopoiesis is summarized as follows:

1. Whereas the HSC circulate everywhere, hemopoiesis is limited to the marrow and to a lesser degree to certain other hemopoietic organs. Experimentally, this is evident by the "homing" of transfused marrow cells to the marrow and spleen of irradiated mice [Till and McCulloch, 1961]. An analogy can be made to the soil and seed: A favorable soil is necessary to support the optimal growth of the seed. This indeed is the basic tenet in marrow transplantation wherein a source of HSC is introduced into the circulation: Transient foci of hemopoiesis are formed throughout the microcirculation, but sustained hemopoiesis occurs only in the marrow [Osogoe and Omura, 1950].

2. In the embryo, hemopoiesis begins in the yolk sac, then the site of hemopoiesis switches to the spleen and liver and finally settles in the marrow. As the one organ's hemopoietic stroma becomes unsuitable to support hemopoiesis, HSC move into the circulation and home in other organs, the stroma of which can support hemopoiesis [Moore and Metcalf, 1970].

3. When fragments of marrow and splenic tissues are implanted in ectopic sites, first the stroma of the tissue is reconstituted and then hemopoiesis is resumed [Tavassoli and Crosby, 1968, 1970].

4. Similar stromal regeneration precedes the resumption of hemopoiesis when the marrow cavity is mechanically evacuated [Tavassoli et al, 1974, Patt and Maloney, 1975]. Here an analogy can be made to the succession process in the restoration of the plant population after a forest fire. Repopulation of the burnt-out area is gradual, the consecutive species forming the environments necessary for the successive species.

5. After high-dose local irradiation, a biphasic aplasia is seen. The early phase is attributed to the destruction of the HSC, which circulate from other parts of the body to reseed the marrow. The late and permanent aplasia is the result of the stromal injury [Knospe et al, 1968].

6. An occasional case has been reported in which transfused marrow cells from an identical twin failed to "take" and grow in the other twin with aplastic marrow disease, suggesting stromal disease [Fernbach and Trentin, 1962].

7. It is now possible to reconstitute the interactions of stroma and HSC in vitro [Dexter and Testa, 1978; Dexter et al, 1977; Tavassoli and Taka-

hashi, 1982]. These methods are based on growing an adherent stromal layer serving as the "soil" upon which a source of HSC can be "seeded." The adherent stroma can then support the proliferation of HSC.

8. Intraperitoneally inserted cellulose acetate membrane becomes coated with a supporting layer of macrophages and fibroblasts [Seki, 1973; Turner et al, 1978]. This layer, after irradiation and intraperitoneal introduction of a source of stem cell, can support hemopoietic colonies. This potential is remarkably enhanced when the membrane is precoated with hemopoietic stroma [Knospe et al, 1978].

9. The stroma cells can form fibroblast colonies (CFU-F) in cultures [Friedenstein et al, 1970; Friedenstein, 1976]. By repeated in vitro passaging, the descendants of CFU-F give rise to fibroblast strains. Heterotopic transplantation of such stromal fibroblasts leads to the formation of hemopoietic organs in which microenvironments characteristic of the donor organs are maintained [Friedenstein et al, 1974].

THE DUAL NATURE OF HEMOPOIETIC STROMA AND THE STEM CELL

Certain qualities of the hemopoietic stroma make it distinguishable from the HSC:

1. Differential radiosensitivity of stroma and stem cell with the stroma being somewhat more radioresistant [Knospe et al, 1968; Tavassoli, 1982b,c]. The survival curve of clonogenic stromal fibroblasts (CFU-F) following exposure to gamma rays is characterized by $Do = 200$ rads and $n = 1.5$ (the extrapolation number) [Kuzmenko et al, 1972; Friedenstein et al, 1981]; for HSC, then, values are 100 rads and 1.0, respectively.

2. Chromosome studies in cross-transplanted stroma indicate that the stroma is of donor origin but that HSC are of recipient origin [Tavassoli and Khademi, 1980]. Immunological and chromosome analyses in heterotopic marrow transplant and in radiochimeras have indicated that stromal fibroblasts and hemopoietic cells are derived from different cell lines [Friedenstein et al, 1968, 1978; Friedenstein and Kuralesiva, 1971]. In heterotopic marrow, the stromal fibroblasts are of donor and hemopoietic cells of recipient origin. The opposite is true of radiochimeras.

3. The two mutant mice $S1/S1^d$ and W/W^v serve as experimental models for the two components of hemopoiesis [Bernstein et al, 1968]. Both mutants are anemic: In $S1/S1^d$ owing to a defect in stroma, whereas in W/W^v the HSC is defective. The two systems are cross-correcting both in vivo and in vitro [Tavassoli et al, 1973a; Dexter and Moore, 1977].

4. HSC are circulating cells, but the stromal cells are fixed tissue cells. Recent evidence, however, indicates that these cells may have limited

mobility and can be transplanted by intravenous infusion [Keating et al, 1982; Piersma et al, 1982].

5. In vitro, the hemopoietic progenitor cells including the pluripotential stem cell can form distinct colonies in a supporting medium, but they need a stimulating factor to do so. Stroma, on the other hand, forms an adherent layer in liquid culture and, when the explantation density is low, may appear as fibroblastic colonies (CFU-F) [Friedenstein et al, 1970, 1974; Friedenstein, 1976].

THE NATURE OF INTERACTION

Little is known of the nature of the interaction between hemopoietic cells and their supporting stroma. Earlier observations on splenic colonies (CFU-S) indicated that the frequency of types of colonies (erythroid, granulocytic) formed in the spleen and marrow differ greatly [Trentin, 1971; Tavassoli, 1975a; Wolf, 1979], suggesting different microenvironmental qualities in the marrow and spleen. Moreover, each colony, although differentiated along only one cell line, still contained pluripotential stem cells as indicated by retransplantation experiments. This indicated that the hemopoietic organs contain microareas with different environmental qualities. As is the case with the yolk sac [Moore and Metcalf, 1970], each microarea is permissive only to differentiation of one cell line and precludes differentiation in other lineages. Several observations support this view:

1. As the splenic colonies expand with time, they encroach upon another microarea with different microenvironmental quality and then a second line of differentiation appears [Trentin, 1971].

2. Application of modern electromicroscopic (EM) techniques has permitted the appreciation of the extent of close association between hemopoietic cells and the stroma [Shaklai and Tavassoli, 1979; Tavassoli and Shaklai, 1979]. Almost three-fourths of the surface of every single developing hemopoietic cell is covered by thin processes of stromal cells which embrace the hemopoietic cells.

3. Both in the marrow and in splenic colonies, the line of differentiation appears to be associated with specific stromal cells type [Westen and Bainton, 1979; LaPushin and Trentin, 1977].

4. The donor stroma, or its fibroblasts, appears to instruct the recipient hemopoietic cells as to what line of differentiation they should take. Thus, transplantation of stroma from $S1/S1^d$ mice leads to normal myeloid and defective erythroid differentiation. Transplantation of single clones of marrow fibroblasts can establish heterotopic marrow organs in which all lines

of hemopoiesis are realized [Chajlakjan et al, 1978]. In the case of thymus, the stromal instruction not only covers the development of T cells, but it also displays the range of its immunological response: Thymus stroma from donors that are strong responders to a given antigen may instruct the recipient lymphoid cells to exhibit a strong response even when the recipient belongs to a low-responding line [Zinkernagel et al, 1978].

How the transfer of information between the stromal and hemopoietic cells comes about is unclear. Several studies in recent years have dealt with junctional structures in hemopoietic tissues [Tavassoli and Shaklai, 1979; Campbell, 1980]. Typical gap junctions are not present in these tissues. In other cell systems, these distinctive structures are means of information transfer by permitting intercellular exchanges of ions and molecules. Small desmosomelike junctions are occasionally seen between the cells in the bone marrow (Figs. IV.3, 4), but these structures may serve as temporary adhesive devices rather than serving as a means of information transfer. In this context it is necessary to point out that the hemopoietic cells in the marrow have a transient presence. Upon the completion of their maturation cycle they must move out in the blood, where they carry out their function. Structures such as tight junction that hold the cells tightly together may be detrimental to the function of hemopoiesis because they do not permit rapid release of cells into the circulation. Such junctions have been described in certain pathologic states associated with packed marrow and pancytopenia, suggesting that hemopoietic cells are not permitted to be released into the circulation. Thus, small desmosomelike junctions may be the only type of junction that can provide temporary adhesion between stromal and hemopoietic cells without interfering with the subsequent release of the latter cells.

Short-range stimuli [Wolf, 1979] are said to be necessary for cellular proliferation, but their nature is unclear. Pits and vesicles are common findings in the hemopoietic tissues both in vivo and in vitro (Figs. IV.3, 4). These structures are involved in endocytosis. Elaboration and local release of substances in the interstitium may be one means of short-range information transfer. Such substances can be removed locally by endocytosis. Direct transfer of vesicles between cells has also been documented [Tavassoli and Shaklai, 1979]. Here the exocytic vesicles in one cell are directly "pinched off " and internalized by another (Fig. IV.3). It is not known how widespread this occurrence is. Local release and uptake of substances as a means of information transfer may be similar to the hypothalamic-pituitary axis. Two hypotheses have been advanced concerning the principles of stromal regulation [Tavassoli and Friedenstein, in press]. The first assumes that the stroma emanates influences inducing expression of differentiation genes in the HSC; this determines which type of committed precursors is to be recruited in a given hemopoietic organ or in its zones. The second hypothesis maintains that HSC differentiate in all possible directions, but that the stromal influence is responsible for the selection of certain types of the committed precursors. More work in this area is needed to clarify the nature of dependence of hemopoiesis on its stromal support.

THE RELATION OF MARROW AND BONE

The developing of marrow is closely related to the formation and remodeling of bone. Thus, in humans, the hemopoietic marrow first appears during the second month of intrauterine life in the clavicles, which are the first bones to ossify. Marrow tissue can form bone [Tavassoli and Crosby, 1968, 1970; Amsel et al, 1969; Sahebekhtiari and Tavassoli, 1978]. The relationship of osteogenesis to hemopoiesis has been demonstrated in ectopic transplants of marrow tissue. When marrow tissue is transplanted autologously or isologously to ectopic sites, during the first 24 hours all hemopoietic cells move out of the implant, leaving only the scaffolding of the marrow stroma. Stromal cells then undergo dedifferentiation to form a mesenchymelike tissue with monotonous primitive cells. Some of these cells redifferentiate into osteoblasts and begin to lay down osteoid tissue. In the interstices of this osteoid tissue, primordial marrow cavity is formed and soon the organization of marrow appears. This marrow is seeded by circulating hemopoietic stem cells which then proliferate. Using chromosome markers in cross-transplanted tissues, it has been demonstrated that the hemopoietic cells are of recipient origin whereas the marrow stroma and osteogenic tissue are of donor origin [Tavassoli and Khademi, 1980]. Expansion of hemopoiesis in these implants is associated with bone resorption, so that the final product is a marrow nodule surrounded only by a shell of bone (see also Chapter VII and Figs. VII.3, 4).

A similar histogenetic pattern is seen when the marrow tissue is evacuated from tubular bones [Sahebekhtiari and Tavassoli, 1976]. Here again the regeneration of marrow tissue is preceded by osteogenesis. The bone undergoes resorption as the hemopoietic tissue expands and the resorption of the new bone is complete, as the preexisting tubular bone provides a shell for the newly regenerated marrow tissue.

Several points must be considered in regard to the close association of marrow and bone:

1. The bone provides a rigid confine for the marrow, where the marrow volume must remain fixed. Any change in the volume of active marrow

must then be compensated for by the development of a space-occupying component. One such component is the marrow adipocyte, which serves as a cushion to compensate for variations in the volume of active marrow. These variations are inevitable if the marrow is to respond to the variability in demand for hemopoiesis. With enhanced marrow activity, adipocytes undergo resorption, providing more space for the expansion of hemopoiesis. The reverse is true when the hemopoietic activity of marrow is reduced.

Another component of the marrow that can compensate for variations in the volume of active marrow is the vascular space. This factor is particularly dominant during the early life, when the marrow adipocyte has not been completely formed. Expansion of hemopoiesis is associated with a reduction in the size of the vascular space. In ectopic marrow implants, this inverse relationship is particularly dominant. In the course of histogenesis of these implants, the newly formed marrow sinuses have a large caliber. They appear to undergo considerable narrowing with the expansion of hemopoiesis.

2. There exists a close vascular connection between the bone and the marrow. Nutrient vessels of the bone enter the marrow to make anastomoses with marrow vessels. In addition, small arteries of the marrow enter the bone, making a loop and returning to the marrow. These anatomical features have been detailed in Chapter V. One consequence of these vascular interconnections is to maintain the anatomic standing of the loose marrow tissue within the hard bone. Otherwise, the marrow could collapse. Other consequences may be functional. It has been suggested that the Haversian canals of the bone may serve as a reservoir of cells that are responsible for marrow regeneration [Patt and Maloney, 1975]. These canals can also harbor hemopoietic stem cell and other progenitor cells. When needed, these cells can be supplied to the marrow through the vascular interconnections. Moreover, several findings suggest that the intensity of hemopoiesis may be related to the bone metabolic activity (see Chapter V). As mentioned above, the intensity of hemopoiesis within the marrow cavity follows a gradient with the peak near the bone. Heightened bone resorption and remodeling are associated with heightened hemopoetic activity [Little, 1969]. The distributions of skeletal blood flow and marrow activity have a similar pattern when studied by double-isotope technique [Van Dyke, 1967]. During the space expeditions, a total inhibition of bone formation has been found [Morey and Baylink, 1978]. This has been associated with a suppression of erythropoiesis [Tavassoli, 1982a], and it is possible that the two findings are related [Tavassoli, 1982a]. These observations all suggest a possible relationship between the metabolic activity of the bone and the

intensity of hemopoiesis. The nature of such interrelationship is not clear, but calcium may have an important role to play. Van Dyke [1967] has postulated a portal circulating pathway between the bone and marrow analogous to that of the hypothalamus-pituitary axis. It is entirely possible that some humoral factors may be produced as a result of bone remodeling and transmitted to the marrow. Such factors could locally alter the rate of hemopoiesis.

3. The limitation of hemopoiesis to the bone in adult primates has led to the question whether the bone is needed for the function of hemopoiesis. This question can be conclusively answered only if the hemopoietic marrow tissue can be grown in the absence of the bone. Ectopic implantation of marrow tissue generally leads to the formation of a marrow associated with bone and usually surrounded by a shell of bone. However, the implantation bed may favor the formation of one or the other component. A subcutaneous site, for instance, appears to favor osteogenesis whereas an omental site, particularly if the host is irradiated before implantation, favors hemopoiesis [Meck et al, 1973]. By implantation of dispersed and recompacted marrow tissue, Mack et al [1973] have been able to obtain hemopoietic modules free of bone, and they concluded that the osteogenesis is not an obligatory prerequisite of hemopoiesis in the marrow. This question, however, is not completely settled as the hemopoietic nodules so obtained are predominantly granulocytic and may not exactly fulfill the organizational criteria of the marrow tissue.

V.

Marrow Circulation

INTRODUCTION

The blood supply of the bone marrow presents a number of distinctive features that make the marrow circulation unique. All three major constituents of the vascular tree—arteries, sinusoids, and veins—exhibit modifications in their morphology that are presumably structural adaptations to the functional needs of the bone marrow, directed to maintaining optimal conditions in the sinusoids. It is in the sinusoids that the essential functions of the bone marrow are discharged, namely to permit the constant passage throughout life of plasma and large numbers of cells—even, at times, cells of the size of megakaryocytes [Tavassoli and Aoki, 1981]—mainly from marrow into blood. Cells leaving the marrow to enter the blood are *myelofugal*; those entering the marrow from the bloodstream are *myelopetal*.

It is true that capillaries in many parts of the body permit the passage of an occasional leukocyte or erythrocyte, but this is a very different phenomenon from the vast numbers of cells that constantly traverse the sinusoidal endothelium throughout life. When one contemplates the extremely thin and apparently delicate endothelium of the sinusoid, one wonders how it maintains its integrity. A full account of the structure of the sinusoidal endothelium is given in Chapter VI. Some interesting data will also be found in the review by Lichtman [1981].

In addition to the specialized structure of its blood vessels, the fact that the marrow is situated within a rigid and inexpansible bony cavity presents problems which in some ways are very similar to those arising in connection with the intracranial vessels. In both situations, one of the first essentials is that venous outflow should not be obstructed. In the case of the intracranial vessels, this objective is attained through the special structure of the venous sinuses, which renders them virtually incompressible, while in addition a system of emissary veins provides a further safeguard.

THE STRUCTURE OF THE MARROW VEINS

In contrast, in the case of the marrow veins, the walls are extremely thin, a fact first noted by Bizzozero as far back as 1868, and later confirmed by numerous observers [eg, de Marneffe, 1951; Yoffey, 1962; Tavassoli, 1974a]. In addition to possessing thin walls, the veins of the marrow are disproportionately large. They are easy to see in section, and they have also been demonstrated in situ by the technique of microradiography [eg, Brookes and Harrison, 1957; Ecoiffier et al, 1957]. The vein wall consists of a single layer of endothelium, exactly like that of the sinusoids, so that it is difficult to decide at what point a sinusoid becomes a vein. Apart from the difference in caliber, the walls of the sinusoids and so-called veins seem to be identical. This led DeBruyn et al [1970, 1971] to refer to the main marrow vein as the "central sinusoid"; the tributary veins they referred to as the "collecting sinusoids."

As far as the thickness of their walls is concerned, therefore, the veins of the marrow are easily compressible. However, they are relatively very large. Rindfleisch [1880] estimated that in the guinea pig the cross section of the marrow veins is about 20 times that of the arteries. Yoffey [1965], working with the same animals, thought the ratio was near 1:30. This very large venous caliber obviously admits of very considerable narrowing of the lumen before the stage of obstruction is reached.

In the guinea pig, the single layer of endothelium which constitutes the wall of the veins has been shown to resemble the sinusoidal endothelium not only in its structure, but also in its phagocytic properties. India ink injected IV is ingested with equal rapidity by both the sinusoidal and the venous endothelium of the marrow [Hudson and Yoffey, 1963]. It is therefore not surprising that one finds in the literature such terms as "venous sinusoids" [Doan, 1922] or "Venensinus" [Bargmann, 1930]. DeBruyn et al [1970, 1971], in addition to the "collecting sinusoid" and "central sinusoid," introduced the term "primary sinusoid" for the start of the sinusoidal pathway.

Ecoiffier et al [1957] illustrated the "centro-medullary vein" running longitudinally in the femur of a rabbit, with many small veins entering it at right angles, a picture not too dissimilar from that obtained by Rindfleisch in 1880, and later observers [cf Hashimoto, 1936; Fliedner et al, 1956; Brookes and Harrison, 1957; Yoffey, 1962; Tavassoli, 1974a]. Venous blood is drained from the marrow both by the main vein, which traverses the nutrient foramen, and through a varying number of additional veins, sometimes quite large, near the ends of the bones. These latter function in the same way as the emissary veins of the skull. Michelsen [1967] made use of an emissary vein for the purpose of measuring the medullary venous pressure.

Because of the extreme thinness of their walls, the medullary veins respond rapidly to changes in the general venous pressure. Furthermore, they transmit these changes to the surrounding marrow tissue [Gilfillan et al, 1957; Cuthbertson et al, 1964], so that the pressures in the medullary vein ("medullary venous pressure") and in the bone marrow are nearly equal [Michelsen, 1967]. The bone marrow pressure, sometimes referred to as the tissue pressure, is measured by means of a needle inserted blindly into the marrow tissue through a hole in the cortex of the bone. Michelsen [1967] found that the intramedullary venous pressure was generally between 25 and 50 cm saline, whereas the pressure in the emissary vein outside the bone ranged between 5 and 25 cm saline.

Although the main vein is relatively very large while actually in the marrow cavity, it narrows down very abruptly as it passes out of the marrow cavity through the nutrient foramen, within whose rigid confines it is capable of only very slight dilation. Consequently, if there is a greatly increased outflow of blood from the marrow, it cannot all escape via the nutrient vein, beyond whose limited capacity other channels of outflow come into action, the most abundant of these being the metaphyseal emissary veins [Breuer et al, 1964]. Furthermore, as these last-named authors point out, "from the outflow through the vena nutritia, which is cannulated at the foramen nutritium, the total flow through the marrow cannot be calculated. The outflow from the cannulated vena nutritia does not proportionately increase with the total blood flow through the femoral bone marrow." Their experiments were performed on rabbits.

Post and Shoemaker [1964], working with dogs, tried to obtain a more accurate measurement of the total venous outflow by dissecting out all the veins draining the femur. The figure thus obtained includes blood-draining bone as well as marrow, but this objection may also apply to an unknown extent to measurements of blood flow in the nutrient vein. In the case of the canine femur this problem does not usually arise, since according to Post and Shoemaker [1964] there was no nutrient vein in 23 out of 27 dogs examined, and in the four animals in which a vein was present, it was very small. In the canine tibia, on the other hand, a well-marked nutrient vein may be found [Drinker et al, 1922].

Another consequence of the great thinness of the walls of the veins and sinusoids is that blood or saline readily enters the general circulation if injected into the marrow at even moderate pressure [Tocantins and O'Neill, 1941]. Furthermore, the tenuous walls of the vessels are easily torn in injuries such as fractures, and under these circumstances the open ends of the larger veins allow easy entry into the bloodstream of cell clumps, including fat cells. If the marrow concerned is fatty, large numbers of fat cells may enter the circulation and give rise to fat embolism [Rappaport et al, 1951; Havig and Gruner, 1973; McCarthy et al, 1977].

THE ARTERIAL SUPPLY

The blood supply of the bone marrow appears to depend primarily on the nutrient artery [Rindfleisch, 1880], but is supplemented to a variable extent by periosteal arteries [Brookes and Harrison, 1957; Branemark, 1959; Gothman, 1960; Tavassoli, 1974a; Lichtman, 1981]. According to Brookes and Harrison, the nutrient artery in the rabbit femur also supplies the compact bone of the shaft, which they regard as receiving virtually no blood from the periosteal arteries. The passage of vessels from the medulla into the compact bone of the shaft and then back to the medulla has been emphasized in varying degrees by a number of workers [eg, Drinker et al, 1922; Johnson, 1927; de Marneffe, 1951; Laing, 1953; Gothman, 1960; Fliedner et al, 1956; Branemark, 1959; Tavassoli, 1974a; Lichtman, 1981]. Rohlich [1941] suggested that blood flowing from the marrow into Haversian canals and then returning to the marrow might in its passage through the bone acquires some hemopoietic stimulus. The nature of such a possible stimulus has been the subject of considerable speculation (see also Chapter IV).

One possible stimulus is calcium. The interchange of calcium between bone and blood may turn out to have some bearing not only on calcium metabolism per se, but also on the possible role of calcium in hemopoiesis. Perris et al [1967] noted that the intraperitoneal injection of calcium and magnesium chloride stimulated the entry into mitosis of cells both in marrow and thymus. However, parathyroid hormone increased mitosis in marrow, but not in thymus, and they attributed this difference to the increased outflow of calcium from the bone. The highest concentration of calcium would be found in the blood vessels immediately on their emergence from the bone, and this could explain the greater hemopoietic activity of the peripheral as opposed to the more centrally situated myeloid tissue of the long bones. Morton [1968] investigated the effect of calcium on the mitosis of bone marrow cells in vitro, and found that the use of calcium-enriched serum produced marked mitotic stimulation. He suggested that the action might be on cells "normally in a dormant state," and noted that the stimulated cells might have a mean generation time of 4 hours.

Hunt and Perris [1973] observed that subcutaneous injections of eryth-ropoietin increased both the plasma calcium concentration and the mitotic activity of the bone marrow. They concluded further that this activity was a specific property of the erythropoietin molecule itself, and was not due to any impurities. The increased mitosis and hypercalcemia consequent upon erythropoietin injection in normal rats did not occur in animals whose parathyroids had been removed. The mitotic changes were measured by counting the number of cells arrested in metaphase at various times after colchicine injections.

The in vivo observations of McCluggage et al [1971] suggest that eryth-ropoietin causes vascular dilation in the marrow, and it is conceivable that its effect on calcium mobilization is secondary to vascular changes. How calcium stimulates mitosis is not clear. But it is pertinent to note that, in the case of lymphocyte proliferation, Tsien et al [1982] reported that lectins which stimulated T lymphocytes caused a rise in cytoplasmic calcium within minutes. They raised the possibility that an increase in cytoplasmic free calcium might trigger the succession of intracellular processes needed for proliferation. The concentration of calcium would presumably be at its highest in the blood first emerging from the Haversian canals into the marrow cavity. It is therefore in the outer part of the marrow that cell growth should be most active if calcium acts as a powerful proliferative stimulus. Conversely, the central part of the marrow cavity, furthest from the bone, should be the least active. This may explain why fat cells tend to develop in the central portion of the marrow.

It is generally assumed that there is free communication in the cortical bone between the branches of the periosteal arteries on the outside of the cortex and the branches of the nutrient artery on the inside. This view is further reinforced by observations such as those of DeBruyn et al [1970], that the vessels of the bone marrow can be injected even if the nutrient artery is completely blocked.

Thick-Walled and Thin-Walled Arteries

There is one respect in which the arteries of the marrow appear to be quite distinctive. Arteries with walls of normal thickness abruptly become thin-walled [Hashimoto, 1936; Yoffey, 1962; Tavassoli, 1974a], so that the walls then consist of only two layers of cells (Fig. V.1). The thin-walled arteries then pass into the single-layered sinusoids. The thin-walled arteries often run for a considerable length in the medulla, and as Tavassoli [1974a] has emphasized, they have the further peculiarity that they give off branches at right angles. It would appear that Bargmann [1930] was also observing the thin-walled arteries when he described the thicker-walled arteries as ending in what he termed arterial capillaries, which then opened into a "Venensinus"—the sinusoid of present-day terminology [cf Burkhardt, 1962]. The thin-walled arteries often run for a considerable distance by the side of the thin-walled veins [Yoffey, 1962].

The precise role of the thin-walled arteries is not clear. From the thinness of their walls, they must be readily distensible. Their distension with every

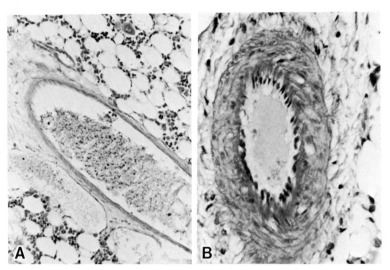

Fig. V.1. The wall structure in diagonally sectioned thin-walled (A) and horizontally sectioned thick-walled (B) arteries of rabbit tibia. Both stained with PAS and hematoxylin. From Tavassoli [1974a]. Both ×45.

heartbeat in a closed and rigid cavity must result in correspondingly repeated increases in medullary pressure which could be a major driving force in expelling cells from the marrow parenchyma into the blood through the endothelium of the sinusoids and veins.

Plasma Skimming

Another possible role of the thin-walled arteries may be to give rise to *plasma skimming* [Yoffey, 1977]. In observations on the sinusoids of living marrow one frequently sees sinusoids which appear to contain hardly any or no cells [Kinosita and Ohno, 1961; Branemark, 1959], so plasma skimming must presumably occur. It seem unlikely that the thin-walled arteries can constrict as completely as normal arteries, but if they can constrict with moderate severity along a fair length, they might conceivably keep back most of the blood cells and thus allow only plasma to flow into the sinusoids. Tavassoli [1974a] has suggested that the occurrence of plasma skimming is accentuated by the peculiar emergence of branches at right angles from the thin-walled arteries.

THE SINUSOIDS IN VIVO

A number of observations have been made on the circulation in the living marrow. The first we owe to Kinosita et al [1956], who made two parallel windows in the lower part of the rabbit tibia, and after removing the bone marrow observed its regeneration and restoration to normality after 5 weeks. The living marrow could then be studied by phase-contrast microscopy. Many of the sinusoids were seen to be arranged in approximately hexagonal units. Kinosita and Ohno [1961] reported a similar procedure in the lower end of the rabbit femur. They confirmed the earlier work, and noted that the sinusoids were often disposed in groups of three or four in which there was a "seemingly circular movement of blood." Erythropoiesis was invariably extravascular, and the maturing erythrocytes were seen traversing the sinusoidal wall and entering the lumen, often very characteristically in line, one after another, through an aperture which closed as soon as the passage ceased. The flow of blood through the sinusoids was sometimes stagnant, and they commented that "momentary stasis of blood flow and distension of the wall in a particular portion of sinusoids appear necessary for the movement and liberation of mature erythrocytes." They noted further that the blood in the sinusoids showed alternate movement and stagnation.

Branemark [1959, 1961] devised a technique for examining the circulation in normal (ie, not regenerating) marrow. The compact bone in a small area of the diaphysis of the rabbit fibula was ground down in two small areas on opposite sides of the bone, on one side to tissue-paper thickness. This provided a transparent window through which the marrow could be studied when transilluminated from the opposite side. Branemark's technique made possible the repeated examination of a segment of normal marrow. He confirmed the presence of hexagonal sinusoids, but also saw some that were spindle-shaped. The sinusoids ranged from 15 to 60 μm in diameter and showed rhythmic dilatation and emptying. The phase of dilatation usually lasted for 1–2 min, during which time the flow either slowed down or else stopped completely. The emptying phase was somewhat shorter. The bone marrow arterioles divided "dichotomously into capillaries," and these ran into either hexagonal or spindle-shaped sinusoids [see Branemark, 1959, Fig. 46, p 75], which were drained by venules into collecting veins.

There is no clear definition of what was meant by "capillaries" in these in vivo studies. It is not certain to what extent the term "capillary," as normally understood, can be applied to the vessels of the marrow. Doan [1922] described intersinusoidal capillaries in the bone marrow of the pigeon, but it is not certain that these "capillaries," apart from being often collapsed, were fundamentally different in structure from the sinusoids. The existence of intersinusoidal capillaries has not been confirmed either in man [Schleicher, 1946] or in the guinea pig [Zamboni and Pease, 1961; DeBruyn et al, 1971]. It is possible that the capillaries described by Branemark are the thin-walled arteries already mentioned.

Branemark observed that in normal fibular marrow, which was relatively fatty, there were only a few narrow vessels, whereas if erythropoiesis was stimulated by bleeding, a complex vascular network developed with many dilated sinusoids. The approximate diameters of the various vessels were as follows: arteriole, 10 μm; capillary, 8 μm; sinusoid, 15–60 μm; and venule, 12 μm. Measurements of the corpuscular flow velocity were the following: arteriole, 1–1.5 mm/sec; capillary, 0.5 mm/sec; sinusoid, 0–0.2 mm/sec; and venule, 0.1–0.3 mm/sec. Thus the rate of flow was slowest in the sinusoids and venules, and as already noted it is impossible to say where the sinusoid ends and the venule begins.

Branemark emphasized that in the spindle-shaped sinusoids one may often see a collection of blood cells, usually leukocytes, "hugging" the wall of the sinusoid in the bulge of the spindle, whereas blood flowed normally through its central portion. The significance of this "hugging" phenomenon is not clear. It could be a stage in the process by which blood lymphocytes leave the circulation to enter the marrow. However, the identity of the leukocytes involved has not been established.

Branemark was also able to see branches from the marrow arterioles entering the Haversian canals and then swinging back into the marrow. The blood flow in the bone was comparatively steady, and the corpuscular rate of flow was fairly high, being 0.8 mm/sec in the capillaries and 0.2 to 0.5 mm/sec in the venules.

McCuskey et al [1971] developed a technique involving the insertion of a chamber into the proximal end of a rabbit's tibia. This technique has the advantage of permitting the examination of living marrow for periods of up to 1 year. In addition, they could employ monochromatic light with a wavelength in the specific absorption wave band of hemoglobin (4,046), thereby greatly facilitating the identification of mature red cells, and some of the earlier stages of the nucleated erythroid series. In the main, they confirmed the findings of previous workers, including the direct passage of arterioles into sinusoids without an intervening capillary. Occasionally, capillaries were seen to bypass a sinusoid and shunt blood from an arteriole into a postsinusoidal vessel, but they were unable to observe the intersinusoidal capillaries of Doan [1922].

McCluggage et al [1971] examined the changes in normally hypocellular bone marrow following the stimulation of erythropoiesis by phlebotomy or erythropoietin. The most striking change seems to have been the great increase in dilated or polygonal networks of sinusoids. This change in vascularity was accompanied by increased numbers of hemopoietic cells, together with some degree of absorption of bone spicules.

MARROW BLOOD FLOW

Cumming and Nutt [1962] measured the flow of blood through the femoral marrow of rabbits by collecting the venous outflow from the nutrient vein. "Mean rate of blood flow through the femoral marrow was 0.41 ml/g/min. Erythroid marrow, which represents 1.7% of the body weight of rabbits, receives 7.6% of the cardiac output." This is a striking observation, but it is possible that the actual blood flow is even greater, since the method would miss other veins which might be draining the marrow, especially in the region of the metaphyses. Post and Shoemaker [1964], working with dogs, devised a technique whereby they could measure the outflow of blood from the entire femur, draining the blood from both ends of the bone (the "upper and lower venous efflux"). In most of the canine femora they examined, a nutrient vein was absent, so that the main venous outflow would be represented by the metaphyseal veins.

Some of the venous outflow would represent circulation through the bone, not the marrow. The problem may be further complicated by the existence of communications between the medullary veins and the veins in the muscles immediately adjoining the bone. Shaw [1964] drew attention to this in studies on the cat femur. When the quadriceps muscle was stimulated to contract, there was an increase in medullary blood flow and pressure. If the quadriceps stimulation is repeated a number of times, there is an increase in the medullary blood flow and a fall in the muscle blood flow, suggesting a shunting of blood from muscle into bone and medulla. If this interpretation is correct, then blood might be capable of flowing in the reverse direction when muscle contraction ceases. We do not know how extensive this osseomuscular circulation may be, but the mere possibility of its occurrence suggests that one should accept with caution any estimates of medullary blood flow which are based on the amount of blood escaping through the nutrient vein. In all probability such estimates give only a minimal figure, in which case the flow of blood through the marrow could be appreciably greater.

Age Variation in Medullary Blood Flow

Normal animals show considerable variation in the amount of blood flowing through the marrow [Drinker et al, 1922; Cumming, 1962; Cumming and Nutt, 1962; Held and Thron, 1962; Breuer et al, 1964; Breuer and Hirsch, 1964; Michelsen, 1968, 1969b]. Cumming [1962] thought that the differences in blood flow were due to variations in the content of red marrow, so that in those bones in which red marrow is progressively replaced by fatty marrow, the differences in blood flow are a function of age. In other words, the red marrow of younger individuals has a richer blood supply than the fatty marrow of older subjects. Michelsen [1967] found that not only the blood flow, but also the intramedullary pressure, showed considerable variation. As a rule the two vary directly, as noted by Shaw [1964] in 90% of his experiments.

Another aspect of the changes in marrow circulation with age was noted by Ecoiffier et al [1957], who reported that both the centromedullary vein and its tributaries were appreciably smaller in old than in young rabbits. In view of what has previously been written about the relationship between the blood supply of marrow and bone, it seems reasonable to speculate that the progressive narrowing of the medullary blood vessels with age is associated with a diminished blood supply to the bone. This could be an important contributory factor in the development of senile osteoporosis. The changes in the bone might therefore be secondary to changes in the marrow.

Changes in Marrow Activity and Blood Flow

If the greater blood flow in the marrow of young animals is a reflection of its hemopoietic activity, it should be possible to reverse the normal age change and to increase the blood flow by stimulating the marrow activity. The experimental production of such an increase has been demonstrated by several observers. Thus, Michelsen [1969b] found a greatly increased blood flow in rabbits made anemic by phenylhydrazine. The mean blood flow through the rabbit femur rose from 0.47 to 1.21 ml/min g wet marrow tissue. Breuer and Hirsch [1964], again with rabbit femoral marrow, found a rate of flow of 0.15 to 0.25 ml/min g in yellow marrow, and 0.9 to 1.3 ml/min/g in red marrow. Linke et al [1965] also recorded an increased blood flow after bleeding. This may be correlated perhaps with the marked dilatation of the sinusoids so evident on erythropoietic stimulation [Slavin et al, 1981].

Branemark [1959], who examined the bone marrow directly in vivo, had previously drawn a distinction between what he termed "high-activity" and "low-activity" marrows. The high-activity marrow was the result of repeated bleeding: 'The capillaries form a complex network and dilated sinusoids dominate the picture." In low-activity marrows, on the other hand, "the vascular bed is made up of a few long narrow capillaries with the cells traveling mainly in single file. Only few sinusoids are seen, and most of them are relatively narrow." However, Branemark took care to emphasize that the vascular bed is never completely uniform, so that even in a high-activity marrow one can always find some fields with only scanty vessels and single sinusoids.

McCluggage et al [1971] also observed vascular dilatation in marrow stimulated by bleeding or erythropoietin, and they further noted that small spicules of bone were actually absorbed during the period of increased vascularity. Almost 50 years previously, Drinker et al [1922] had noted that the tibiae of dogs which had been bled a number of times showed "diminution of cancellous bone and a relatively smooth-walled cavity filled with marrow." Findings of this nature suggest that one of the reactions to bleeding—or other forms of erythropoietic stimulation such as the administration of erythropoietin or prolonged hypoxia—might be to induce the absorption of bone on a scale sufficient to enlarge the marrow cavity, with resultant increase in the volume of erythropoietic tissue. However, the experiments of Hudson [1960b] appear to argue against this, at least in the case of moderately sustained hypoxia. By means of an accurate technique for the measurement of marrow volume, Hudson was able to show that there was no significant increase in the total marrow volume in guinea pigs hypoxic from birth and killed when several weeks old.

Nervous Control of Blood Flow

Since the observations of Gros [1846], a number of investigators have confirmed the presence of nerves, both myelinated and unmyelinated, in the bone marrow [Variot and Remy, 1880; de Castro, 1929a,b; Ottolenghi, 1902; Calvo, 1968]. That some of the fibers may be sensory is suggested by the unpleasant sensation sometimes evoked by marrow biopsy in the conscious patient. But most of the fibers seem to terminate in the vicinity of blood vessels and are presumably vasomotor in function. Drinker and Drinker [1916] stimulated what they termed the "nerve to the marrow." This is a small nerve, a branch of the tibial, which lies in close relation to the nutrient artery and accompanies it into the medullary cavity. They noted that stimulation of this nerve results in a diminished outflow of blood from the marrow. Drinker et al [1922] also observed the vasoconstrictor effect of adrenalin on the marrow vessels. Michelsen [1968] compared the action of acetylcholine and of noradrenaline, and noted that "the predominant effect of the former was to dilate, and of the latter to constrict the arteries of the marrow." Recent observations [Brown and Adamson, 1977] on the stimulation of erythroid colony formation by β-adrenergic agonists (isoproterenol), and the inhibition of this effect by the global β-blocker, propranolol, raise the question whether there may be a more direct action on erythropoiesis resulting from nervous stimulation than has hitherto been thought. One is reminded of observations such as those of Feldman et al [1966] and Medado et al [1967], who implanted electrodes into the posterior hypothalamic region and midbrain, and found that electrical stimulation was associated with a marked increase in erythropoietic activity. There was no increase in the secretion of erythropoietin. Erythropoietin-independent factors such as the burst-forming factor had not yet been described.

RETICULOENDOTHELIAL CELLS IN THE MARROW

For over a century numerous investigators have demonstrated the uptake by the bone marrow of particulate matter from the bloodstream [Hoffman and Langerhans, 1869; Hoyer, 1869; Ponfick, 1869; Cousin, 1898; Kiyono, 1914; Evans, 1915; Nagao, 1920, 1921; Wislocki, 1921, 1924; Hashimoto, 1936; Huggins and Noonan, 1936; Patek and Bernick, 1960]. However, the illustrations accompanying these reports are remarkably few in number and show very little detail. Hudson and Yoffey [1963, 1968] reinvestigated the uptake of particulate matter by the marrow, using a nontoxic suspension of colloidal carbon. The distribution of carbon particles was followed in the bone marrow of normal guinea pigs at intervals from 5 min to 28 days after IV injection.

In light-microscopic studies [Hudson and Yoffey, 1963] particles of carbon were first seen in the parenchyma after 15 min. After 30 min, macrophages

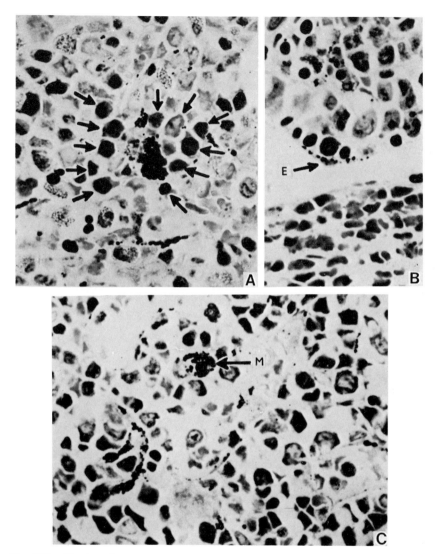

Fig. V.2. Uptake of carbon particles, after IV injection, by reticuloendothelial cells of guinea pig bone marrow. A) Sixty minutes after injection, a parenchymal macrophage is full of carbon and surrounded by a number of erythroblasts (arrows). This is a typical erythroblastic island. ×1,000. B) Endothelium of a vein 90 min after injection. The lower part of the figure is occupied by a mass of blood cells lying within the lumen of a large vein. A number of carbon particles are present in an endothelial cell (E), some in the region of the nucleus. ×1,050. C) Parenchymal macrophage 90 min after injection. The arrow indicates the nucleus of a macrophage (M) laden with carbon particles. From Hudson and Yoffey [1963]. ×850. Courtesy of the Journal of Anatomy.

containing carbon could be identified readily in teased preparations, whereas at 60 min heavily labeled macrophages could be seen in erythroblastic islands (Fig. V.2). By 3 hours after injection, ink-containing macrophages are to be found diffusely scattered throughout the marrow. The spacing between these ink-laden macrophages is of the same order as between erythroblastic islands, though in fact one sometimes sees ink-laden macrophages without surrounding erythroid cells. The finding of carbon particles in the parenchyma 15 min after IV injection compares with the observation of Zamboni and Pease [1961], who found that colloidal thorium dioxide in the bloodstream became dispersed throughout the marrow parenchyma within 10 min.

Ultrastructural examination shows that 5 min after the IV injection of ink, caveolae and vesicles containing carbon particles may be seen (Fig. V.3). It is not clear whether these vesicles represent the normal mechanism for the transport of particles across the endothelium [Palade 1953, 1961; Moore and Ruska, 1957; Florey, 1964], or whether the particles can pass through very fine ad hoc fenestrations in the endothelium as suggested by Zamboni and Pease [1961] in their experiments with colloidal thorium dioxide, or whether in fact both these processes can occur. At any rate, the injected particles can find their way through the endothelium in a very short time. Once through the endothelium, their movement might be effected by the transparenchymal plasma flow, only to cease when they are ingested by macrophages, most of which seem to be in the erythroblastic islands.

TRANSPARENCHYMAL PLASMA FLOW

The endothelium of the sinusoids is freely permeable to large molecules such as the plasma proteins, and even to particulate matter [Hudson and

---

Fig. V.3. Upper figure is a low-power electron micrograph of a sinusoid of guinea pig bone marrow 5 min after IV injection of carbon particles. E, endothelium. Large numbers of carbon particles are present in the lumen of the vessel where several cells, mostly lymphocytes, are also seen. Small accumulations of particles are present in vesicles (V) in the endothelium. P is the cytoplasmic process of a cell protruding into a fenestration in the endothelium, but no particles are seen either in or outside this fenestration. From Hudson and Yoffey [1963]. ×6,800. Lower figure is a high-power view of the endothelium of a sinusoid 5 min after IV injection. The lumen is at the top of the picture. Several caveolae (C) are present, one of which contains carbon particles. Particles are also present in intracytoplasmic vesicles (V). In the vesicle to the right, the particles lie peripherally while the central part contains amorphous material. From Hudson and Yoffey [1968]. ×37,400. Courtesy of the Journal of Anatomy.

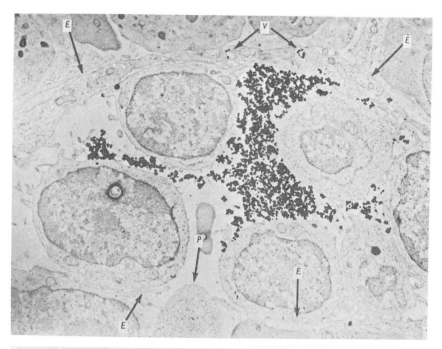

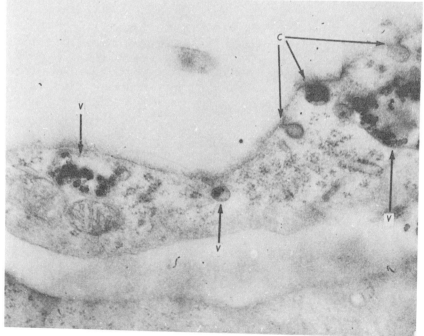

Yoffey, 1963, 1968]. The plasma proteins can pass rapidly both from the blood into the marrow parenchyma and from the parenchyma back into the bloodstream [Michelsen, 1969a]. This obviates any necessity for lymphatic drainage, and explains why the marrow does not require lymphatics for the removal of extravascular protein. The free flow of plasma through the marrow parenchyma is referred to as the *transparenchymal plasma flow* [Yoffey, 1977]. Because of this transparenchymal flow, it should be possible for a sinusoid, even with complete stasis of blood flow, to receive a considerable amount of plasma percolating through the surrounding parenchyma after traversing the endothelium of many neighboring sinusoids in which blood is flowing freely. The marrow pressure [Michelsen, 1967] would constitute a driving force perfectly adequate to ensure the passage of plasma from the marrow parenchyma through the endothelium of the sinusoid—temporarily deprived of its own blood supply—into its lumen and on into the vein.

Plasma flowing through the marrow parenchyma could well be an accessory factor in aiding the egress of nonmotile cells, such as erythrocytes, from the marrow into the bloodstream. In the case of rebound marrow, containing here and there dense accumulations of small lymphocytes, the transparenchymal plasma flow could accelerate their entry into the sinusoids and be largely responsible for the phenomenon of loading.

LYMPHOCYTE MIGRATION

The general problem of the passage of cells through the sinusoidal endothelium is discussed in Chapter VI. Lymphocyte migration has some special features that can be appropriately considered in relation to the marrow circulation.

The vast majority of the cells produced in the marrow are *myelofugal*, leaving the marrow to enter the blood stream. In the case of the lympho-

---

Fig. V.4. A) A lymphocyte (L) lying partly within and partly outside the lumen of a sinusoid (S) in guinea pig bone marrow. There is a narrow waist lying within a gap in the endothelium. Another gap (E) is shown on the opposite side of the sinusoid. Most of the cytoplasm of the lymphocyte and all its mitochondria (M) are at the parenchymal pole. ×7,800. B) A lymphocyte in the bone marrow of a guinea pig. The lymphocyte (L) lies within the lumen of a sinusoid (S) and has a pseudopodium (P) which projects through a gap in the sinusoidal endothelium (E). Mitochondria (M) are concentrated at the pole opposite the pseudopodium. The appearance is consistent with the view that this lymphocyte is entering the marrow from the sinusoid. From Hudson and Yoffey [1966]. × 11,700. By courtesy of the Royal Society.

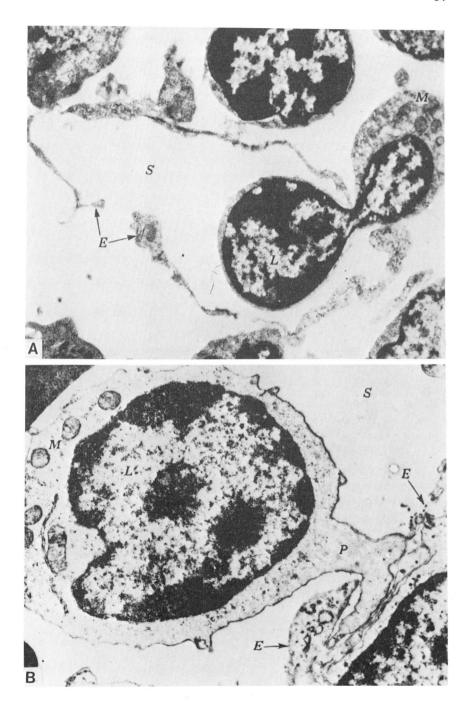

cytes one has to take into account a relatively small number of *myelopetal* cells, entering the marrow from the bloodstream. Figure V.4 contains micrographs of what we conceive to be the two types of lymphocyte, myelofugal and myelopetal, though one cannot be sure, on the basis of a static figure, in which direction a cell is actually moving. Panel A is the appearance one would expect to find when lymphocytes are leaving the marrow, the nucleus characteristically in front, and the cytoplasm with organelles behind. Panel B depicts the less frequent appearance of what could be a myelopetal lymphocyte entering the marrow from the blood stream. It is true, of course, that all inferences concerning lymphocyte movement which are based on static figures must to some extent be speculative, and more conclusive evidence concerning the direction of movement must be sought in other ways. In addition to the evidence for myelopetal lymphocyte migration presented in Chapter VI, a further discussion of the problem will be found in the reviews by Rosse [1976] and Osmond [1980].

If some lymphocytes can pass from the bloodstream into the marrow, there must presumably be a mechanism whereby the cells can first be anchored to the wall of the sinusoid before they traverse it. This would seem to be most likely to occur in temporarily stagnant sinusoids.

LYMPHOCYTE LOADING

If newly formed cells were leaving the marrow in large numbers, their presence in the sinusoids should readily be observed in marrow sections. This is true of all the major cell types produced by the marrow—erythrocytes, granulocytes, and lymphocytes. In the case of the erythrocytes, for example, in the normal steady state only an occasional reticulocyte may be seen in the lumen of the sinusoid. Most of the erythrocytes in the lumen are mature postreticulocytic cells. However, as has already been noted, powerful erythropoietic stimuli, such as hypoxia or bleeding, may stimulate a massive reticulocyte discharge, so that not infrequently one finds sinusoids predominantly containing reticulocytes. Similar considerations apply to the discharge of granulocytes from the marrow after a granulopoietic stimulus. A sinusoid that contains an unusually high proportion of newly discharged cells we describe as "loaded." Sinusoids loaded with platelets have also been described [Tavassoli and Aoki, 1981].

Lymphocyte loading is seen not infrequently in normal marrow, but is more likely to be found in rebound marrow, when lymphocytes are present in unusually large numbers [Yoffey, 1977]. In many instances of lymphocyte loading, the sinusoids may contain almost exclusively lymphocytes, without any other blood cells. This puzzling phenomenon has been attributed to a combination of plasma skimming, resulting in sinusoids containing only plasma, followed by subsequent occlusion of the presinusoidal arteries, leaving a plasma-filled sinusoid into which lymphocytes can enter from the parenchyma.

VI.

Marrow-Blood Barrier

INTRODUCTION

The concept of the marrow-blood barrier is a logical derivation of the compartmentalized hemopoiesis: Mammalian blood cells are produced in the extravascular compartment of the bone marrow. To enter the vascular compartment, they must migrate through the wall of specialized vascular sinuses which forms a barrier between the hemopoietic compartment and the circulation: the marrow-blood barrier (MBB) [Tavassoli, 1978c, 1979b]. The magnitude of cell traffic across this barrier gives an indication of its physiological significance: In an adult man, every day some 2×10^{11} erythrocytes, 1×10^{10} granulocytes, and 4×10^{11} platelets cross this barrier to enter the circulation [Tavassoli, 1979b]. This is in addition to lymphocytes and monocytes and other cell types that may have a steady traffic across this barrier. In addition, cells entering the marrow must traverse this barrier. Such cells include the hemopoietic stem cell (HSC). HSC that are present in the extravascular compartment of the marrow, are also present in circulation. There appears to be a gradient between the two compartments, with a high concentration of HSC being present in the extravascular compartment and a relatively low concentration in the circulatory compartment. The cells in the two compartments may be in a steady state of equilibrium. Therefore, the gradient must be maintained and its maintenance is a function of the marrow-blood barrier. The HSC in the circulatory pool are selectively trapped by marrow sinus endothelium, permitting them to enter the hemopoietic arena. This selective trapping is evident during bone marrow transplantation when a relatively high concentration of HSC is introduced in the circulation. The cells circulate in the entire vascular bed only to be trapped by the marrow (or other hemopoietic organs) where hemopoiesis proceeds and is sustained [Osogoe and Omura, 1950]. The high concentration of HSC in the marrow relative to blood indicate that the marrow-blood barrier maintains a gradient between the two compartments.

The traffic across the barrier is not limited to cellular elements. Such molecules as transport proteins and hormones have their first interactions with the endothelium of the marrow sinus and perhaps of other vascular structures. Through such interactions, they enter the marrow providing necessary nutrients and stimuli for hemopoiesis and other functions. The requirement of marrow for certain nutrients and humoral factors may exceed that of other organs, and the MBB may be selective in removing these substances from the circulation. Whether the bone marrow also secretes certain humoral factors into the circulation, and the MBB may be instrumental in their excretion, is not known.

EVIDENCE FOR THE EXISTENCE OF THE BARRIER

Several observations suggest that the barrier serves to control cellular traffic in and out of the marrow:

1. Vascular sinuses of the marrow, the site of cell traffic, display unique structural features suggesting that they have evolved in adaptation to the special function [Shaklai and Tavassoli, 1979; Weiss, 1970; Zamboni and Pease, 1961; Hudson and Yoffey, 1966; DeBruyn et al, 1971; Campbell, 1972].

2. Cellular migration is transcellular (transendothelial) rather than inter-cellular [Tavassoli and Crosby, 1973; DeBruyn et al, 1971; Campbell, 1972]. This mode of migration is characteristic of selective transvascular migration [Farr and DeBruyn, 1975], and implies an interaction between endothelium and migrating cells. In this manner, vascular endothelium can screen the cell traffic, retaining immature or defective cells and permitting passage only of suitable cells.

3. When a nucleated erythrocyte migrates through this barrier, its nucleus is removed [Tavassoli and Crosby, 1973]. This "pitting" function of MBB involves deformability on the part of the migrating cell. The cytoplasm can squeeze through, and the rigid nucleus remains behind. Mature granu-

locytes have segmented nuclei. They can migrate out by aligning their nuclear segments, as they are deformable [Lichtman, 1970]. Cellular inter-actions may be required for the migration of other cells [Tavassoli, 1978c].

4. A related observation is the difference between erythropoiesis in birds and mammals. Whereas mammalian erythropoiesis is extravascular, in birds this is intravascular [Campbell, 1967]—ie, involving no MBB. The circulat-ing erythrocyte displays the stamp of this difference. Thus, in birds eryth-rocytes are nucleated; in mammals they are not.

5. In certain human diseases, intravascular erythropoiesis occurs, again avoiding the MBB. Agnogenic myeloid metaplasia is the best-known exam-ple [Tavassoli and Weiss, 1973]. Here again, nucleated red cells appear in the blood and their numbers may serve as a crude index of intravascular erythropoiesis [Gardner and Nathan, 1966].

6. In infiltrative diseases of the marrow, both neoplastic and nonneo-plastic, a leukoerythroblastic blood picture may be present. It is believed that in this situation the function of MBB is compromised. In some hyper-proliferative states such as hemolytic diseases, immature cells may escape the marrow and enter the blood. Here, the MBB may function maximally but it cannot keep pace with a proliferation which has the potential of expanding to more than eight times its normal activity [Crosby, 1975]. In newborn children a few immature cells escape through the MBB. Here, immaturity of the barrier may permit the immature blood cells to escape. Similarly, in severe hypoxia (cardiopulmonary) failures, severe blood loss, and shock), the MBB may be metabolically damaged [Tavassoli, 1975b].

These observations indicate that the sinus wall controls the traffic of cells coming into the blood.

FUNCTIONAL ANATOMY OF THE BARRIER

Cell traffic across the MBB occurs in specialized vascular sinuses. These are the first efferent elements of the marrow vascular system. Cell traffic also occurs in collecting sinuses and the central vein sometimes known as the central sinus. Collecting sinuses receive the content of vascular sinuses and in turn lead to the central vein. Despite minor structural variations, these three elements form a single functional unit involved with the traffic of cells and molecules across the MBB.

The two distinct anatomic features of these vessels (Figs. VI. 1–4) are the relatively large caliber and the relatively thin wall. The in vivo microscopic studies of Branemark [1959] suggest that the caliber of these vessels may vary considerably as the vessels undergo rythmic contraction and dilatation. Nonetheless in histologic preparations [Campbell, 1972; DeBruyn et al,

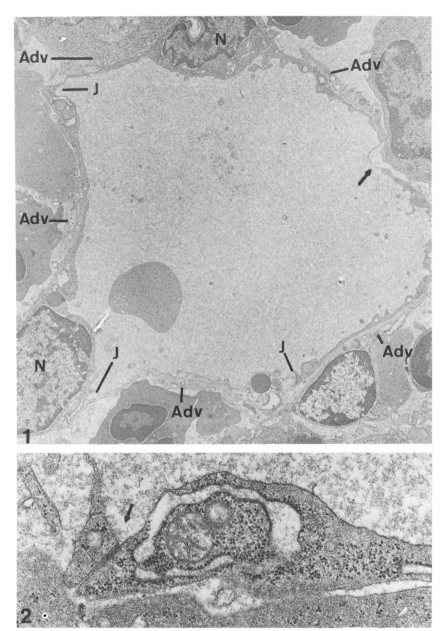

Fig. VI.1. Electron micrograph of a marrow sinus in the rat. The endothelial cells, of which the nuclei (N) are identified, have either dense or light cytoplasm but the relative density remains constant in any one cell. This density may reflect the functional state of the cell. The areas where endothelial cells come into contact are identified (J). Note that the endothelium is remarkably thin and although it is a continuous layer, there are diaphragms in the wall (arrow). The abluminal surface of the endothelium is partly covered by an inconstant layer of adventitial cells (Adv). From Shaklai and Tavassoli [1979]. Courtesy of Academic Press. ×43,000.

Fig. VI.2. Higher magnification from one of the areas where endothelial cells are in contact. Note the intercellular distance indicating absence of tight junctions. From Shaklai and Tavassoli [1979]. Courtesy of Academic Press. ×43,000.

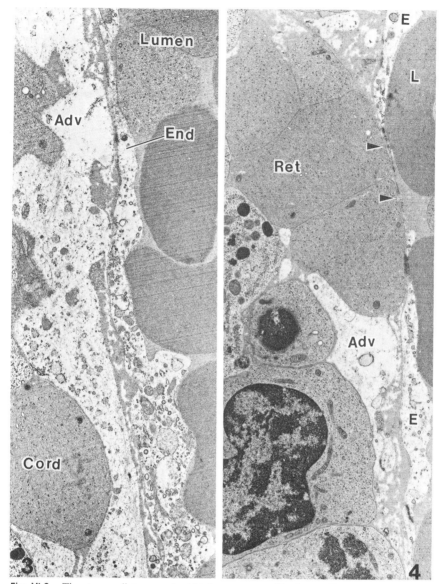

Fig. VI.3. The sinus wall in normal rabbit bone marrow. The lumen (L) is on the right and contains several mature red cells and two reticulocytes. The wall consists of endothelium (End) containing a number of vesicles and in some areas is remarkably thin. The adventitial cell (Adv) covers the entire abluminal surface of the endothelium. Note the microfilaments within the cytoplasm of the adventitial cell. A basement membrane is not seen and the distance between the two layers of the wall is occupied by a relatively electron dense substance indistinguishable from the ground substance. The hemopoietic cord is on the left. From Tavassoli [1977a]. ×9,000.

Fig. VI.4. The field is contiguous with that in Fig. VI.3. Again the lumen (L) is on the right. A process of adventitial cell (Adv) covers the abluminal surface of endothelium (E) only in the lower half of this figure. Note a group of young red cells (Ret) pressing between the two layers of the wall appearing to lift the adventitial cell process. At this point the endothelial layer is extremely thin and its continuity is barely perceived. Evidently these reticulocytes are in the process of migration into the circulation. From Tavassoli [1977a]. ×9,000.

1971; Shaklai and Tavassoli, 1979; Zamboni and Pease, 1961], vascular sinuses stand out because of their large caliber. The vascular wall is remarkably thin. Except in the perinuclear region of its endothelium, the thickness seldom exceeds 2–3 μm. In its fullest development, the wall consists of two cellular layers (Fig. VI.1, 3, 4), a continuous endothelium and a discontinuous adventitial layer. Between the two layers a thin film of extracellular proteinaceous substance may be present. This appears to be simply a condensation of the ground substance and lacks the definitive form of the basal lamina.

Adventitial Layer

The adventitial cell has been classified as a reticular cell with a perisinal topography [Weiss, 1970; Shaklai and Tavassoli, 1979]. This is a branched fibroblastic cell which elaborates argentophilic fibers and extends its slender, long cytoplasmic projections deep into the hemopoietic cords (see also Chapter IV and Fig. IV.2). Thus, the adventitial cell merges with other reticular cells in the hemopoietic cord to form a reticular meshwork which supports the hemopoietic cells. Morphologically too, this cell is similar to other reticular cells and is characterized by its rarefied cytoplasm which may even appear "empty" and indistinguishable from the extracellular space except through the use of tracer techniques. The adventitial cell contains ribosomes and rough endoplasmic reticulum as well as bands of microfilaments usually in the submembranous location. No junctional structures are seen between these cells and endothelial cells [Tavassoli, 1977a].

Adventitial layer is discontinuous (Figs. VI.1, 4). It covers a variable proportion of the abluminal surface of the endothelium. In rat this amounts to 60% [Weiss, 1970], whereas in rabbits it does not exceed 30% [Tavassoli, 1977a]. Moreover, this proportion depends on the functional state of the MBB. In developing marrow where there is no cell traffic across the MBB, only negligible proportion of endothelium is covered by the adventitial cells [Tavassoli and Weiss, 1971]. In well-developed marrow, this proportion increases but it has an inverse relationship with the magnitude of cell traffic across the MBB. When the cell traffic is experimentally stimulated by induced hemolysis, phlebotomy [Tavassoli, 1977a], or injection of endotoxin [Weiss, 1970], there is a remarkable decrease in the extent of this coverage and this is associated with an increase in the rate of cell traffic across the MBB. Under these experimental conditions, the bands of microfilaments in adventitial cells are more noticeable and this has been interpreted as evidence of contraction of adventitial cells "retracting" from the abluminal surface of endothelium so that more endothelial surface could be available to interact with the mature cells in exit [Tavassoli, 1977a]. In fact, this "retraction" leaves a subcompartment, 10–12 μm in diameter, just underneath the endothelium where mature cells accumulate (Fig. VI.5). This retraction and the formation of a subcompartment are possible only because of the absence of adhesive junctions between endothelial and adventitial cells. In those parts of the sinus wall where the adventitial cell is absent, two cell types may subserve this function: the marrow adipocytes and megakaryocytes. Marrow adipocytes (see Chapter VII) are thought to originate from adventitial layer by accumulation of lipid and, therefore, should be considered as the product of modulation of adventitial cells. Megakaryocytes are typically located in the subendothelial region (Fig. VI.6) inserting short, cytoplasmic processes into the endothelium [Tavassoli 1979a, 1980a; Tavassoli and Aoki, 1981]. These processes are organelle-free and probably serve to anchor the cell to the wall. They could also serve as the receptor of certain information from the circulation. Subsuming the function of the adventitial layer, megakaryocytes may then be considered as a component of the sinus wall and the MBB. Evidence for this concept comes from the observation that megakaryocytes often display the phenomenon of emperipolesis—ie, wandering of a small cell into a larger one (see Chapter XI). In those states associated with blood loss, emperipolesis of megakaryocytes relative to nucleated red cells and reticulocytes is pronounced [Sahebekhtiari and Tavassoli, 1976], suggesting that the reticulocytes may take a transmegakaryocytic route in their path across the MBB [Tavassoli, 1981a].

Endothelium

In contrast to the adventitial layer, the endothelial layer is continuous (Figs. VI.1, 3, 4). It has an elongated nucleus with considerable peripheral heterochromatin. Its thickness in the perinuclear region may be up to 6–7 μm, and in this region the cytoplasm contains many organelles including mitochondria, ribosomes, rough endoplasmic reticulum, granules, and many vesicles.

Cytoplasmic processes of endothelial cells may extend into the hemopoietic cords and participate in the formation of the reticular meshwork. This however, is not a common finding, and when it is seen it is usually in the perinuclear region. The cytoplasm tapers off laterally extending for a long distance, forming the only continuous element of the wall. In these segments the endothelial layer is, then, usually 1–2 μm.

The salient feature of the cytoplasm is the presence of numerous endocytic pits and vesicles (Figs. VI.3, 4) on both luminal and abluminal sides, many but not all bristle-coated. Three types of membrane structures are

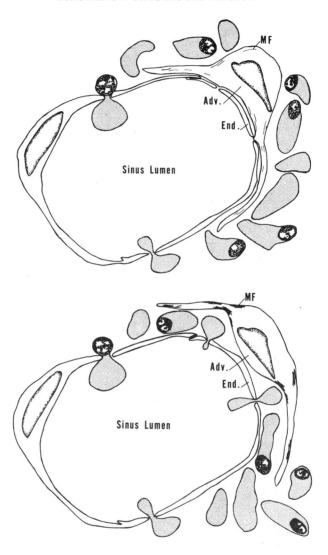

Fig. VI.5. Conceptual representation of the mechanism whereby the sinus wall can modu-late the rate of cell delivery into the circulation. The top represents normal state of the sinus wall. A proportion of the sinus wall is covered by an adventitial cell which does not permit erythroid cells (shaded) to gain access to the endothelial (End) surface for passage. Migration of cells into the lumen can occur only in those parts of the wall not covered by the adventitial cell. Normally this is adequate to respond to the body's demand for cell delivery. Loosely-arranged microfilaments (MF) are present in processes of adventitial cells (Adv). When the demand for cell delivery is enhanced, the microfilaments contract thereby withdrawing the adventitial cell processes. A subcompartment between the two layers of the wall is created, which permits erythroid cells to gain access to a larger area of endothelium. More erythroid cells are therefore able to migrate into the lumen. From Tavassoli [1977a].

particularly noteworthy (Fig. VI.7): diaphragmed pits, diaphragmed channels and diaphragmed fenestrae. They are all spanned by diaphragms and
all are involved in controlling the permeability of the endothelium. Diaphragmed pits or vesicles are similar to other coated or noncoated pits but are

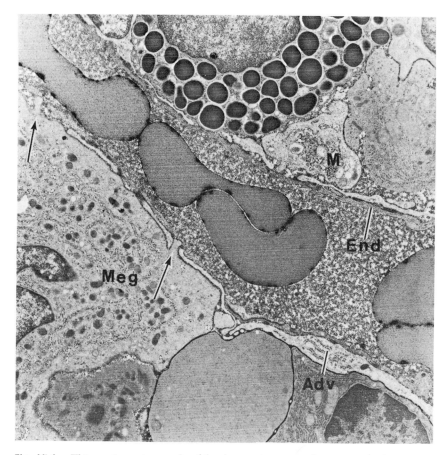

Fig. VI.6. Thin-section micrograph of lanthanum-impregnated marrow. A sinus passes
diagonally in this figure and contains many red cells. Endothelium has either dense (End) or
light cytoplasm in the area where it is in contact with a magakaryocyte (Meg). Adventitial
layer (Adv) is lucent and covers most of the abluminal surface of the endothelium. Note that
the adventitial layer is absent where the megakaryocyte is located on the abluminal surface
of endothelium. This is the typical location for megakaryocytes which penetrate the endothelium (arrows) and are in contact with the lumen. Portion of what may be a perisinal
macrophage (M) has also penetrated the wall. From Shaklai and Tavassoli [1979]. Courtesy
of the Academic Press. ×6,200.

spanned by a diaphragm. Diaphragmed channels are vesicles that span across the endothelium facing both sides of the endothelium and their mouth is on both sides covered by diaphragms, thereby providing a diaphragmed channel across the vessel wall. Diaphragmed fenestrae are fenestrations spanned by a diaphragm, again providing a channel across the vessel wall. These fenestrae are considerably larger [Bankston and DeBruyn, 1974] in diameter (85–150 nm) than those found in other fenestrated endothelia (45–68 nm). Nondiaphragmed channels across the wall are not seen, and earlier reports are now considered to be the result of fixation artifacts.

Endothelial cells in the same sinus appear, in TEM, either dark or light (Fig. VI.1), suggesting they may be in different functional states [Shaklai and Tavassoli, 1979]. The density of a single endothelial cell remains relatively unchanged, and abrupt changes in the density occur only at the juncture of two cells where the cells often overlap and sometimes extensively interdigitate. In these overlapping areas, patchy submembranous areas are sometimes seen but the intracellular space is wide (Fig. VI.2) and freely open to extracellular tracers which permeate the space without delineating junctional structures [Tavassoli and Shaklai, 1979]. Nor are such junctions seen in freeze-fracture preparations. The absence of such junctional structures as tight junctions may permit the endothelial cells to slide over each other in the overlapping areas and therefore change the caliber of the vessel. Such a mechanism is consistent with the rhythmic dilatation of sinuses observed by Branemark [1959] in his vivo microscopy. The presence of contractile filaments in the endothelium [Aoki and Tavassoli, 1981a] may provide an anatomic basis for this rhythmic change in the caliber. On the other hand, the submembranous densities seen in the overlapping area may represent adhesive devices that limit such motions in endothelial cells not permitting them to come far apart.

The functional significance of this rhythmic dilatation may be in controlling the cell traffic across the MBB: Mature cells accumulate in the subendothelial region. Within the rigid confines of bone where the volume is fixed, sinus dilatation can only lead to the displacement of cells into the lumen and from there into general circulation. During the subsequent contraction, new cells can accumulate in the subendothelial region to be displaced again into the lumen during the subsequent dilation. Thus, the entry of blood cells into the circulation may occur in bursts.

In agreement with this concept are the morphometric studies after single phlebotomy [Aoki and Tavassoli, 1981b]. In this experimental situation the overlapping parts of the sinus endothelial cells are reduced, often to points of end-to-end contacts suggesting maximal dilatation of sinuses which can displace all the mature cells from the extravascular into the vascular compartment. In hypertransfused plethoric animals, the sinuses are also maximally dilated, but this is due to the packing of the sinus lumen with red cells, and this limits the traffic of cells across the MBB. Few if any red cells can be delivered under these conditions [Aoki and Tavassoli, 1981c].

PERMEABILITY AND THE MODES OF TRANSPORT

Marrow sinuses provide an example par excellence of fenestrated endothelium [Simionescu et al, 1981a; Clementi and Palade, 1969]. These vessels, most commonly encountered in liver, spleen, marrow, and a few other organs, have in common an endothelium which displays large pores or fenestrae (up to 100 nm) and a basal lamina which is either discontinuous or entirely missing. Considerable information has come about with regard to structural-functional correlates in this type of endothelium using probe molecules such as graded size dextrans. Basically, two types of pores can be recognized: small pores with a diameter or approximately 9 nm, and large pores with a diameter of 50–70 nm. Unlike large pores, the small pores restrict diffusion with increasing molecular size.

In the marrow sinuses particulate materials are removed from the circulation and transported by both intracellular and transcellular routes. Earlier work by Hudson and Yoffey [1963, 1968] established the ability of such particles to permeate the endothelial barrier. Bankston and DeBruyn [1974] subsequently demonstrated that carbon particles with a mean diameter of 28 nm can penetrate the extravascular space within 3 minutes. They demonstrated that the transport was transcellular, occurring through diaphragmed fenestrae. Despite the absence of tight junctions, particles were not transported between the endothelial cells. DeBruyn et al [1975] subsequently demonstrated an intracellular mode of uptake of particulate substances. They used both carbon (28 nm) and ferritin (11 nm) particles. By injection of these particles they were able to induce an increase in the

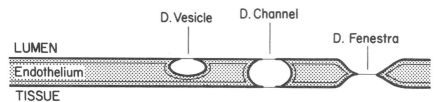

Fig. VI.7. Diagrammatic representation of the 3 types of diaphragmed structures (pits, channels, and fenestrae) in the endothelium. The luminal and tissue sides are identified.

number of bristle-coated pits and vesicles on the luminal surface of endothe-lium. The particles were removed by these vesicles. The vesicles subse-quently fused with each other to form phagosomes, or alternatively, fused with smooth-surfaced "transfer tubules" that transferred the particles to multivescular bodies. The lysosomal enzyme acid phosphatase was demon-strated in the latter tubules, indicating that they were lytic bodies. There was considerable difference between carbon and ferritin in their mode of deposition. Carbon was generally sequestered in the phagosome whereas ferritin was transferred primarily to the lytic bodies. The nature of this selectivity is not clear. This may be a function of particle size (as is the case with graded probe molecules in other fenestrated endothelial cells), or the biological nature of the molecules.

Little is known of the transport of biologically active molecules across the endothelium. It is not known, for instance, how hormones such as erythropoietin or transport proteins such as transferrin or transcobalamin are transported to the hemopoietic cords. Undoubtedly these molecules must cross the MBB in order to fulfill their biological function.

CELLULAR PASSAGE

Cellular passage across the endothelium is transendothelial rather than interendothelial [Tavassoli and Crosby, 1973; DeBruyn et al, 1971; 1977; Campbell, 1972; Aoki and Tavassoli, 1981b,c]. There are no preformed pores, and each passing cell opens a new pore which is immediately closed after the passage is completed. The evidence for this view is derived from both scanning electron microscopy and serial sectioning transmission elec-tron microscopy. The process is essentially a variation of fusion-fission reorganization of membrane [Tavassoli, 1979]. A cell entering the sinus must press against the abluminal membrane of the endothelium bringing it into contact with the luminal membrane (Fig. VI.4). The two membranes then fuse in one direction and, under the pressure of the passing cell, undergo separation in a direction perpendicular to the first. This opens a pore through which the cell enters the lumen [Tavassoli,, 1981b]. Immedi-ately after the passage is completed, a fusion-fission in a reverse direction leads to the closure of this pore. Scanning electron microscopy indicates the presence of numerous pores, morphologically indistinguishable from dia-phragmed fenestrae at the site of penetration. This suggests the formation of multiple fenestrae, one of which the passing cell uses for the entry [DeBruyn et al, 1977]. This mode of entry suggest that biological rather than purely mechanical factors are involved.

It is of interest that the cell migration, while not occurring at the juncture between the endothelial cells, usually occurs very near the juncture. This may be related to the presence of microdomains on the endothelial cell surface (vide infra). But it also could be related to the deformability of endothelium at these sites. Such deformability may be related to lability of endothelial cytoplasm. Studies on transmural cell egress after phlebotomy [Aoki and Tavassoli, 1981b] have indicated the presence of large number of cytoplasmic granules which are thought to be of lysosomal nature. Local release of these granules within the cytoplasm may lead to the formation of unstable areas of the cytoplasm, rendering these areas suitable for cell migration.

The pores through which the cells must pass are generally 2–3 μm in diameter [Tavassoli and Crosby, 1973], and the largest diameter reported is 6 μm which entire megakaryocytes can traverse [Tavassoli and Aoki, 1981]. Thus, the cells must negotiate these marrow pores and this calls for the deformability of the cell. Only cells that are deformable can exit [Lichtman and Weed, 1972; Lichtman et al, 1978a,b]. Most cells including their nuclei of granulocytes can align their lobes to exit. That is not, however, the case with nucleated red cells. Normally such cells lose their nuclei and only reticulocytes enter the circulation. Yet, when a nucleated red cell attempts to enter the lumen, the malleable cytoplasm can negotiate the pores and enter the lumen as a reticulocyte; the nucleus is rigid and, unable to negotiate the pores, remains in the hemopoietic cords (Fig. VI.8): The cell thus becomes anucleated [Tavassoli and Crosby, 1973]. This phenomenon, known as the "pitting" function of bone marrow, prevents the entry of nucleated red cells in the circulation.

CONTROL OF CELL TRAFFIC

Delivery of cells into the circulation is linked to the requirement of the body which, in the long term, modulates the production rate. In the short term, however, whatever cell reserve is present in the marrow can be delivered into the circulation upon demand. Thus, after a single phlebotomy, there is a biphasic reticulocytosis; the first, a small peak, appearing within a few hours, and the second, a marked peak, appearing after 3 days and signifying an increase in production [Tavassoli, 1977a].

The signals for both events are probably humoral to reach the widely dispersed marrow. To modulate production, there are glycoproteins; erythroprotein, colony-stimulating factor, and thrombopoietin. These glycoproteins not only enhance cell production but appear to enhance cell

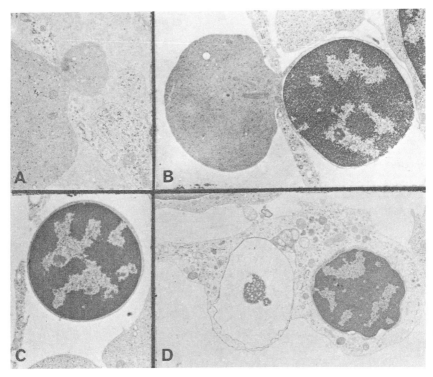

Fig. VI.8.   Sequential steps leading to nuclear elimination and delivery of the reticulocyte into the circulation. (A) A reticulocyte, in passage through the sinus endothelium, has undergone deformation to conform to the size of the opening. (B) A nucleated red cell in passage through the wall of a marrow sinus. The cytoplasm is completely within the lumen. The nucleus, however, cannot conform to the size of the opening. The cell is, thus, enucleated (nuclear pitting). (C) A red cell nucleus located in an area adjacent to an endothelial opening may have been lost from a passing erythroid cell. (D) A red cell nucleus is still recognizable within a perisinal macrophage. The remnant of another nucleus is seen within a phagosome. In A, B, and C the lumen is on the left. From Tavassoli and Crosby [1973]. Courtesy of the American Association for the Advancement of Science. A, B, and C: ×8,500; D: ×6,800.

delivery, although with somewhat different kinetics [Tavassoli, 1979]. Thus, the signal for cell delivery is either a different function of the same glycoprotein or that of a biochemically similar molecular which is present in preparations of these glycoproteins and may explain "impurities" in these preparations. This relation is far more clear for erythropoietin [Chamberlain et al, 1975] than for the signals to the other cell lines.

For granulocytes, apart from the glycoprotein colony-stimulating factor which essentially promotes the production rate in vitro, a number of humoral substances have been found to induce acute, short-lasting leuocytosis by promoting the migration of granulocytes across the MBB. Expectedly, inflammatory effusions are rich sources of these "leuocytosis inducing factors" (LIF). One such factor studied by Gordon et al [1964] was found to be a heat-labile, nodialyzable globulin, precipitable by 35–75% ammonium sulphate. Substances reported by others [Boggs et al, 1968] appear to be similar in nature and are probably identical [Metcalf and Moore, 1971]. Substances of bacterial origin such as endotoxins can also . cutely enhance the migration of granulocytes across the MBB [Weiss, 1970], and this effect may be mediated by LIF [Boggs et al, 1968]. By contrast, there are hormones and other substances of bacterial origin [Rice, 1966] capable of inducing leuocytosis more slowly. These subtances appear to speed up primarily the maturation rather than the delivery or proliferation of granulocytes.

Tryptic digestion of human C_3 has yielded as acidic fragment with a molecular weight of 10–12×10^3, containing 101 amino acid residues. This molecule can mobilize leuocytes upon the perfusion of isolated rat femur. Its intravenous injection in rabbits is rapidly followed by leuocytosis reaching a peak in 60 min and lasting for 2 h [Ghebrehiwet and Muller-Eberhard, 1978].

For platelets, there is little reserve in the marrow. This is indicated by a "recovery lag" after experimentally induced thrombocytopenia [Craddock et al, 1955]. Megakaryocytes are typically located on the abluminal surface of the sinus endothelium subsuming the function of adventitial cells (see Chapter XI). They extend projections into the lumen and are in contact with blood circulation (Fig. VI.6). Some even move in toto in the lumen and lodge in the pulmonary vascular bed, where they are fragmented into platelets [Tavassoli and Aoki, 1981].

PHAGOCYTIC FUNCTION OF MBB

The two major components of MBB are the endothelium and adventitial cells. As discussed above, megakaryocytes and marrow adipocytes can subserve the adventitial function as adventitial cells are absent where these two cells types are present.

Macrophages abound in the vicinity of marrow sinuses (Fig. VI.6). They are known as perisinal macrophages and may be considered as the third component of MBB [Tavassoli 1974d, 1977b]. A function of these cells is to remove the extruded nuclei of mature erythroid cells (Fig. VI.8). Nuclear extrusion occurs in the hemopoietic cord [Campbell, 1968; Tavassoli, 1974d] in a process that bears many similarities to cytokinesis [Tavassoli, 1978c], in which the cell divides but the nucleus does not. The bulk of the cytoplasm forms the reticulocyte. The nucleus, surrounded by a thin rim of hemoglobinized cytoplasm and a membrane, remains in the hemopoietic cord and it is phagocytized by perisinal macrophages. Campbell [1968] has suggested that the nucleus is directly transferred to the macrophage and that the latter cells are necessary for nuclear extrusion. However, since nuclear extrusion can occur in vitro [Bessis, 1973] in the absence of macrophages, this view is not tenable. The recognition of the extruded nucleus by the macrophage may be through a nonimmunologic mechanism [Hibbs, 1973] where the cell surface charge may be involved [Stutelsky and Danon, 1969; 1972]. In contrast to the reticulocyte, the membrane of the extruded nucleus is positively charged and can be attracted to macrophages that bear strong negative surface charge. The difference between the membranes of the reticulocyte and the portion containing its extruded nucleus has gained further support in recent studies of Zweig et al [1981], who demonstrated that various membrane components segregate during the extrusion. Almost all spectrin goes with the reticulocyte, whereas the membrane surrounding the nucleus-containing portion is spectrin-free.

In addition the extruded nuclei, perisinal macrophages can also phagocytize defective cells in their path into the circulation. This includes reticulocytes, immature nucleated red cells as well as granulocytes. It is estimated [Tavassoli, 1974d] that about 2% of the cells produced in the bone marrow are defective. Their phagocytosis by perisinal macrophages is another control mechanism by MBB that prevents the entry of these defective cells into circulation (ineffective hemopoiesis). Degradation of hemoglobin contained in these cells may contribute to early appearing peak of bile pigment 3 days after the administration of labeled hemoglobin precursors [London and West, 1950]. Also contributing to this peak is the hemoglobin contained in the rim of the cytoplasm surrounding the extruded nucleus as well as in the nucleus itself [Campbell, 1968; Orlic et al, 1965; Simpson and Kling, 1967; Tavassoli, 1974d].

In certain species such as the rabbit, perisinal macrophages penetrate the endothelium sending cytoplasmic processes into the lumen [Tavassoli, 1977b]. This penetration is again transendothelial rather than interendothelial. In this position the macrophages monitor the circulation, and recognize and remove senescent red cells (Fig. VI.9). Morphometric studies indicate that as much as 83% of circulating red cells can be removed by this mechanism in the bone marrow [Tavassoli, 1977b]. This mechanism, how-

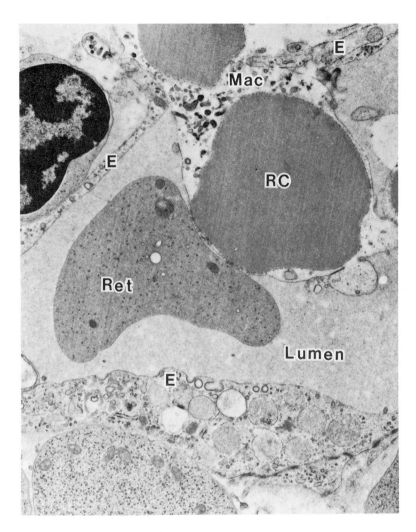

Fig. VI.9. A marrow sinus in the rabbit. The lumen is identified. Endothelium (E) shows numerous pits and vesicles, some coated. A perisinal macrophage (Mac) has penetrated the endothelial wall sending its cytoplasmic process into the lumen. In this position, it can monitor the circulation to remove senescent red cells. Note a red cell (RC) is completely engulfed by the intraluminal portion of the macrophage. Another red cell is already phago-cytosed and is moving into the cordal compartment. By contrast a newly released reticulocyte (Ret) is not engulfed. ×12,000.

ever, may not be operative in all species as radioactive studies have demonstrated that whereas in the rabbit the bone marrow is the site of destruction of senescent red cells [Ehrenstein and Lockner, 1959; Hughes-Jones, 1961], the spleen may perform this function in the rat.

SELECTIVITY OF THE MBB

Cellular traffic across the MBB is a selective phenomenon. This is true both for mature cells entering the circulation and for such cells as hemopoietic cells entering the hemopoietic arena. Moreover, it is probable that many molecules such as erythropoietin and other factors involved in the regulation of hemopoiesis are also selectively transported across the MBB. Although the nature of this selectivity is not well understood, recent evidence has pointed toward the presence of certain surface recognition mechanisms.

In considering the nature of the selectivity of the MBB, it seems most probable that this selectivity resides in the endothelium. In favor of this concept is the fact that the endothelium is the only continuous component of the MBB with which the cells and molecules must interact for their traffic. Moreover, all cells entering the circulation do so by transendothelial (transcellular) rather than interendothelial passage. This is also true of the cytoplasmic processes of perisinal macrophages entering the lumen. Transendothelial cell passage, a form of "emperipolesis" [Humble et al, 1956] is a characteristic of selective passage. It is also seen in the case of lymphocyte passage across the wall of the postcapillary venules in the lymph node [Marchesi and Gowan, 1964; Messier and Sainte-Marie, 1972; Farr and DeBruyn, 1975; Cho and DeBruyn, 1979; Farr et al, 1980]. This mode of traffic permits an interaction between the endothelial membrane and that of the passing cell, and thereby permits the endothelium to be selective.

It should also be emphasized that the marrow sinus endothelium is highly polarized, with its luminal and abluminal membranes displaying different structural characteristics [Shaklai and Tavassoli, 1978b]. Though most capillaries are so polarized, this is more so in the case of sinus endothelium. This polarization permits different interactions by the endothelial cell membrane on the luminal and abluminal sides. This polarization is indicated by freeze-fracture studies where the density of the intramembraneous particles significantly differs in the two sides of the endothelium. There exists also a layer of glycocalyx on the luminal side which is not noted on the membrane of the abluminal side [Shaklai and Tavassoli, 1979]. Moreover, as will be discussed below, there are considerable differences in the distribution of the surface glycoproteins on the two sides of the endothelium.

DeBruyn and Michelson [1981] studied the changes at the surface of marrow cells involved in this selective transcellular migration. They found that an anionic substance accumulates at the advancing margin of the migrating cell. As the migration into the lumen continues, this anionic aggregate disappears either through intravascular shedding or through distribution over the entire surface of the cell. Thus, the migrating cell seems to be polarized into an active anterior pseudopodial front and a more or less passive tail. These authors advanced the hypothesis that this anionic substance might be involved in either a discriminative recognition event or with the formation of the migrating pore or both. The significance of this finding relative to the selectivity of the barrier remains to be better defined.

In recent years the anionic sites (recognizable by their ability to bind cationic probes) have defined microdomains on the fenestrated capillary endothelia in general. The distribution of these sites is nonrandom, indicating differences in the functional state of various parts of endothelial cell membrane [Simionescu et al 1981a,b, 1982a]. On the luminal side, while every part of the plasmalemmal membrane shows some anionic sites, their density is particularly high in fenestrated diaphragms and coated pits. Diaphragmed transendothelial channels and the diaphragmed pits apparently do not have anionic sites. Whereas the anionic sites on the plasmalemmal membrane are sensitive to neuraminidase (suggesting, at least in part, the sialic acid nature of these sites), those of the coated pits and the fenestrated diaphragms are not. Using specific hydrolases, Simionescu et al [1981b] have sugested the presence of sulfated glycosaminoglycans, primarily heparan sulfate, in these membrane domains. On the abluminal side, the plasmalemmal membrane and coated pits show high density of anionic sites whereas the diaphragms of transendothelial channels and diaphragmed pits are free of these sites. In contradistinction to the luminal side, the diaphragmed fenestrae of the abluminal side do not show anionic sites, further supporting the polarization of the endothelium [Simionescu et al, 1982a]. The chemical nature of the anionic sites on the abluminal surface remains to be elucidated.

In considering the functional significance of these anionic domains in transendothelial transport, it should be emphasized that they are expected to discriminate against the anionic molecules. Is is noteworthy that the majority of plasma proteins are anionic, but the size range at which charge discrimination becomes effective is not known.

As in the case with other fenestrated endothelia, marrow sinus endothelium also shows a nonrandom distribution of anionic sites on its luminal surface. Anionic molecules are excluded from the site of coated pits [De-

Bruyn et al, 1978] and diaphragmed fenestrae [DeBruyn and Michelson, 1979], suggesting that these anionic substances are antagonistic to the uptake of molecules by these routes or at least not essential to their uptake. The anionic sites on the marrow sinus endothelium are made mostly by sialoglycoprotein, although there exists evidence that other anionic molecules are also present. The distribution of anionic sites on the abluminal surface of marrow sinus endothelium has not been studied.

It is of interest that the receptors for various lectins show a similar nonrandom distribution on fenestrated endothelia (unpublished data). Soybean, peanut, retinis communis, and wheat germ agglutinins all show diffuse binding to the plasmalemma proper whereas Con A and lotus agglutinin display binding in patches. But receptors for all lectins appear to be absent or considerably less concentrated on diaphragmed fenestrae. Pits and transendothelial channels are particularly rich in residues recognizing retinis communis, peanut, and wheat germ agglutinins. A similar pattern with some variations has been found in bone marrow sinus endothelium.

Although these studies have not firmly established the basis of selectivity of the endothelium, they have indicated cell surface domains that may lead to better understanding of the selective nature of the transendothelial transport.

VII.

Marrow Volume and Distribution

INTRODUCTION

Although the bone marrow functions as a single organ, the diffuseness of its distribution makes its study difficult. For the quantitative study of the bone marrow as an organ, we need to know the total numbers of various cell types it contains. This information has been obtained (1) by measuring the hemopoietic marrow volume, (2) by estimating the total cellularity per unit volume, and (3) by performing differential counts. The marrow in each of the various bones may be uniform in composition, though not in absolute cellularity. Bone marrow also appears to react uniformly in all its scattered parts.

An obvious difficulty in attempting to measure the total size of the bone marrow as an organ is that a variable amount of the marrow consists of fat. This is true even for red marrow, where there is always some fat, though this diminishes when erythropoiesis is stimulated. The proportion of the marrow occupied by fat varies in different species. This may be a function of total marrow volume in relation to what is needed for the hemopoietic activity. Thus, in man a small proportion of marrow volume is adequate to provide for all the hemopoietic needs. The remaining volume is occupied by fat. In small animals, such as the mouse, marrow fat is scarce as all the marrow volume is needed for the hemopoietic requirements of the body to which the spleen may also contribute in part.

Moreover, the fat content of the marrow varies with its functional state and especially with age. Thus, measurements of marrow volume designed to throw light on cell content and production must always be made with this point in mind. This is one of the main reasons for choosing animals of similar age in making quantitative studies.

It would perhaps be more accurate to state that the fat content of the marrow varies with growth. During the growth period, the marrow has not merely to keep pace with the normal wear and tear of the circulation, but also to contribute additional cells to the growing blood volume. The differing amounts of fat in red marrow give rise to varying shades of red and pink, so that a very rough estimate of the degree of cellularity may be made by observing the color of the marrow [Custer and Ahlfeldt, 1932].

Techniques for the measurement of marrow volume are usually designed to measure the total space occupied by the marrow, both red and fatty. In order to measure the volume of active marrow, three corrections are required: The most important correction is for fatty marrow, the second is for the blood contained in the marrow vessels, and the third correction results from the agar impregnation technique by which most of the data have been obtained. This technique involves weighing the thoroughly cleaned and dried bones, impregnating them with agar, and weighing them again. Since most of the agar is in the marrow cavities, the difference in weight depends mainly on the marrow volume, but in addition, a small amount of agar enters the vascular channels in the bone.

TOTAL MARROW VOLUME

Three methods have been used for the measurement of total marrow volume: marrow displacement, marrow replacement, and incineration.

Marrow displacement was the method used by Mechanik [1926] in his study of marrow volume in the human adult. The freshly cleaned bones were weighed, macerated, and weighed again. The loss of weight was attributed mainly to the marrow, which disappeared during maceration. Mechanik was able to show that maceration of bone itself resulted in only slight loss, and when the marrow-containing bone was macerated, virtually all the loss of weight was due to the removal of the marrow.

Dietz [1944] employed an incineration technique which depends on the large difference in ash content between bone and bone marrow after incineration. He concluded that the bone marrow in the adult rabbit is about one-third the weight of the skeleton, and about 2.2% of the body weight. This is the figure for the *total* marrow volume. Dietz estimated that in his series of five rabbits the active red marrow constituted 85—90% of the total marrow, compared with Nye's [1931] estimate of 75% of active marrow. Without precise information as to age, it is difficult to institute comparisons between the two series.

It may be noted that both Mechanik's [1926] technique of marrow displacement, and Dietz's [1944] method of incineration require a lengthy process of tedious dissection, involving the complete removal of soft tissue and cartilage from most bones in the skeleton. Even though time and effort can be saved, as in the case of Mechanik's studies, by cleaning the bones on one side only, the work involved is still very time-consuming.

Besides these two techniques, the method most frequently employed has been that of marrow replacement by a substance whose volume can then be determined. Friedrich [1890] is stated to have used Wood's metal to determine marrow volume in the limb bones of two human cadavers. Wetzel [1910] obtained data on the marrow content of the human vertebral column by means of gelatin replacement. Nye [1931] used agar to determine the marrow volume in two rabbits, and since then agar seems to have become the method of choice. It was used by Fairman and Whipple [1933] on two dogs, and by Fairman and Corner [1934] on four rats. The most extensive studies on marrow volume are those of Hudson on the guinea pig [1958a], cat [1960a], and human fetus and newborn [1965]. In addition, Hudson [1958a, 1960b] investigated the effect of hypoxia on marrow volume. From these latter observations it appears that even prolonged hypoxia does not have any measurable effect on marrow volume.

Miller and Osmond [1973] have used the replacement method to measure the marrow volume in the mouse femur.

Marrow Volume in the Standard Guinea Pig

In a series of 25 guinea pigs, with body weights ranging from 350 to 450 g, the mean total marrow volume was found [Hudson, 1958a] to be 7.014 ± 0.358 ml; of this the red marrow formed by far the greater part, viz 6.249 ml. In the 400-g guinea pig, about one-seventh is fatty, and the remainder red. Fatty marrow was found only in the distal portion of the limbs and in some animals in the last two or three pieces of the coccyx. In the case of the tibia, a characteristically sharp dividing line was found between the proximal red marrow and distal fatty marrow, just over half-way down the length of the bone.

Marrow Volume in Relation to Body Weight

In addition to determining the marrow volume in a standard guinea pig with a mean weight of 400 g, Hudson [1958a] also estimated the total marrow volume in a further 120 guinea pigs ranging in body weight from 85 to 1,250 g. The findings are summarized in Figure VII.1, from which it will be seen that there is a rapid increase in marrow volume after birth until the weight reaches about 200 g, after which the rate of increase gradually diminishes. The correlation between total marrow volume and body weight is so close that for aminals anywhere in this weight range the marrow volume can readily be ascertained from the body weight.

Anatomical Distribution of Marrow

Hudson [1959] investigated the relative distribution of total marrow volume between skull, trunk, and limb bones in 50 animals. Approximately 50% of the total marrow volume was in the limbs, 30% in the trunk, and

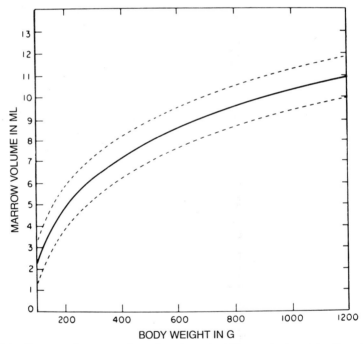

Fig. VII.1.   Forecast of marrow volume for guinea pigs of known body weight. From Yoffey [1957]. The graph was drawn from the data of Hudson [1958]. The broken lines indicate 95% confidence limits.

20% in the skull. In the rabbit, Dietz [1944] estimated that 47% of the total marrow volume was in the hind legs; 18% in the forelegs; 6% in the ribs, sternum, and clavicles; 9% in the head; and 20% in the vertebrae.

Bone Marrow Volume in Man

For human marrow we rely in the main on the data of Mechanik [1926], who measured the marrow volume in 13 adults ranging in age from 16 to 68 years. Several of the subjects suffered from wasting diseases, so that the mean body weight in the series was only about 55 kg. The total marrow volume, at 4.6% of the body weight, would have been lower had the subjects not been subnormal in weight. But even allowing for an average body weight of 70 kg, the total marrow volume would still have been about 3.5% of the body weight, well above the figure obtained in laboratory animals.

Mechanik found that about half the marrow volume in his subjects was red, half fatty. Furthermore, as in the guinea pig, about half the total marrow was in the limb bones. It is preponderantly the marrow of the limbs that becomes fatty with advancing years. Though the limbs as a whole contain about 50% of the total marrow volume there is a striking difference between the contribution of the upper limb (11.44%) and the lower (38.76%). Mechanik thought that from the marrow of a single bone one could calculate with approximate accuracy the total amount of marrow in the entire skeleton. A summary and analysis of Mechanik's extensive data has been given by Woodard and Holodny [1960] and Ellis [1960].

FETAL MARROW

For information on bone marrow volume in the human fetus and the newborn we are also indebted to Hudson [1965], who made careful measurements on 16 fetuses and infants, ranging in age from an estimated 29 weeks of intrauterine life to full term. On average, the bone marrow was 1.4% of the body weight, a figure much lower than that obtained by Mechanik [1926] for adults. But this low figure is not surprising, since throughout fetal life the marrow cavities are not fully developed, and the limbs at birth have not yet attained their normal size in relation to the rest of the body. Furthermore, throughout fetal life (though to a diminishing extent as full term approaches) the marrow contains numerous large thin-walled veins [Hammar, 1901; Yoffey and Thomas, 1964; Kalpakstoglou and Emery, 1965]. In fetal marrow, therefore, much greater allowance needs to be made for contained blood than in the marrow of the adult.

DISTRIBUTION OF RED AND FATTY MARROW

Two features may differentiate marrow hemopoiesis from its extramedullary counterpart. First, there is present in the marrow a large component of fat cells not present in association with extramedullary hemopoiesis (Figure VII.2). Second, marrow hemopoiesis takes place within the confines of a rigid frame of bone. These two features may be related. The volume contained within the frame of bone is fixed, whereas the hemopoietic tissue expands and shrinks in response to the fluctuating body requirement for blood cells; the adipose component of the marrow may serve as a "cushion," having a reciprocal relationship with the hemopoietic component. Thus, in aplastic anemia, biopsy of the marrow may reveal that the fatty component has replaced entirely, or almost entirely, the hemopoietic tissue.

An intriguing phenomenon, however, is that this association is not uniform. The more peripherally located marrow consists entirely of adipose tissue, imparting a yellowish color (yellow or fatty marrow); whereas in the axial skeleton the adipose tissue coexists, in a variable but roughly equal proportion, with the hemopoietic tissue. Heme chromogen in the latter

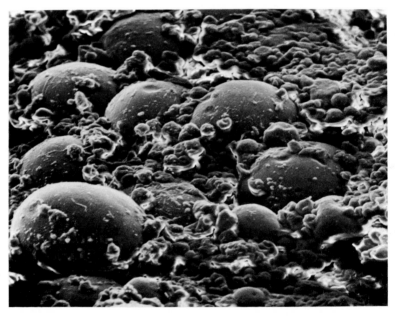

Fig. VII.2. Scanning electron micrograph of rabbit tibial marrow. Note the presence of numerous large round adipose cells interspersed with considerably smaller hemopoietic cells. × 580.

imparts a reddish color (red marrow). The relative proportion of these two types of marrow may vary from one species to another and, indeed, in some smaller animals yellow marrow may not exist at all.

Development of Fatty Marrow

In his classical contribution published in 1882, Neumann noted that at birth all bones contain red marrow. With age, however, hemopoiesis undergoes regression in a centripetal direction so that in adults, the more peripherally located marrow consists entirely of adipose tissue and does not participate in hemopoiesis. During the ensuing 50 years, other investigators substantiated this observation, which is now sometimes referred to as Neumann's law [Neumann, 1882a,b; Askanazy, 1927; Peabody, 1926; Oehlbeck et al, 1932; Hashimoto, 1962; Custer and Ahlfeldt, 1932; Uchida, 1958; Nagahama, 1959; Tateno, 1957; Higuchi, 1959; Piney, 1922]. Askanazi [1927] suggested that premature vascular senescence of marrow may be responsible for its subsequent fatty involution. According to Emery and Follett [1964], fatty marrow begins to appear even before birth, the change starting in the toes. But whether or not the first traces of fatty marrow appear before birth, all observers seem to be agreed that fatty marrow begins peripherally and then gradually spreads centripetally. By the time the adult stage is reached, virtually all the marrow of the limb bones is fatty, whereas that in the bones of the trunk and vertebral column remains red throughout life. However, the caudal vertebrae are exceptional in that they become fatty, as was first noted by Ranvier [1874] in the tails of dogs, rabbits, and cattle. Huggins and Blocksom [1936] found the same state of affairs in the tail of the rat, in which the yellow marrow begins 1–2 vertebrae beyond the last trunk segment.

In the case of the long bones, the change from red to fatty marrow seems to be more complete in large animals. Furthermore, the smaller the animals, the more obvious is the hemopoietic activity of the spleen. A characteristic feature of the marrow of the long bones is that the fat shows a predilection for the central part of the marrow, whereas the red marrow is found surrounding this fatty core—ie, nearer the surface (Fig. VII.3). This has been noted repeatedly by many observers. Drinker et al [1922], commenting on this pattern of marrow distribution in the dog, attributed it to the fact that the marrow nearer the endosteum has a richer blood supply than the central portion by reason of the additional blood reaching it from the periosteal arteries. Huggins [1939] confirmed the more central location of fatty marrow in dogs and rabbits; Tavassoli [1976a], in addition to confirming the central location of the fatty marrow, noted a histochemical difference between the central and peripheral fat cells.

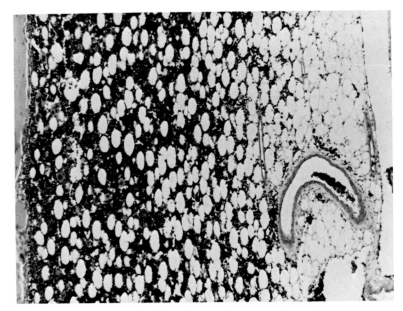

Fig. VII.3. Horizontal section of bone marrow in lower femur in the rabbit. The bone is at left and the central artery and vein are at right. Note the increasing gradient of the fat cells toward the center of the cavity, and the increasing gradient of hemopoiesis toward the bone. With permission from Tavassoli [1976]. ×45.

When fatty marrow forms and extends, a sharp line of demarcation is often present between the two types of marrow. This was observed by Hudson [1958a] in the tibia of the guinea pig, and by Huggins and Blocksom [1936] in the tail of the rat, concerning which they comment: "The transition is exceedingly sharp, indeed often in the proximal end of one vertebra the marrow will be mostly red, while the distal end contains mostly fat and all distal vertebral marrows are fatty." Hudson [1958a] draws attention to one additional fact—that in the tibia of the guinea pig "the red marrow does not extend as far distally in the centre of the section as it does at the periphery," recalling the histochemical observations of Tavassoli [1976a].

Interconversion of Red and Fatty Marrow

In 1936, Huggins and co-workers [Huggins et al, 1936] observed that at birth, marrow temperature is comparable in all bones, but with maturity a cooling of 4–8°C develops in a centrifugal direction. The parallelism with fatty transformation of the marrow immediately suggested a relationship: Thermal conditions in bones of the extremities is not optimal for hemopoiesis; thus hemopoiesis regresses to be confined only to the central parts of body where thermal conditions favor hemopoiesis. To test this hypothesis the researchers "looped" a rat tail and implanted it in the peritoneal cavity where the temperature was higher. The vertebrae in the adult rat tail normally contains yellow marrow, but after this experimental manipulation, hemopoiesis resumed in the tail vertebrae, and the marrow tissue assumed the appearance of red marrow [Huggins and Blocksom, 1936; Huggins and Noonan, 1936].

The thermal effect on hemopoiesis was supported by the fascinating comparative observations of Weiss and Wislocki [1956] in the nine-banded armadillo (*Dasypus novemcinctus*). Hemopoietic activity of the marrow in the dermal bones of these animals undergoes seasonal variation. In the winter months hemopoiesis ceases, the marrow being replaced by adipose tissue. As warmer weather returns in spring, hemopoiesis resumes, and during the summer months the entire marrow cavities of the dermal bones are hemopoietic. Further support for this hypothesis is provided by an earlier observation of Barcroft et al [1923] regarding an increase in blood reticulocytes in two men kept for several days in a glass chamber at 32–35°C. Huggins and Blocksom also cited an observation indicating that the recovery from hemolytic anemia is more rapid in tropical than in temperate climates.

The "temperature-gradient" hypothesis is both attractive and plausible. Nonetheless, when Petrakis [1966] measured directly the temperature of tail vertebrae in the rat, he found that the temperature gradient did not exactly coincide with the transition zone from red to yellow marrow. Furthermore, several investigators [Peabody, 1926; Oehlbeck et al, 1932; Hashimoto, 1962; Hamazato, 1958; Sheard, 1924] have shown that under conditions of intense hemopoietic stimulation, hemopoiesis does expand into areas where normally the yellow marrow resides. With the advent of modern radiotherapy in ablative doses for malignant lymphomas, a similar observation has been made when the normally hemopoietic areas of marrow are ablated [Knospe et al, 1976]. Were the local temperature of the marrow the sole determinant of hemopoietic activity, one would have not expected extension of red marrow into the areas where yellow marrow normally resides and where thermal conditions are presumably suboptimal.

The observations of Emery and Follett [1964] further indicate that the first appearance of fatty marrow can be noted in utero during the last month or so of fetal life, in the toes, before any question of cooling arises. The formation of fatty marrow after birth may then be as much a function of a diminishing growth rate as of cooling. We have already noted that red marrow can be transformed to a large extent into fatty marrow during rebound, when the animal is polycythemic, in the course of a few days

[Slavin et al, 1981]. Here there is no question of an external temperature change, though it is true that a diminished blood flow through the marrow may have an effect on the actual marrow temperature. The reverse change is equally true, in that a good deal of the fatty marrow can be converted into red, in a matter of days by stimulating erythropoiesis. However, the increase or decrease of fat content in hemopoietic red marrow indicates a capacity for change that seems to be absent in marrow once it has become completely fatty.

Moreover, the experiments of Huggins and Blocksom [1936] have not been confirmed. Maniatis et al [1971] repeated and extended the tail implantation experiments and found that transplantation alone increased the cellularity only slightly, but that the addition of phenylhydrazine treatment led to a great increase in cellularity. They concluded that there was an "inherent determinant" of the cellularity of marrow in different sites, though this could be modified to some extent by the phenylhydrazine treatment.

Tavassoli et al [1974] then performed experiments on the tibial marrow of the rabbit. They first observed that a normal fatty tibia did not become hemopoietic in an animal treated with phenylhydrazine. They then noted that if the marrow was first evacuated, there was a phase during its regeneration when it became hemopoietic, but this phase was transient, for after 6 months the marrow was fatty again. If, however, phenylhydrazine was given three times per week for the duration of the study, the marrow remained hemopoietic.

Tavassoli et al [1979] subsequently carried out tail loop implantation in both newborn (where the tail still contains red marrow) and adult rats (in whom the tail contains fatty marrow). They implanted the tail in the abdomen and found that the fatty transformation could be prevented in newborn rats. They concluded that the adipose cells are fairly stable in the fatty marrow and, once developed, they can be displaced only with difficulty. Here again systemic stimuli such as phlebotomy and phenylhydrazine-induced hemolysis acted in concert with the temperature increment in preventing the fatty transformation. Tavassoli et al [1979] suggested that the observations of Huggins and Blocksom [1936] might have resulted from the presence of a compensated hemolytic state due to Bartonella infection in experimental rats. Bartonella-free strains of experimental rats were not available before 1944.

Ectopic Implants of Yellow Marrow

When bits of marrow tissue are removed and autotransplanted in various ectopic sites, a sequence of histogenetic events take place, leading to the formation of a marrow nodule (Fig. VII.4) surrounded by a shell of bone [Tavassoli and Crosby, 1968]. The regenerating process is reminiscent of marrow ontogenesis, where the formation of bone and marrow stroma preceeds the proliferation of hemopoietic cells. Tavassoli and Crosby [1970] studied the behavior of peritoneal implants taken from marrow of the extremities of adult rabbits, which are normally fatty. Such implants undergo the same recapitulation of marrow ontogeny to become actively hemopoietic nodules. Then the recapitulation goes full circle, and hemopoietic tissue is again replaced by fatty tissue (Fig. VII.5). This difference in the behavior of red and yellow marrow appears to be unrelated to the supporting bed: Implants of red marrow in the subcutaneous tissue of the extremities remain actively hemopoietic, whereas the implants of yellow marrow in the abdominal cavity undergo fatty involution. When bits of red and yellow marrow were implanted [Tavassoli, 1978a] side by side, the hemopoietic activity of the regenerated implant always reflected that of its site of origin, irrespective of the supporting bed.

This varied behavior of the two tissues, placed in similar environments, represents a fundamental intrinsic difference between them. This fundamen-

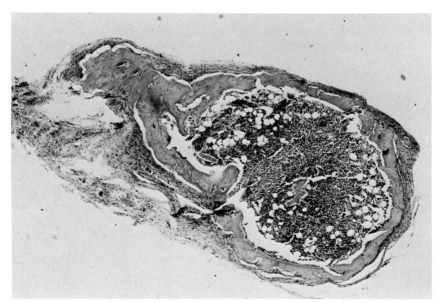

Fig. VII.4. Subcutaneous implant of red marrow after 8 weeks. The regenerated marrow nodule is surrounded by a shell of bone. The marrow is intensely hemopoietic and contains only a few fat cells. ×36.

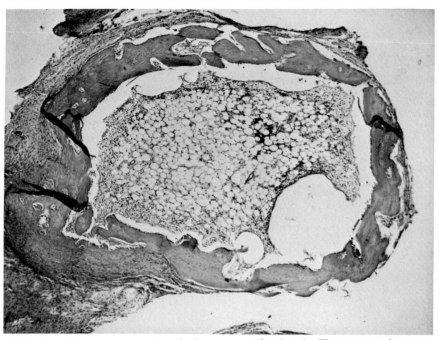

Fig. VII.5. Subcutaneous implant of yellow marrow after 8 weeks. The regenerated marrow nodule is surrounded by a shell of bone. The marrow is devoid of hemopoiesis, consisting only of adipose tissue. ×36.

tal intrinsic difference is further substantiated in the work of Patt et al [1982]. These authors have cultured fibroblasts from the two types of marrow. Upon reimplantation of these in vitro grown fibroblasts in the subcapsular area of the kidney, they observed the formation of marrow nodules. Red marrow–derived fibroblasts gave rise to a red marrow nodule; fatty marrow–derived fibroblasts gave rise to a fatty marrow nodule. Because the tissues are of similar genetic constitution (both are of the same genotype), Abercrombie [1967] used the term "epigenetic" to refer to this fundamental difference. Epigenotype is defined as a self-reproducing regulatory mechanism that characterizes each of the differenct tissue types of an organism. It is of interest that when the sequence of events during this period of fatty transformation is closely followed, one may observe the development of adipose cells in both red and yellow implants (Figs. VII.4, 5). In both types of implants fat cells develop after hemopoietic cell proliferation has already been established. In the implant of yellow marrow, however, the fatty component totally replaces the hemopoietic tissue, whereas in the implant of red marrow relatively few adipose cells develop interspersed with hemopoietic tissue. Systematic study of the postnatal development of rabbit marrow in different medullary cavities indicates that the process is similar: At birth most bones are in the process of ossification from the preexisting cartilage (cartilaginous osteogenesis). Few foci of marrow are seen, and none contains adipose cells. These cells begin to develop 2–3 weeks after birth in the areas of marrow already formed, while the process of cartilaginous osteogenesis continues in other bones. This developmental process takes place both in the axial bone (prospective sites of red marrow) and in the bones of extremities (prospective sites of yellow marrow). As the animal grows, the development of adipose cells in the marrow cavities continues. In the distal bones, it completely overtakes the hemopoietic tissue, whereas in the axial bones it does not, and remains side by side in coexistence with hemopoietic tissue.

These observations suggested that there exists an inherent (epigenetic) determinant of the cellularity of marrow in different sites, although this can be modified to a certain extent by environmental factors and by physiological stimulation. This epigenetic determinant appears to reside in the adipose cell component of marrow.

Marrow Adipose Cells

Investigations on white adipose tissue generally have centered upon extramedullary adipose tissue, presuming a functional unity of adipose cells throughout the body [Zakaria and Shafrir, 1967]. The primary function of extramedullary adipose tissue relates to energy conservation, its development and degradation being controlled by the nutritional state of the organism through a complex endocrine and neuroendocrine control. Thus, in starvation this adipose tissue atrophies, and with refeeding it is rebuilt [Tavassoli, 1974b]. By contrast, Cohen and Gardner [1965] observed that a population of marrow adipose cells is resistant to the effects of starvation. We have confirmed and extended their findings in rabbits [Tavassoli, 1974b]. With total food deprivation, epididymal adipose tissue undergoes characteristic cellular changes resulting in fat mobilization, whereas tibial marrow adipose tissue remains unchanged (Fig. VII.6). With partial food deprivation, extramedullary fat behaves in a similar manner, while the adipose marrow undergoes characteristic gelatinous transformation [Tavassoli et al, 1976]. On the other hand, with hemopoietic stimulation over a short period of time (blood-letting, phenylhydrazine-induced hemolysis), the extramedullary adipose tissue remains unchanged, whereas the marrow adipose cells, or at least the component associated with red marrow, undergoes cellular changes resulting in fat mobilization [Tavassoli et al, 1972].

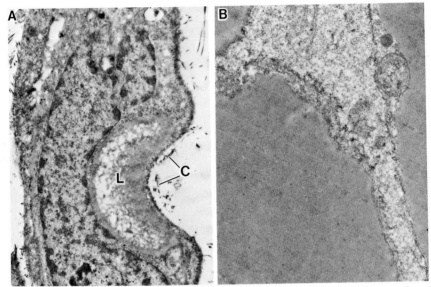

Fig. VII.6. Epididymal and marrow adipose tissue in the rabbit after 10 days of total starvation. A) Epididymal adipose cell undergoes lipid resorption. As a result, the cell size shrinks. Only a small fat vacuole (L) displaying a "fluffy" appearance remains in the vicinity of the nucleus. Note also the association of the cell with collagen fiber (C). B) In contrast, bone marrow adipose cells do not undergo lipid mobilization and the central lipid vacuoles are retained, maintaining their homogeneous appearance. From Tavassoli [1974b]. Both ×17.500

Other differences appear to exist between a marrow adipose cell and its extramedullary counterpart [Slavin, 1972]. Structurally, extramedullary adipose cells are associated with a large amount of collagen (Fig. VII.6), whereas their marrow counterparts are not [Tavassoli, 1976b, 1974b,c; Oberling et al, 1972]. The progenitor of the extramedullary adipose cell is a fibroblastlike cell containing numerous strands of rough endoplasmic reticulum evidently forming collagen. The progenitor of the marrow adipose cell appears to be a "reticulum cell" closely resembling the adventitial cells of the marrow [Tavassoli, 1976b]. This cell contains but few profiles of rough endoplasmic reticulum, and is not associated with extracellular collagen. In the course of their development, extramedullary adipose cells contain large amounts of glycogen; this feature is absent in the marrow adipose cell [Tavassoli, 1976b].

Marrow fat cells are generally smaller than their extramedullary counter-parts [Bathija et al, 1978]. Trubowitz and Bathija [1977] observed metabolic differences in the behavior of marrow and extramedullary adipose cells in culture. There are also differences in enzymatic content of the two cell types, particularly with respect to esterases [Tavassoli, 1978b].

Therefore, it appears that marrow cells and extramedullary adipose cells are two distinctly different cell types, having in common intracellular accu-mulation of lipid in the form of lipid vacuoles. This should not be surprising, since lipid accumulation is not a hallmark of a single cell type. A variety of cell types—monocyte, granulocyte, lymphocyte, hepatocyte—can all accu-mulate lipid in normal and pathological conditions. The mere possession of lipid inclusions cannot be considered as a marker of a cell type.

In a recent study of rat marrow, by light and electron microscopy, Slavin et al [1981] observed a great reduction in both number and size of marrow adipocytes during 7 days of hypoxia at 17,000 feet, while at the same time there was a general dilatation of sinusoids (Fig. VII.7). After 7 days of hypoxia most of the adipocytes had lost their spherical shape, and contained lipid droplets of varying size and fingerlike extensions to the cytoplasm (Fig. VII.8). During rebound, the lipid-depleted adipocytes showed little change, but by 5 days the smaller lipid droplets were coalescing with one another or with larger lipid droplets as the cell assumed a more spherical shape and the nucleus was pushed peripherally. By 7 days of rebound, though many adipocytes had resumed a normal appearance, a number of cells were still small (Fig. VII.7).

The decrease in marrow fat during hypoxia, however produced, has been reported by a number of observers [eg, Evans et al, 1955; Hudson, 1958b; Tavassoli et al, 1972], but care must be exercised in distinguishing between the reduction in the number of fat cells in marrow that is already hemo-poietic and the conversion to red marrow of marrow that is already com-pletely fatty. Some of the factors affecting the conversion of yellow to red marrow have been discussed by Maniatis et al [1971].

Moreover, there is evidence to indicate that within the adipose cell population of marrow there exist two different subpopulations, and the distribution of these two subpopulations is congruent with the distribution of red and yellow marrow. Cohen and Gardner [1965] reported that the yellow marrow fat partially defends itself against starvation, whereas the red marrow fat is mobilized as readily as extramedullary fat. Tavassoli et al [1974] have reported that after intense hemopoietic stimulation, using phle-

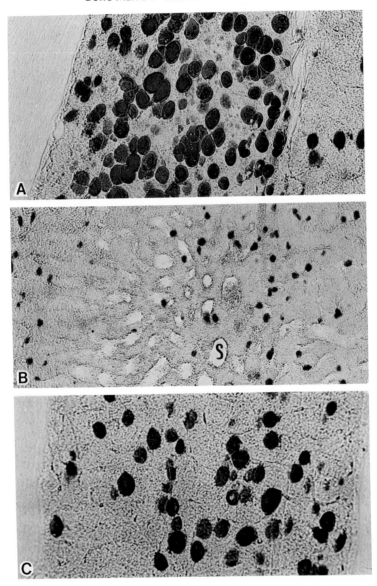

Fig. VII.7. A) Bone marrow of normal rat. Densely stained spherical cells are adipocytes stained for neutral fat with oil red O. B) Bone marrow of hypoxic rat. Note the drastic reduction in number and size of adipocytes. Also, note dilated sinusoids (S). C) Rat bone marrow in rebound following hypoxia. Adipocytes reaching normal dimension. All figures stained with oil red O. Slightly reduced from ×275. From Slavin et al [1981].

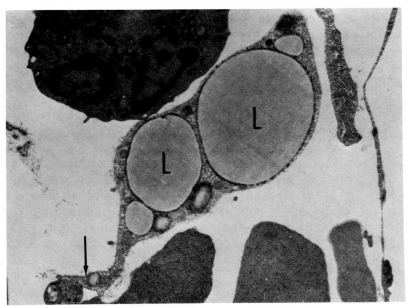

Fig. VII.8. Electron micrograph of marrow adipocyte following 7 days of hypoxia in a guinea pig. Note the oval shape of the cell and fingerlike cellular extensions (arrow). Lipid droplets (L) of various sizes are seen. From Slavin et al [1981].

botomy or phenylhydrazine-induced hemolysis, yellow marrow adipose cells are not mobilized as readily as their counterparts in the red marrow [Tavassoli et al, 1974]. The latter readily yield to expanding hemopoietic tissue.

Furthermore, in the course of studying lipid histochemistry of marrow, it was noted that the performic acid-Schiff reaction (PFAS) can be used to differentiate between two populations of adipose cells: The lipid substance in one gives a positive reaction, and that in the other, negative. The distribution of these two populations is congruent with distribution of red and yellow marrow. After hemopoietic stimulation, using phenylhydrazine-induced hemolysis, only PFAS-negative cells remain [Tavassoli, 1976a]. This observation suggested a relation between the chemical composition of lipid contained within adipose cells and their relative stability during the expansion of hemopoietic tissue. The bulk of lipid contained within marrow fat cells consists of triglycerides. Therefore, gas chromatographic analysis of fatty acids in the fat cells of red and yellow marrow was carried out [Tavassoli et al, 1977]. There was a consistent and highly significant shift from myristate and palmitate (in red marrow) to myristoleate and palmitoleate (in yellow marrow), with an intermediate pattern in the tibia.

Although there is no evidence that these differences bear any relationship to hemopoietic activity of red and yellow marrow, the good correlation may suggest more than a chance relationship. It is possible that the lipid composition of marrow adipose cells may determine their relative stability during the expansion of hemopoiesis.

The presence of two populations of adipose cells of different stability permits the formulation of a coherent hypothesis to explain the apparently contradictory experimental findings. The total volume of hemopoietic tissue is controlled by the requirement of the body. Marrow adipose tissue, serving as a "cushion," has a reciprocal relationship with hemopoietic tissue within the marrow cavity. The stability of adipose cells, however, is governed by the thermal environment; therefore their potential as a "cushion" varies according to their thermal environment. To induce hemopoiesis in otherwise aplastic yellow marrow, two factors are required: First, hemopoiesis must be stimulated to expand; second, the adipose tissue must be made labile in order to yield to the expansion of hemopoietic tissue. The latter condition can be brought about by an increment in temperature. In the absence of an increment in temperature, adipose tissue, being relatively stable, is not easily displaced by expanding hemopoietic tissue.

This hypothesis can explain the experimental results described above. Thus, when rats are subjected to hemopoietic stimuli, induction of hemopoiesis cannot be attained in the yellow marrow of the tail vertebrae. With an increment of temperature, but in the absence of hemopoietic stimuli, adipose cells—now labile under new thermal conditions—nevertheless remain in the marrow cavity, for there is nothing to displace them.

The Marrow Reserve

The extent to which fatty marrow can become converted into red marrow is important from the point of view of reserve marrow capacity. In man, according to Mechanik's [1926] figures, red and fatty marrow are each 2% of the body weight in the adult. If most of this fatty marrow can become red when the need arises, then it is clear that fatty marrow is in effect a reserve space for the development of additional red marrow. In that case adult human marrow could be considered a "high-reserve" marrow, whereas the standard 400-g guinea pig, in which only about one-seventh of the marrow is fatty, would possess a "low-reserve" marrow. However, the comparison is not altogether a valid one, since the 400-g guinea pig is still young and not yet fully developed, whereas Mechanik's data were obtained from fully developed adults. In younger subjects, and even more so in the fetus, the fatty marrow forms a much smaller proportion of the whole, and hence the reserve is lower.

The concept of high-reserve and low-reserve is based on the assumption that, in case of need, all the fatty marrow can become red. But this may not be the case. Hudson [1958b] observed that in guinea pigs at a stimulated altitude of 20,000 feet, the fatty marrow was not converted entirely to red even after 4 or 5 weeks. However, as skeletal growth was also imparied by this degree of hypoxia, he thought this might in some way be a factor in retarding the change from fatty to red marrow. He therefore repeated his studies at 14,000 feet—an altitude that does not seem to impair skeletal development—and examined the marrow in guinea pigs subjected to hypoxia from birth. The resulted was unexpected: "A notable finding was that fatty marrow occupied its normal centrifugal position in the skeletons of the hypoxic animals. Assuming that all the marrow of the newborn mammal is hemopoietic, it may be concluded that the original red marrow of the distal limbs and coccyx had actually been converted into inactive, fatty marrow even in the presence of a potent erythropoietic stimulus." This finding would fit in with the concept of an "inherent determinant" suggested by Maniatis et al [1971], though as yet we have no idea what this determinant might be.

VIII.

Quantitative Studies of Bone Marrow

INTRODUCTION

In postnatal life the bone marrow is the central organ of the lymphomyeloid complex (LMC). As discussed elsewhere in this volume (see Chapter III), in prenatal life, before the bone marrow acquires it definitive status, its place is taken first by the yolk sac and then by the liver and spleen. The LMC has six constituent parts: bone marrow, thymus, spleen, lymph nodes, lymphoepithelial tissues, and connective tissues. In the connective tissues, we include the serous cavities, blood and lymph.

Not only is the bone marrow the tissue in which many of the blood cells are produced, it also controls, to a varying extent, the activities of the other members of the LMC. The thymus resembles the bone marrow in being a very active site of cell production, but differs from it in two important respects. The bone marrow not only produces its own cells throughout life, but also continually replenishes the stem cell compartment of the thymus. Furthermore, whereas the bone marrow gives rise to a variety of cells, the thymus seems to be concerned primarily with the production of T lymphocytes, even though on occassion it, too, may be the site of limited production of other blood cells.

The constituents of the LMC are integrated throughout life by streams of migrating cells [Yoffey et al, 1959]. It seems likely that we are not yet fully aware of all the cellular migration streams, but a sufficient number are known to make us realize the importance of their intensive study. However, quantitative data on cell production in the marrow provide a useful starting point for an initial approach to the study of some of the major cellular migration streams. These streams consist of a variety of cells, including lymphocytes, monocytes, and granulocytes. In the case of lymphocytes, the recognition of specific subgroups has led to the study of functionally specific migration streams. One of the more recent migration streams to claim increasing attention is that of the various stem cells, and here too one has to consider the migration pattern of the various types of stem cell and their ultimate destination.

In quantitative terms, the three major cell groups in the marrow are lymphoid, erythroid, and myeloid cells. There are also smaller numbers of monocytes and monocyte precursors. The lymphoid cells are composed predominantly of B cells and their precursors, as also T-cell precursors, null cells, and natural killer (NK) cells. The megakaryocytes, which give rise to the blood platelets, are generally believed to remain for the most part within the marrow parenchyma, though some may enter the bloodstream [Tavassoli and Aoki, 1981].

Since the early days of hematology, the marrow has been known to possess erythropoietic and granulopoietic activities, but it is only since the studies of Osmond and Everett [1964] that we have come to appreciate its fundamental importance as a major source of lymphocytes.

Finally, in the case of both the marrow and other constituents of the LMC, an important factor in cell growth and differentiation is thought to be connected with the stromal cells [Tavassoli, 1975]. Recent studies raise the possibility that substances stimulating or inhibiting the growth and differentiation of stem cells may be formed within the marrow, in addition to the extrinsic factors which reach the marrow via the blood stream.

QUANTITATION OF MARROW CELLULARITY

From a historical point of view, the quantitative study of bone marrow is a relatively recent phenomenon. We owe the pioneer quantitative studies, not only of bone marrow but of several major components of the lympho-myeloid complex, to Kindred [1940, 1942]. His extensive studies of the hemopoietic tissues of the rat, involving mitotic counts on serial sections, involved an enormous amount of work, and have not been repeated. When one compares Kindred's data with those of subsequent workers, one cannot fail to be impressed by the way his main conclusions were right. He drew attention to the very large myeloid reserve in the marrow and, on the basis of his data, concluded that granulocytes could have only a short (30 min) life-span in the blood. He suggested that the thymus was continually supplying cells to the lymph nodes, and disputed the role of reticulum cells as stem cells—at that time almost a sacred dogma for most hematologists.

After Kindred's work, more than a decade elapsed before a burst of renewed interest came about in quantitative studies of bone marrow. Yoffey [1954] published the first of a series of quantitative investigations, in collaboration with colleagues at the University of Bristol. These investigations were based on the direct study of the bone marrow in order to analyze experimentally induced changes, mainly in the guinea pig. The technique, and some of the main results, are described in several chapters in the present volume. As the work progressed, interest was directed increasingly to the interrelationships between the various cell groups. These studies focused attention repeatedly on the transitional cell compartment, and led to the conclusion that it was this compartment that contained the various stem cells—committed and uncommitted. One of the early examples of this was the work of Harris [1956] on sublethal irradiation, where a marked increase in transitional cells preceded the regeneration of the other marrow constituents.

Though the Bristol studies constitute the most extensive series of quantitative investigations of bone marrow, the literature contains occasional quantitative estimates or actual measurements of bone marrow for specific purposes [eg, Fand and Gordon, 1957; Fruhman and Gordon, 1955a,b]. For human marrow a number of scattered estimates have also been made [eg, Osgood, 1954; Donohue et al 1958a,b].

Experimental Animals

Quantitative marrow studies have been performed by a number of workers, mainly on the smaller laboratory animals. The most extensive studies have been made in guinea pigs, and in these studies interesting comparisons have been made of changes in marrow and blood. A number of studies have been made on rat marrow [Kindred, 1942; Fruhman and Gordon, 1955a,b; Burke and Harris, 1959; Ramsell and Yoffey, 1961]. Among quantitative studies of murine bone marrow one may note those of Chan et al [1966], Beran and Tribukait [1971], and Miller and Osmond [1974, 1975]. The studies on murine bone marrow are of special interest because of the light they can throw on the spleen colony-forming units [Thomas et al, 1977].

The most extensive quantitative studies have been made in guinea pigs, using a standard experimental animal—a healthy male guinea pig of the Dunklin-Hartley strain weighing approximately 400 g. The use of such a standard animal avoids the variations due to age, species, and sex. With increasing experience it has become evident that even with such a standard animal the response to a given stimulus may show considerable variation.

The use of a standard animal has a number of advantages, but care must be exercised in applying the results thus obtained either to other animals or to man. It is evident, for example, that there may be varying stem cell requirements between different animal species, while even in the same species stem cells requirements are made greater in the embryo and in early postnatal life than in the adult [Yoffey, 1966, 1980; Yoffey et al, 1961].

Quantitative Techniques

In the guinea pig studies, on which the following pages are largely based, the quantitative technique is a simple one and has been repeatedly described [Yoffey, 1966]. A marrow plug of known volume is placed in a given volume of serum, and shaken up so that the marrow disintegrates and forms a uniform suspension of cells which can be counted by standard hemocytometric techniques. Counts can finally be expressed as absolute numbers of cells per μl of marrow. The figure obtained is almost but not quite a true volume dilution of marrow in serum, since allowance has to be made for the blood in the marrow vessels, which Osmond and Everett [1965] estimated to range between 4.90% and 6.96% of the total marrow volume. Brookes [1965], working with rats, obtained a somewhat lower figure, and for the rabbit femur Michelsen [1969b] obtained a higher figure—8.9 ml per 100 g of wet marrow tissue.

The technique employed for the guinea pig is equally applicable to the bone marrow of the rat. In the case of the mouse, Miller and Osmond [1974] developed a technique that enabled them to obtain quantitative data on the cell content of femoral marrow. The marrow was flushed out of the femur, and the cleaned and dried bone was then filled with paraffin of known specific gravity, so that the marrow volume could be determined.

Reproducibility of Results

Despite the possible sources of error, it has been established repeatedly that in the hands of experienced workers the results of the technique are fully reproducible. This problem was specifically investigated by Hudson et al [1963]. Two completely independent groups of experiments were performed. Of 25 experiments, 12 were performed by one investigator, and the remaining 13 by the other two. The results of the two groups were not compared until the conclusion of the series. The results are given in Table VIII.1, which presents the total nucleated cell counts, and the counts of the three major cell groups—lymphoid, myeloid, and erythroid. In a statistical comparison of the two groups no significant differences were found.

Cellularity in the Marrow of Different Bones

It is usually assumed that the composition of red marrow is uniform throughout the body. In man, the cellularity of the marrow in different parts of the body has been investigated by a number of workers [eg, Custer

TABLE VIII.1. Counts of Nucleated Cells and Main Cell Groups in Normal Guinea Pig Bone Marrow

Total nucleated cells	Lymphocytes	Myeloid	Erythroid	Damaged forms
1,810	469	695	326	132
2,130	503	739	398	239
1,620	389	531	397	136
1,920	409	634	516	163
2,040	596	563	443	296
1,990	589	700	398	151
2,100	588	554	628	218
1,680	511	415	423	170
1,800	292	680	488	189
1,980	511	735	358	210
1,900	367	524	720	150
1,870	568	671	318	116
1,684	448	515	451	209
1,839	581	588	412	195
1,670	711	511	193	157
1,751	620	347	557	193
2,279	479	579	830	255
2,027	677	482	612	174
2,030	593	512	560	288
1,571	336	559	418	167
1,129	312	332	366	65
2,068	558	542	711	103
2,245	440	907	633	216
1,868	390	504	691	116
1,965	607	605	428	193
Mean 1,880	502	577	491	180
SD 243	114	125	151	55

From Hudson et al [1963].

and Ahlfeldt, 1932; Van den Berghe and Blitstein, 1945], but the results have been conflicting. A quantitative study seemed an excellent way of tackling the problem, and this was undertaken on two occasions. Harris et al [1954] compared the marrows of right and left humerus in 17 guinea pigs. While in individual experiments there were on occasion appreciable differences between the two sides, the differences between the mean values of the two sides were not significant, except in the case of the monocytes. It is difficult to know how much importance should be attached to this difference in a small group of cells showing rather wide fluctuations in the different specimens. The results of the comparison between the two sides are presented in Table VIII.2.

Hudson [1959], in 16 guinea pigs weighing between 370 and 450 g performed total nucleated cell counts on marrow from five differenet sites—sternum, ribs, humerus, femur, and upper end of tibia (Table VIII.3). The mean values per μl were 2.06, 2.01, 1.93, 1.83, and 1.76 × 10^6 respectively. The counts obtained from the humerus were significantly lower than those obtained from sternal (t = 3.1), costal (t = 2.4), and upper tibial marrow (t = 4.1). The mean differences between humeral and other marrow do not exceed ± 8% [cf Hulse, 1964] in the rat. The humerus gives counts intermediate between the higher and lower values, and it would appear that, at any rate in the standard guinea pig, calculations of total marrow cellularity are least likely to be in error if they are based on humeral marrow.

TABLE VIII.2. Comparison of Right and Left Humeral Marrow in Guinea Pigs

	Mean	Standard deviation	Standard error of the mean
Right			
Erythroid	272,218	96,073	23,240
Myeloid	389,687	130,000	31,464
Lymphocytes	301,131	170,470	28,460
Monocytes	19,941	12,570	3,049
Damaged	316,792	117,730	28,554
Total abs. count	1,402,217	240,500	58,330
M:E ratio	1.526	0.657	1.59
Left			
Erythroid	273,163	74,250	19,158
Myeloid	386,802	132,000	34,082
Lymphocytes	326,000	101,600	26,232
Monocytes	30,952	20,000	5,164
Damaged	291,427	116,000	30,131
Total abs. count	1,383,810	266,000	66,500
M:E ratio	1.452	0.475	0.123

From Harris et al [1956].

TABLE VIII.3. Cellularity of Hemopoietic Marrow of Various Sites

Body wt (g)	Total nucleated cells $\times 10^6$ per mm^3				
	Sterum	Ribs	Humerus	Femur	Upper tibia
450	2.42	1.84	1.91	1.74	2.04
445	1.58	1.47	1.45	1.46	1.35
440	2.10	1.88	1.90	1.88	1.69
435	1.99	2.20	2.13	1.80	1.77
430	1.81	2.01	1.87	1.73	1.62
425	1.71	1.92	1.63	1.43	1.44
420	2.06	1.93	1.84	1.79	1.43
410	2.01	2.23	1.85	1.97	1.73
410	2.36	2.19	2.23	2.01	2.05
405	1.87	2.09	1.93	1.55	1.64
405	2.27	2.01	1.93	1.85	1.90
400	2.10	1.95	2.10	1.87	2.05
400	2.07	2.00	2.10	1.87	2.03
395	2.04	1.89	1.80	2.01	1.70
390	2.15	2.16	2.04	2.02	2.11
370	2.37	2.31	2.12	2.26	1.87
Mean	2.06	2.01	1.93	1.83	1.78

From Hudson [1959].

Coggle and Gordon [1975] studied the distribution of CFU-S in the marrow of three strains of mice. They examined the marrow in seven different sites: sternum, ribs, humerus, vertebrae, iliac crest, femur, and tibia, and found that in all these the number of CFU-S ranged from 9.53 to 11.56 per 10^5 marrow cells. However, there were marked differences in the absolute numbers of CFU-S in the three different strains.

TOTAL CELL POPULATIONS IN THE MARROW

Using Hudson's [1958] figure for total volume of red marrow, and taking the cell count of humeral marrow as most representative of the marrow as a whole, one may calculate from the absolute counts per ml the total body populations, in the guinea pig, both of the nucleated marrow cells as a whole and of the various subgroups. The total body population of nucleated marrow cells would on this basis be $118 \pm 17 \times 10^8$. The corresponding figures for the main cell groups are as follows: lymphocytes, $31 \pm 7 \times 10^8$; myeloid cells, $36 \pm 9 \times 10^8$; erythroid cells, $31 \pm 10 \times 10^8$.

Although these figures for total marrow population can be regarded as only approximate, they are of the same order as the values estimated in a variety of ways in other species. Expressed in relation to body weight, the total nucleated marrow cell population in the guinea pig is 2.9×10^9 cells per 100 g. For the 200-g rat, using Ramsell and Yoffey's [1961] figure of $2.25 \pm 0.34 \times 10^6$ nucleated cells per ml marrow, and Kindred's [1942] figure of 1.176 ml per 100 g for marrow volume, one arrives at a figure of 2.6×10^9 per 100 g. Donohue et al [1958], using a different method, obtained figures of $1.3-2.2 \times 10^9$ in the rat, $0.9-1.8 \times 10^9$ for the rabbit, and $2.2-4.4 \times 10^9$ in the monkey. In man, corresponding figures have been obtained of 1.6 [Suit, 1957], 1.4 [Patt, 1957], 1.1–3.0 [Donohue et al, 1958], and 1.0–1.1 [Harrison, 1962]. In view of the sources of error in all these estimates, the figures indicate a considerable measure of agreement over a number of different species. Table VIII.4 presents the results obtained by different observers for total marrow populations of erythroid and myeloid cells, and these are of the same order as those found in the guinea pig.

The Normal Myelogram

Table VIII.5 presents the normal myelogram for guinea pig bone marrow. A small group of miscellaneous cells (plasma cells, macrophages, "reticulum" cells, megakaryocytes, also damaged cells) has not been included. There are three major groups: myeloid (ie, granulocytes, preponderantly neutrophil), erythroid, and lymphoid. The term "lymphoid" is usually applied to the combined "lymphocyte" and "transitional cell" population, but they are

TABLE VIII.4. Absolute Numbers of Nucleated Marrow Cells in Different Species. Total Marrow Cells/kg $\times$ 10^9

Author	Species	Erythroid	Myeloid
Kindred [1942]	Rat	10.0	14.6
Yoffey [1954]	Guinea pig	6.7	9.6
Osgood [1954]	Man	8.6	25.7*
Fruhman and Gordon [1955]	Rat	6.3	15.5
Suit [1957]	Man	4.6	10.6
Patt [1957]	Rat	22.0	27.0
	Dog	6.7	11.5
	Man	3.4	8.3
Donohue et al [1958]	Rat	5.6	6.7
	Rabbit	5.8	4.8
	Monkey	9.2	15.4
	Man	5.0	11.4
Burke and Harris [1959]	Rat	14.0	12.1
Bierring [1960]	Rat	10.5	10.6
Ramsell and Yoffey [1961]	Rat	5.3	10.1
Hudson et al [1963]	Guinea pig	7.5	9.1
Hulse [1964]	Rat	8.4	10.6

*Excluding mature granulocytes. Modified from Donohue et al [1958].

TABLE VIII.5. Absolute Counts (Thousands per mm³) of Main Cell Groups in Guinea Pig Marrow

Cell group	Counts[a]
Early neutrophils[b]	49 ± 21
Late neutrophils[c]	405 ± 120
Total eosinophils	73 ± 22
Total basophils	17 ± 9
Myeloblasts	25 ± 13
Proerythroblasts	18 ± 9
Basophilic erythroblasts	50 ± 27
Polychromatic erythroblasts	358 ± 128
Orthochromatic erythroblasts	53 ± 31
Reticulocytes	197 ± 58
Lymphocytes	502 ± 114
Transitional cells	48 ± 16
Monocytes	93 ± 17

[a]Mean ± SD.
[b]Early neutrophils-promyelocytes and myelocytes.
[c]Late neutrophils-metamyelocytes, band and segmented forms.

fundamentally different, and are listed separately in Table VIII.5. The transitional cells comprise the stem cell compartment of the bone marrow, and are discussed in detail elsewhere in this volume (Chapter XIII).

As seen with the light microscope, both the erythroid and myeloid cells consist of a graded series in which there are numerous intermediate forms, and in which a clear line of demarcation between the different stages is difficult to establish. This difficulty arises from the very outset of the developmental pathway. It is often difficult to decide at what stage a transitional cell becomes a proerythroblast or a myeloblast, and this is true whether the cells are examined by light or electron microscopy. A typical proerythroblast is clearly distinguishable from a typical basophilic erythroblast, and similarly, a typical polychromatic erythroblast is readily distinguishable form the basophilic erythroblast from which it has developed and from the orthchromatic erythroblast into which it subsequently changes. But in between the characteristic cells of each stage, there are intermediate cells which one attempts to classify on the basis partly of fine tinctorial differences, and partly of changing nuclear morphology. Since neither of these criteria may be very precise, the classification can only be approximate. In addition, bone marrow can show marked biological variations, and this, added to the difficulties in cell classification, accounts for the variable results obtained by different workers. Depending on the type of study, it is useful at times to record fewer cell groups—eg, to grade proerythroblasts and basophilic erythroblasts as early erythroid cells, and polychromatic and orthochromatic as late. Similarly with myeloid cells.

Age Changes

The data in Table VIII.5 are based on a standard animal—a healthy male guinea pig of the Dunklin-Hartley strain, weighing approximately 400 g. Even the standard animal can show quite a range of variation. One of the most important variables eliminated by the use of a standard animal is that of age.

That the marrow cellularity diminishes with age has been noted by a number of observers [eg, Fand and Gordon, 1957; Hudson, 1959]. Fand and Gordon [1957] found that the marrow of younger guinea pigs not only possesses a higher total nucleated cell count, but in addition has a higher lymphocyte content. Elson et al [1958] reported a similar finding in the rat, adding that there was a marked increase in the lymphocyte population of the marrow in the first fortnight of life, followed by a steady decrease. Burke and Harris [1959] performed quantitative cell counts of the nucleated cells of rat bone marrow, and in addition to confirming the postnatal increase in marrow lymphocytes, they also emphasized the presence of "lymphocyte-like" cells, which were evidently transitional cells.

The marrow in the human fetus has a fairly high lymphocyte content before birth [Yoffey et al, 1961], the average lymphoid cell content (including transitional cells) being 29% (range 10–45%) as against 5–20% in the human adult [Whitby and Britton, 1963]. Leitner [1949] summarized the myelograms of normal adults recorded by 20 different workers.

Gairdner et al [1952] employed a semiquantitative technique to study the marrow of 25 normal infants ranging in age from a few minutes after birth to 3 months. They noted that the content of "lymphoid" cells, expressed as a percentage of total marrow nucleated cells, varied with age as follows: 0–24 h, 12.1%; 3–5 days, 22.9%; 8–10 days 37.3%; 26–33 days, 55.6%; 55–62 days, 48.5%; 82–99 days, 47.0%. They emphasized the presence of considerable numbers of damaged cells ("smear" cells), "ignored by the standard authorities, probably because no interest has been taken in absolute values of the marrow cells." Though they did not recognize the distinctive morphology of transitional cells, it appears likely from the studies of Rosse [1969] that the smear cells were for the most part transitional cells. Rosse et al [1977] also noted the rapid postnatal increase in marrow lymphocytes, which rose to 40–58% of the total nucleated marrow cells at 1 month, and were 43.55% even at 18 months. They clearly identified the transitional cells, 1% at birth, and thereafter around 2% up to 18 months.

Miller and Osmond [1974] have provided important quantitative data on age changes in murine bone marrow. They found that the nucleated cell content of the marrow was maximal at 8 weeks (2.25×10^6/ml), and fell to 1.66×10^6/ml at 12–16 weeks. Granulocytes and their precursors increased sharply to reach a plateau at 8–16 weeks. Small lymphocytes reached a peak at 2–4 weeks, 626–648×10^3/ml, but fell to about half this number by 12–16 weeks. In the mouse, too, one finds the characteristic postnatal lymphocyte peak. The large transitional ("lymphoid") cells fell steadily from 2 to 12 weeks. Miller and Osmond [1975] made use of continuous ^{3}H-thymidine infusion to investigate the kinetic changes in the marrow lymphocytes in the bone marrow of young, pubertal, and adult C3H mice. Their results are discussed in relation to the transitional cell compartment elsewhere in this volume (Chapter XIII).

QUANTITATIVE RELATION BETWEEN MARROW AND BLOOD

In the case of the guinea pig, sufficient quantitative data are available to enable us to compare the total populations of the various cells in the bone marrow with the cells present in the blood stream. Comparisons of this nature are most easily made with the erythrocytes, a relatively stable blood population. In the case of the granulocytes, which remain in the blood for a much shorter time, the comparison involves a consideration of variations in the length of time the cells remain in the blood. Similar considerations apply to the monocytes. The lymphocytes present a problem of special complexity because of their movement through the blood between the various parts of the lymphomyeloid complex in the cellular migration streams [Yoffey et al, 1959].

The total cell population of the blood may readily be calculated if one knows the count per ml and the blood volume. Table VIII.6 gives representative blood counts for the normal healthy guinea pig. Edmondson and

TABLE VIII.6. Blood Cells in Normal Guinea Pig

Erythrocytes ($\times 10^6$ per mm^3)	5.02 ± 0.28
Reticulocytes (per mm^3)	$65{,}000 \pm 20{,}000$
Total leucocytes (per mm^3)	$5{,}020 \pm 711$
Lymphocytes	$3{,}710 \pm 802$
Neutrophil granulocytes	$1{,}150 \pm 336$
Eosinophil granulocytes	67 ± 39
Basophil granulocytes	19 ± 16
Monocytes	74 ± 40
Haematocrit (%)	44 ± 1.9

Wyburn [1963] estimated the erythrocyte life-span, red cell mass, and plasma volume of normal guinea pigs by means of [51]chromium and [32]phosphorus-labeled diisopropylfluorophosphate (DFP). Their figure for the life-span of the guinea pig circulating erythrocyte was 79 days, very close to the 83 days estimated by Everett and Yoffey [1959], who followed the percentage of ^{59}Fe-labeled cells in the blood over a period of 8 days in autoradiographs of blood smears. For purposes of calculation we have taken 80 days as the life-span of the circulating red cell in the normal animal. For blood volume we have the data of Osmond and Everett [1964], who obtained a figure of 6 ml/100 g, so that in a 400-g guinea pig the total blood volume would be 24 ml.

The Erythroid Equation

On the basis of a blood volume of 24 ml, a red cell count of 5,020,000 per μl of blood, and a red cell life of 80 days:

$$\text{Total circulating RBC} = 120 \times 10^9$$
$$\text{Daily loss of red cells} = 1/80$$
$$= 1.5 \times 10^9$$

This, therefore, is the number of red cells the marrow is daily called upon to produce in the normal steady state. In the adult guinea pig, splenic erythropoiesis comes seriously into play only under abnormal conditions. Taking Hudson's [1958] figure for red marrow volume as 6,250 μl, (6.25 ml), a daily production of 1.5×10^9 red cells would require the production of 240,000 per μl of marrow.

The erythroid compartment as a whole contains approximately 480,000 nucleated cells per μl, and if these can double in the course of 48 hours, they would just meet the requirements for steady-state red cell production. The kinetic data seem to fit in with this [Rosse and Trotter, 1974b; Starling and Rosse, 1976; Prothero et al, 1978]. The last-named authors summarize the earlier work in a mathematical model in which the transit times for the four major erythropoietic compartments (proerythroblast, basophilic erythroblast, polychromatophilic erythroblast, and orthochromatic erythroblast) are 13.7, 13.2, 12.9, and 14.0 hours respectively, a total of around 54 hours in all. These data indicate that in the steady state red cell production keeps pace with requirements, but there is nothing corresponding to the massive granulocyte reserve.

The Reticulocyte Reserve

Though erythropoiesis in the normal steady state seems to be finely balanced, and there is virtually no reserve of nucleated erythroid cells, there is a small reserve of reticulocytes that can be rapidly discharged into the circulation [Yoffey, 1966; Tavassoli, 1977a; Aoki and Tavassoli, 1981b,c]. The size of this reserve seems to be somewhat variable. Hudson et al [1963] obtained a count of 197,000 per μl of marrow, whereas Bhuyan [1965] obtained a count of 426,000—the highest count on guinea pig marrow in an extensive series of investigations by different observers. This latter figure is 1.7 times the daily requirement for new red cell formation, and is on the high side. Suit [1957] calculated from the ^{59}Fe uptake that the marrow contains a 24-hour supply of reticulocytes, and possibly a little more. Increased red cell requirements beyond this small reserve necessitate changes in the erythropoietic pathway, which are discussed in Chapter X.

IX.

Granulocyte Production

INTRODUCTION

The majority of the marrow granulocytes are neutrophils. The two other granulocytic groups, the eosinophils and the basophils, not only are very much smaller numerically, but also have different reaction patterns.

NEUTROPHIL REACTIONS

In considering the granulocyte reactions, it is important to emphasize that these cells are primarily tissue cells. They are produced in the marrow, and move into bloodstream in order to enter the tissues. Thus, they are passengers in the blood. Moreover, there is a considerable reserve of granulocytes in the marrow. They are called upon when the body requires them. Mobilization of the marrow granulocyte reserve compartment leads to its depletion which, in turn, stimulates granulopoiesis in the bone marrow to replenish this compartment. These events are described here as granulocyte reactions.

The Myeloid Equation

The neutrophil equation—ie, the relation between neutrophil granulocyte production in the marrow and the blood granulocytes—differs from the erythroid equation in several important respects. In the normal steady state, the life-span of the neutrophil in the bloodstream is measured in hours rather than days. Among various estimates, Patt and Maloney [1964] place it at a maximum of 8 hours. Under abnormal conditions it may be measured in fractions of an hour. The great variability in the blood life-span of the neutrophils depends on the fact that they can migrate through capillary walls and move rapidly out of the bloodstream in response to numerous stimuli. The speed with which this extravascular accumulation may occur can be measured readily in the case of the peritoneal cavity [Spiers and Dreisbach, 1956; Fruhman, 1970] or in skin window exudates [Rebuck and Crowley, 1955].

Within the bone marrow itself there are three major differences between the myeloid and the erythroid cells: 1) There is a larger myeloid reserve; 2) the rate of neutrophil proliferation can undergo more rapid acceleration; and 3) the speed of neutrophil discharge from the marrow can also be greatly increased. All these factors play an important part in enabling the neutrophil granulocytes to function in the response to infection.

The Myeloid Reserve

The total freely circulating neutrophils in the blood of the standard healthy guinea pig range from 27×10^6 [Bhuyan, 1965] to 45×10^6 [Moffatt

TABLE IX.1. Absolute Number of Nucleated Marrow Cells (Total Marrow Cells/kg × 10⁹)

Author	Species	Erythroid	Myeloid
Kindred [1942]	Rat	10.0	14.6
Yoffey [1954]	Guinea pig	6.7	9.6
Osgood [1954]	Man	8.6	25.7*
Fruhman and Gordon [1955]	Rat	6.3	15.5
Suit [1957]	Man	4.6	10.6
Patt [1957]	Rat	22.0	27.0
	Dog	6.7	11.5
	Man	3.4	8.3
Donohue et al [1958]	Rat	5.6	6.7
	Rabbit	5.8	4.8
	Monkey	9.2	15.4
	Man	5.0	11.4
Burke and Harris [1959]	Rat	14.0	12.1
Bierring [1960]	Rat	10.5	10.6
Ramsell and Yoffey [1961]	Rat	5.3	10.1
Hudson et al [1963]	Guinea pig	7.5	9.1
Hulse [1964]	Rat	8.4	10.6

*Excluding mature granulocytes. Modified from Donahue et al [1958].

et al, 1961]. Intermediate values, obtained by several other investigators, were mostly near the lower end of this range, around 30 × 10⁶. If one takes the circulating and marginating granulocytes as being approximately equal, the total blood granulocytes would be double this figure. The marrow population of late neutrophils has been estimated at 2,530 × 10⁶ [Hudson et al, 1963] equal to 42 times the total blood neutrophils in the guinea pig, or possibly 84 times those which are freely circulating. Evidently the myeloid equation differs fundamentally from the erythroid, as was pointed out by Kindred [1942] and Yoffey [1954]. It is not only in the guinea pig that there is this enormous neutrophil reserve. Table IX.1 indicates that this is true in many species.

Life-Span of Mature Granulocytes in Blood

As already noted, the literature contains many and widely varying estimates of the time taken by neutrophils to mature in the bone marrow, and the length of time they remain in the blood [eg, Boggs, 1967; Lo Bue, 1970; Robinson and Mangalik, 1975]. In man, a blood life-span of about 8 hours has been suggested [Boggs, 1967], and similarly in the dog [Patt and Maloney, 1959], though very much shorter and very much longer blood life-spans have been proposed. An understanding of the relation between marrow and blood neutrophils would be greatly facilitated if quantitative data were available. If we calculate on the assumption that newly formed segmented neutrophils are discharged from the marrow in 4 days, and that the total marrow population of late neutrophils is 2,512 × 10^6 [Hudson et al, 1963], we would expect a daily discharge into the blood of 630 × 10^6, or about 26,000 neutrophils per μl per day. Since the level of the blood neutrophils is 1,150 per μl, this would seem to imply a blood life-span of about 1 hour. These tentative calculations would seem to point to quite a short blood life-span for the guinea pig neutrophils in the normal steady state. Whether this is the case or not, there is no doubt that under abnormal conditions neutrophils can enter and leave the bloodstream with even greater rapidity.

Mitotic Data in Normal Marrow

Patt and Maloney [1964] estimated that in canine marrow every 1,000 cells in the proliferative compartment (ie, myeloblasts, promyelocytes, and myelocytes, with perhaps some early metamyelocytes) can give rise to 80 cells per hour—ie, 1,920 cells per day. If we assume a similar rate of proliferation in the guinea pig, then the proliferative compartment (myeloblasts and early neutrophils in Table IX.2) at 74,000 per μl would give rise to 74 × 1,920 mature neutrophils per day. For the marrow as a whole this would mean 887 × 10^6 per day. If all these cells proceed to maturity and enter the blood, this would amount to about 37,000 neutrophils per μl of

TABLE IX.2. Absolute Counts (Thousands per mm^3) of Main Cell Groups in Guinea Pig Marrow

	Mean ± SD
Early neutrophils	49 ± 21
Late neutrophils	405 ± 120
Total eosinophils	73 ± 22
Total basophils	17 ± 9
Myeloblasts	25 ± 13
Proerythroblasts	18 ± 9
Basophilic erythroblasts	50 ± 27
Polychromatic erythroblasts	358 ± 128
Orthochromatic erythroblasts	53 ± 31
Reticulocytes	197 ± 58
Lymphocytes	502 ± 114
Transitional cells	48 ± 16

Early neutrophils—promyelocytes and myelocytes; late neutrophils—metamyelocytes, band, and segmented forms.
From Hudson et al [1963].

blood per day, and since the normal level of blood neutrophils is 1,150 per μl, this would mean that the neutrophils should remain in the blood for only 48 min. If one assumes, with Patt and Maloney [1964], that there is a substantial loss of cells at the myelocyte stage, then even if this loss is of the order of 50%, we would still have to reckon with a blood life-span of less than 2 hours in the normal steady state. In fact, however, we have been unable to detect evidence of myelocyte loss of this magnitude.

Another calculation may be made on the basis of Patt and Maloney's [1964] conclusion that, even allowing for a substantial loss at the myelocyte stage, one myeloblast normally gives rise to 12 mature neutrophils. This would mean that in the guinea pig (Table IX.2) 25,000 myeloblasts would ultimately produce 300,000 neutrophils per μl of marrow. Assuming that this process requires 4 days for its completion, it would necessitate the daily production of 75,000 mature neutrophils per μl of marrow, equivalent to around 18,000 neutrophils per μl of blood per day, as against a count of 1,150 neutrophils per μl (Table IX.3), a blood span of about 1½ hours. If there is a 3-day maturation period in the marrow, there would be a blood life-span of less than 1 hour.

On the whole, then, in the case of the guinea pig all the quantitative data suggest that the neutrophil granulocyte stays in the blood for 1–2 hours. It is difficult to make the data fit in with a blood life-span of the order of 8 hours.

Methods for the Study of Granulocyte Production

Evidence for the discharge of granulocytes from the marrow can be obtained by direct quantitative study of the marrow itself, in the intact animal. Direct evidence of a different kind may be obtained by perfusion of the isolated marrow [Dornfest, 1970]. Indirect evidence of the discharge of

TABLE IX.3. Absolute Counts of Blood Cells in the Normal Guinea Pig[a]

Erythrocytes ($\times 10^6 \mu$l)	5.02 ± 0.28
Reticulocytes (per μl)	$65,000 \pm 20,000$
Total leukocytes (per μl)	$5,020 \pm 711$
Lymphocytes	$3,710 \pm 802$
Neutrophil granulocytes	$1,150 \pm 336$
Eosinophil granulocytes	67 ± 39
Basophil granulocytes	19 ± 16
Monocytes	74 ± 40
Hematocrit (%)	44 ± 1.9

[a]Based on a study of 25 normal guinea pigs by Dr. R.K. Bhuyan, to whom we are indebted.

granulocytes from the marrow may be obtained by withdrawing leukocytes from the blood and observing their replacement, by the process of leukapheresis in dogs [Craddock et al, 1956] and man [Bierman et al, 1961]. Another indirect method is the mobilization of neutrophils into the peritoneal cavity, or the connective tissues as studied in skin window preparations, but this type of study is essentially of value for studying the *speed* with which neutrophils can leave the bloodstream, and does not give data on total neutrophil production.

Neutrophils in Peritoneal Fluid

Fruhman [1964] made a careful study in the mouse of the extent of neutrophil mobilization following the injection of appropriate stimuli into the peritoneal cavity. Normal peritoneal fluid contains relatively few neutrophils, but they can be made to appear in appreciable numbers in both rat and mouse [Fruhman, 1960, 1964]. In Sprague-Dawley rats, for example, the neutrophil content of the peritoneal cavity rose from 100,000 in the normal peritoneal cavity to almost 50 million after the intraperitoneal injection of 0.1 ml of Piromen, a Pseudomonas polysaccharide complex. Mobilization of 50 million neutrophils would make very modest demands on the bone marrow. If one calculates the total marrow content of late neutrophils, on the basis of Ramsell and Yoffey's [1961] data in the Lister hooded rat, and Kindred's [1942] estimate of red marrow volume in the Wistar rat, the total marrow content of neutrophils is $1,692 \times 10^6$, a figure greatly in excess of the 50×10^6 neutrophils appearing in the peritoneal cavity.

Although from a quantitative point of view the study of neutrophils in peritoneal exudate is of little use in assessing the bone marrow output, it brings out very clearly the speed with which neutrophils can leave the blood stream. Increased numbers of neutrophils are found in the peritoneal cavity within an hour of the intraperitoneal injection of Piromen [Fruhman, 1964].

Leukapheresis

The technique of leukapheresis [Craddock et al, 1955] is essentially a method of determining the myeloid reserve by removing granulocytes from the blood and measuring the number that then enter it. Blood is repeatedly withdrawn, freed of its leukocytes, and then reinjected. It is easy in this way to clear 1.5–2 times the blood volumes per hour for 2–3 hours in the normal dog, and this results in a leukopenia of about 1,000 cells per μl. After a single leukapheresis the blood leukocytes remain at a low level for about 2 hours (phase I). This is followed by a period of 6–8 hours (phase II) during

TABLE IX.4. Changes in Blood Leucocytes 4 Hours After Intraperitoneal Injection of LPF

	Total WBC	Total neutrophils	Total band neutrophils	Total mature neutrophils	Total lymphocytes
Saline					
1st count	5,170 ± 690	770 ± 80	28 ± 6	750 ± 70	4,090 ± 690
2nd count	6,880 ± 770	2,530 ± 430	175 ± 59	2,350 ± 410	3,960 ± 420
	+1,710	+1,760	+147	+1,600	−130
Saline and LPF					
1st count	6,000 ± 500	1,120 ± 150	53 ± 11	1,070 ± 140	4,540 ± 370
2nd count	9,040 ± 560	4,480 ± 470	431 ± 153	4,040 ± 340	4,170 ± 320
	+3,040	+3,360	+378	+2,970	−370

In each case the first count is made immediately before the injection, and the second count 4 hours later, immediately before killing the animal.
From Harris et al [1956].

which the leukocytes rise to as much as 300% above their level before leukapheresis. Once phase II has begun, the entry of leukocytes into the blood proceeds at a greatly increased rate, so that if a second leukapheresis is performed it is difficult to induce a leukopenia even if leukocytes are removed from the blood much more rapidly than during the first leukapheresis.

Does the marrow in fact possess a sufficient number of neutrophils to replace those removed from the blood by leukapheresis? In a single acute leukapheresis 1.5–2 volumes of blood per hour are cleared for 2–3 hours—ie, a maximum of six volumes. If we translate this into quantitative term in the guinea pig leukapheresis of this scale would remove about 180×10^6 neutrophils from the bloodstream, as against $2,512 \times 10^6$ late neutrophils in the bone marrow [Hudson et al, 1963]. In the guinea pig, then, the effective myeloid reserve of mature neutrophils is more than adequate to cope with the requirements of leukapheresis. The studies of Craddock et al [1956] on leukapheresis have confirmed the earlier conclusions of Kindred [1942] and Yoffey [1954] on the large neutrophil reserve of the marrow.

Leukocytosis

The quantitative approach greatly facilitates the study of leukocytosis. In one series of experiments this was induced by means of Menkin's leukocytosis-promoting factor (LPF). Harris et al [1956] examined the marrow and blood changes 4 hours after the intraperitoneal injection of LPF. Following LPF the blood shows a definite leukocytosis (Table IX.4). Whereas neutrophils exhibit a marked increase, lymphocytes diminish slightly. The neutrophil increase involves mainly the segmented forms, but there is also a small rise in the band forms of neutrophils.

The main changes in the bone marrow are shown in Table IX.5. On comparing the control marrow with that of the experimental series, there is little change in the total nucleated cells. However, neutrophils show a significant decrease with the mean falling from 714,000 to 551,000 per μl ($t = 4.05$). A differential count of the marrow neutrophils showed that segmented and band forms were discharged in approximately equal numbers, but since initially there were more of the latter than the former, the ratio in the marrow of the immature band forms (B) to the mature (M) segmented neutrophils underwent a marked change. In the control marrow the B:M (band:mature) ratio averaged 2.73, whereas in the experimental animals it was 5.40.

Masked Leukocytosis

The experiments with LPF provided the first clear evidence of "masked leukocytosis." A comparison of blood and marrow data showed that, following LPF, the total number of neutrophils discharged from the marrow over a 4-hour period was 798×10^6, whereas the total neutrophil rise in the blood was 48×10^6. About 750×10^6 neutrophils that had been discharged from the marrow were unaccounted for. The masked leukocytosis following LPF is quite different from the "masked granulocytosis" later reported by Boggs et al [1965], owing presumably to enlargement of the marginating pool. The number missing in the LPF experiments was far greater than could be accounted for by margination.

TABLE IX.5. Changes in Marrow Cells After Intraperitoneal Injection of LPF

	Total nucleated cells	Total neutrophils	Lymphocytes
Control	1,922,000 ± 102,800	714,700 ± 57,600	396,300 ± 26,000
Experimental	2,033,000 ± 54,700	551,100 ± 41,600	515,600 ± 13,800
	+111,000	−163,600	+119,300

	Changes in the main groups of marrow neutrophils		
	Mature neutrophils	Band neutrophils	Myeloblasts, myelocytes, and metamyelocytes
Control	130,600 ± 13,600	338,900 ± 25,900	245,400 ± 29,100
Experimental	69,600 ± 15,100	279,500 ± 21,700	205,000 ± 19,700
	−61,000	−62,400	−40,400

From Harris et al [1956].

Speed of Granulocyte Discharge

How quickly, and how completely, can granulocytes be discharged from the marrow? With the dose of LPF administered there was still an appreciable number of residual granulocytes in the marrow despite the considerable number that had been discharged. As to the speed of discharge, the "plasma expulsion factor" of Steinberg and Martin [1950] required 2–4 hours before its action on the marrow became evident. Gordon et al [1960] reported a leukocytosis 4 hours after the administration of LPF; in the marrow they noted a significant fall in neutrophils and eosinophils together with a rise in lymphocytes, as had been described by Harris et al [1956]. Plasma from rats given typhoid vaccine also induced leukocytosis 4 hours after injection [Gordon et al, 1964].

These and similar observations seem to indicate that about 4 hours are needed for a clear-cut leukocytosis to become evident. However, with more careful methods of analysis, changes in both marrow and blood become recognizable much sooner than this.

Experiments With Typhoid Vaccine

With injection of TAB vaccine containing 250 million Salmonella typhi, and 125 million each of Salmonella paratyphi A and B [Yoffey et al, 1964], a massive discharge of granulocytes from the marrow occurs. This was injected into an ear vein, and so could immediately reach the bone marrow via the bloodstream. This avoided sites of injection such as the peritoneum or subcutaneous tissues, where absorption might be slow or variable so that the experiments might not be uniform. In addition, there was always the possibility of the elaboration of special tissue factors such as LPF. In relation to the size of the animal the dose of vaccine employed was massive and slightly toxic. But the effect quickly wore off, and within a short time the animal was moving about actively and feeding quite normal.

Table IX.6 gives data on the marrow granulocytes at 15, 30, and 120 min after injection of TAB vaccine. In controls, the total marrow neutrophils were well below the figure usually regarded as normal but, even so, there is no doubt that after 2 hours the mature granulocytes have been almost completely discharged from the marrow.

Blood Changes

Figure IX.1 depicts the changes occurring in the blood during a period of 72 hours. There is a neutrophilic leukocytosis which reaches its peak at 12 hours, and then subsides to levels below normal. An initial lymphopenia is followed by a moderate degree of lymphocytosis. From the marrow volume

TABLE IX.6. Absolute Counts of Neutrophils in Marrow 15, 30, and 120 Minutes After TAB Vaccine IV

Time after injection	Myeloblast	Promyelocyte	Myelocyte	Metamyelocyte	Band	Mature	Total neutrophils
Normal	21,000 ± 15,000	11,000 ± 4,000	33,000 ± 35,000	96,000 ± 39,000	135,000 ± 145,000[a]	63,000 ± 121,000	359,000
15 min	14,000 ± 6,000	20,000 ± 7,000	23,000 ± 13,000	37,000 ± 9,000	148,000 ± 49,000	118,000 ± 49,000	358,000
30 min	14,000 ± 7,000	16,000 ± 8,000	17,000 ± 8,000	29,000 ± 14,000	168,000 ± 107,000[b]	117,000 ± 62,000	365,000
120 min	42,000 ± 12,000	21,000 ± 10,000	21,000 ± 10,000	64,000 ± 35,000	111,000 ± 61,000	8,000 ± 8,000	247,000

[a]Range 24,000–146,000, except for one at 399,000.
[b]Range 79,000–200,000, except for one at 431,000.
Two hours after the intravenous injection of vaccine, most of the mature neutrophils have been discharged from the marrow, and there are hardly any left.
From Yoffey et al [1964].

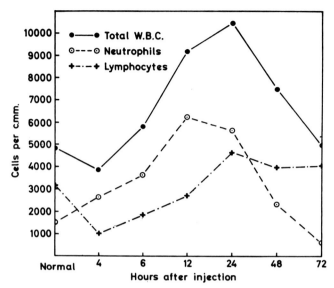

Fig. IX.1. Blood leucocytes (guinea pig) following the injection of TAB vaccine. The neutrophil leucocytosis reaches its peak at 12 hours, after which it steadily falls so that at 72 hours there is a leucopenia. The early fall in the lymphocytes followed by a slight increase at 24 hours is characteristic. Note the inverse relationship between neutrophils and lymphocytes at 4 hours. From Yoffey et al [1964]. Courtesy of the New York Academy of Sciences.

data of Hudson [1958] and the blood volume data of Osmond and Everett [1965], one anticipates that, during the first 2 hours, the discharge of band and mature neutrophils from the marrow (Table IX.6), should give rise to a leukocytosis of about 20,000 per μl of blood, compared with the observed 1,400. During the course of two hours, therefore, not only has the marrow discharged all its mature granulocytes into the blood, but most of them have already left the bloodstream.

Blood Life-Span of Discharged Granulocytes

From Figure IX.1 it might be inferred that increasing number of neutrophils are entering the blood during the first 12 hours, but a more detailed analysis shows that the changes are more complex. By means of a modified Arneth count, in which bilateral indentation of the nucleus was regarded as evidence of commencing lobulation, it was possible to analyze the sequence of events in greater detail. The results, presented in Table IX.7, indicate that after as short a time as 15 min there is already an appreciable change in the ratio of younger to older cells. By 2 hours the pattern has changed so completely that there could have been present in the blood-stream very few of those leukocytes in the blood at the start of the experiment. A comparison of the marrow discharge with the number of granulocytes present in the blood suggests that the blood granulocytes may have been replaced under the conditions of the experiment 10–15 times. This represents a far more rapid rate of passage through the blood than has been previously suggested, but the quantitative data do not seem to be consistent with any other interpretation. It must be borne in mind that the massive dose of vaccine is an exceptionally powerful stimulus, and can presumably give rise to very marked departures from the normal kinetic pattern.

As far as the normal steady state is concerned, the literature contains widely divergent estimates of the length of time granulocytes remain in the blood. The following are some representative examples: In rabbits, Weiskotten [1930] gave neutrophils ("amphophiles") an intravascular life-span of 3–4 days. In rats, Kindred [1942], on the basis of careful quantitative studies of mitotic activity in sections of myeloid tissue and a comparison of these data with the circulating leukocytes, concluded that the neutrophils had a blood life-span of 30 min. Van Dyke and Huff [1951], also working with rats, gave the neutrophils an even shorter intravascular life, 23 min. In man, Kline and Clifton [1952] gave human neutrophils a blood life-span of 9

TABLE IX.7. Arneth Count in Guinea Pig Blood 15, 30, and 120 Minutes After TAB Vaccine IV

Time after injection	Injection	Total neutrophils counted	Band forms	Modified Arneth count:[a] Cells percent of total neutrophils (No. of indentations)					
				1	2	3	4	5	6
15 min	Before	1,135	0.5	3	8	23	32	22	11
	After	387	5	12	18	25	24	12	5
30 min	Before	1,202	1	2	11	25	26	24	11
	After	740	10	19	23	23	20	4	1
120 min	Before	1,075	1	2	9	33	43	12	1
	After	1,427	47	27	16	6	3	1.5	0

[a]Bilateral indentations of the nucleus were regarded as definite evidence of commencing lobulation.

The Arneth count shows some change even in as short a time as 15 min after the intravenous injection of vaccine, whereas after 120 min the change is very marked. During the course of 2 hours the neutrophils originally present in the blood have been almost completely replaced.

From Yoffey et al [1964].

days. Bierman et al [1960] distinguished in man three groups of granulocytes, with intravascular life-spans of 4.4, 7.9, and 12.9 days. Boggs [1967]
concludes that in man, in the normal steady state, the total circulating
blood granulocyte pool is replaced about 2.5 times daily.

Changes in the Erythroid Population

Myeloid stimulation is associated with a sharp drop in the nucleated
erythroid cells of the marrow by 24 hours, and at 48 and 72 hours they are
still only half their normal level (Fig. IX.2). This is an example of interrelated
changes between the different cell types in the marrow. The abrupt fall in
the marrow neutrophils during the first 4 hours is followed by a moderate
increase at 24 hours, and a return to not quite normal levels at 48 hours.

A similar change occurs during erythropoietic stimulation (see Chapter
X): Increased erythropoietic activity is associated with a fall in the myeloid
cells. In both situations, whether the fall in the erythroid cells upon granulopoietic stimulation, or the fall in the myeloid cells upon erythropoietic
stimulation, the most likely explanation would appear to be stem cell
competition.

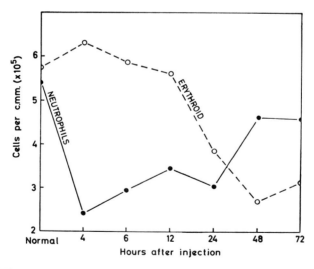

Fig. IX.2. The neutrophil and erythroid populations of marrow following the injection of
TAB vaccine. The effect of the TAB vaccine is to cause a marked discharge of neutrophils
from the marrow, followed by a slow return towards normal, almost complete at 72 hours.
The nucleated erythroid cells in the marrow fall abruptly after the twelfth hour. From Yoffey
et al [1964]. Courtesy of the New York Academy of Sciences.

EOSINOPHIL REACTIONS

The introduction of the differential staining of the blood cells by Ehrlich [1879] marks the starting point of the modern study of the eosinophil granulocytes. Since then, a vast literature has accumulated [reviewed inter alia by Spiers, 1958; Rytomaa, 1960; Archer, 1963; Hudson, 1968; Zucker-Franklin, 1974; Mahmoud and Austen, 1980; Tavassoli, 1981]. For a number of reasons the marrow eosinophils seem to have presented considerable difficulties in classification. Hudson [1968] adopted Downey's [1915] classification, subdividing the marrow eosinophils into three compartments: 1) a compartment of early forms, consisting of promyelocytes and myelocytes; 2) a metamyelocyte compartment; and 3) a compartment of late forms—the band and segmented eosinophils.

According to Hudson [1960], out of 400 marrow eosinophils, 50 were early forms, 50 were metamyelocytes, and 300 band and segmented forms. The ratio of marrow to blood eosinophils was 400:1. The relatively large number of late forms constituted the marrow reserve of eosinophils. These observations were made in guinea pigs.

One frequently sees large accumulations of eosinophils in extramyeloid situations such as the spleen, the submucosa of the intestine, the interstitial tissue of the lung, and lymph nodes. In a survey of the organ distribution of eosinophil granulocytes in the rat, Rytomaa [1960] concluded that "eosinophil granulocytes in the rat could rightfully be regarded as tissue rather than blood cells." In addition to the accepted eosinophil classification, Rytomaa [1960] recognized "small eosinophils" and "large tissue eosinophils." The relation between these two varieties is not clear [cf Padawer and Gordon, 1952].

Maturation Time in Marrow

How long does it take for eosinophils to mature in the marrow? A number of studies have been carried out on the appearance of labeled eosinophils in the blood following the administration of tritiated thymidine. Though the results show some variations, both species and otherwise, the continuous administration of tritiated thymidine in rats [Foot, 1965] resulted in the first appearance of labeled eosinophils in the blood at 3 days, with peak labeling on days 5 and 6. Further data are given by Tavassoli [1981].

Blood Life-Span

How long do eosinophils remain in the blood? The continuous thymidine infusion studies of Foot [1965] give a mean circulating life of 16–23 hours.

This is longer than other estimates. In the case of the guinea pig, Hudson [1968] inferred from the quantitative data that the time spent in the bloodstream can be hardly more than a few hours. Archer [1970] concluded that the blood life-span of eosinophils is shorter than that of neutrophils, and that it is probably somewhere between 1 and 24 hours, most likely about 6 hours.

Quantitative Changes in Marrow Eosinophils

Quantitative changes in marrow eosinophils have been studied in four experimental situations: the reactions to 1) foreign protein, 2) corticosteroids, 3) hypoxia, and 4) parasitic infections.

The foreign protein response. It has been repeatedly observed that eosinophils play an important part in response to foreign proteins, and that increased numbers of eosinophils are present in both blood and marrow after repeated antigenic stimulation [Schlecht, 1910], as also in anaphylaxis [Schlecht and Schwenker, 1912]. Hudson [1963, 1964] has made a careful quantitative study of blood and marrow eosinophils in the foreign protein response, and reviews of the literature will be found by Hudson [1968], Mahmoud and Austen [1980], and Tavassoli [1981].

Hudson [1968], working with guinea pigs, gave three subcutaneous injections of 1 ml of horse serum at intervals of 5 days. Five days after the last of these injections, a further injection of horse serum was given to the test group, and 1 ml of saline or egg albumen to a control group. Twenty-four to 30 hours after the reinjection of specific antigen, there developed a marked circulatory eosinophilia, which did not develop in the controls. The marrow eosinophils in the test group were only half the number of those in the marrow of the controls, which were considerably more numerous than in normal animals. The results appeared to indicate that in the test animals there had been extensive discharge of eosinophils from the marrow into the bloodstream. But since less than 10% of these missing eosinophils were present in the circulation, most of the cells that had been discharged from the marrow had presumably left the bloodstream. This appeared to be another instance of masked leukocytosis. Even allowing for margination of half the cells, the data indicate the rapid disappearance of considerable numbers of eosinophils from the bloodstream. A number of observations have been made on possible sites at which extravascular accumulation of eosinophils may occur. Peritoneum and lymph nodes [Litt, 1961, 1963] are sites in which rapid extravasation of eosinophils has been reported.

Corticosteroid hormones. One of the factors controlling the exit of eosinophils from the marrow may be corticosteroids. Hudson [1966] noted

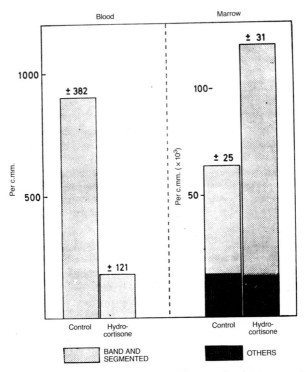

Fig. IX.3. Blood and bone marrow eosinophils 29 hours after foreign protein reinjection. The average blood and bone marrow eosinophil counts are shown for two groups of 10 animals. Each group had received four subcutaneous injections of horse serum at 5-day intervals. At times of 1, 9 and 24 hours after the last of these, either hydrocortisone acetate (hydrocortisone group) or suspending medium (control group) was injected. The difference in the marrow eosinophil counts is accounted for by the difference in the band and segmented forms. From Hudson [1966]. Courtesy of Edward Arnold, London.

that in guinea pigs, after four subcutaneous injections of horse serum, and then an injection of hydrocortisone acetate, the previously observed changes were reversed. In the animals given hydrocortisone, there was no diminution of marrow eosinophils and no increase in the circulating eosinophils (Fig. IX.3).

The simplest explanation of the action of hydrocortisone would seem to be that somehow it directly blocks the discharge of eosinophils from the marrow. But it has been suggested that this explanation may not be correct. The tissue reaction at the site of injection may release an eosinophilotactic substance which enters the bloodstream, and on reaching the marrow stimulates an eosinophil discharge. The action of hydrocortisone might therefore possibly be not on the marrow, but on the tissue whose reaction liberates the eosinotactic materal.

Hypoxia. Changes in marrow and blood eosinophils have also been noted in severe hypoxia. Guinea pigs were kept in a decompression chamber at a simulated altitude of 20,000 ft (approximately 350 mm Hg). A comparison was made not only with normal controls, but also with animals subjected to moderate hypoxia (10,000 ft) [Yoffey et al, 1967]. At 10,000 ft there was a significant fall in the marrow neutrophils but not the eosinophils. At 20,000 ft there was a highly significant fall in the marrow eosinophils, and a rise in blood eosinophils (Fig. IX.4). The fall in the marrow

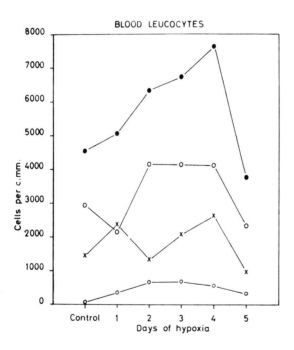

Fig. IX.4. Blood leukocytes of guinea pig during hypoxia at 20,000 feet. Lymphocytes fall on day 1 and then rise significantly on days 2, 3 and 4. Eosinophils are significantly raised from the first day onwards. From Yoffey, Smith, and Wilson [1966]. • Total leukocytes; O lymphocytes; x neutrophils; o eosinophils.

eosinophils affected predominantly the late forms—a depletion of the myeloid reserve.

The eosinophil changes in severe hypoxia are difficult to interpret. The hypoxia in itself is a definite source of stress, and if the eosinophil changes were the response to a stress reaction, the result should be eosinopenia, not eosinophilia. An alternative explanation could be that the rapid expansion of erythropoiesis in a limited space would crowd out the eosinophils from the marrow. Another possibility would be that the erythropoietic changes are associated with increased eosinophil motility, though there is no direct evidence for this.

Parasitic infections. The powerful eosinophilic response associated with many parasitic infections has evoked an extensive literature [Beeson and Bass, 1977], though there have been only limited observations on the bone marrow. Following the work of Basten and Beeson [1970], Spry [1971] examined the marrow changes in rats after the intravenous injection of *Trichinella spiralis* larvae. From 4.7% in normal rats, the marrow eosinophils rose to over 20% by 5 days, and then began to fall, but were still more than 10% at 10 days. Because of the marked shortening of the cell cycle time, from 30 hours in normal rats to 9 hours in infected animals, Spry suggested that there might be as many as 5–6 additional mitoses in the dividing eosinophil compartment.

Ogilvie et al [1977] gave a subcutaneous injection of 4,000 *Nippostrongylus brasiliensis* larvae to rats, and noted that the total eosinophils in the marrow of a femur rose from about 4×10^6 in the normal animals to 14×10^6 in the infected animals 16 days later. In a more recent study, Wertheim et al [1982] made a quantitative examination of rat femoral marrow after the intraperitoneal injection of 300 adult *Nippostrongylus brasiliensis*. Femoral marrow was flushed out of a femur with saline, and after counting the total nucleated cells, the eosinophils were then counted in smears as a percentage of these. The eosinophils rose from $1.35 \pm .063 \times 10^6$ in the control animals to a peak of $4.54 \pm 2.75 \times 10^6$ at 10 days in infected animals. At the same time there was a marked increase in the total nucleated cell content of the marrow (Fig. IX.5), partly because of the increased content of lymphoid cells. A number of observers have assigned a role to T lymphocytes in the eosinophil response [eg, Basten and Beeson, 1970; Ponzio and Speirs, 1975; Tavassoli, 1981], but the number of these lymphocytes in the marrow is not known and such a putative function could originate from the humoral substances produced by extramedullary T cells, reaching the marrow via the bloodstream.

Radiation. The eosinophilogenic effect of ionizing radiation was first recognized in cyclotron workers and served as a parameter indicating expo-

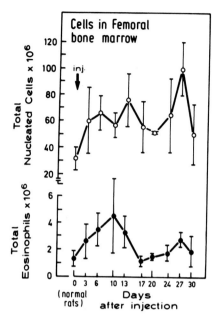

Fig. IX.5. Total nucleated cells O---O and total eosinophils •---• in femoral bone marrow of rats following an intraperitoneal injection of 300 adult *Nippostrongylus brasiliensis*. From Wertheim, Silverman, and Yoffey [1982].

sure [Moses and Platt, 1951]. In experimental systems, ionizing radiation can enhance the eosinophilogenic action of certain agents [Cohen et al, 1967]. It is thought that this effect is mast cell–mediated: Radiation induces mast-cell degranulation releasing factors chemotactic for the eosinophil [Tavassoli, 1981]. Other possible factors are alterations in T-cell function with subsequent alteration in IgE production which can also cause mast-cell degranulation.

BASOPHIL REACTIONS

The basophils, at 17,000 per μl marrow, compare with 73,000 eosinophils and approximately 479,000 neutrophils. The figure for the neutrophils includes 25,000 myeloblasts, the majority of which are in all probability neutrophil precursors.

Basophils are the least numerous of all the marrow granulocytes. In Romanowsky-stained smears the basophil granules are conspicuous by their size and brick-red coloration. Ultrastructural examination [Chan, 1969;

Terry et al, 1969; Zucker-Franklin, 1980] brings out the characteristic appearance of the basophil granules. The fact that the granules stain deeply and metachromatically with toluidine blue or thionin makes it possible to count them directly, in the hemocytometer counting chamber. Because of the small numbers of the marrow basophils, Chan and Yoffey [1960] were particularly concerned about the accuracy of the quantitative estimation, and counted the marrow basophils in three ways—one direct, and two indirect. In the direct method, the basophils alone were counted in the counting chamber, and their numbers calculated from the dilution factor. Two indirect methods were employed. In one method they were enumerated in the counting chamber as a percentage of all the nucleated cells; in the other the total nucleated cell count was obtained in the counting chamber, and the basophils were then counted as a percentage of all nucleated cells in the stained smear.

Basophils in Normal Marrow

Table IX.8 gives the count of marrow basophils obtained by the three different methods in seven normal animals. The differences are not great, and it was thought that the indirect smear count was probably the more accurate. At 12,400 per μl of marrow it compares with 15,400 reported by Winquist [1960] on 51 animals, and 17,000 by Hudson et al [1963] in 25 animals. In normal marrow the basophils seem to be a relatively static population, in which 95.4% are mature, 4.5% are myelocytes, and only 0.1% are in mitosis.

TABLE IX.8. Absolute Counts of Basophils in Normal Guinea Pig Marrow

No.	Direct count	Indirect count (chamber)	Indirect count (smear)
1	7,166	6,820	5,115
2	8,529	9,792	12,246
3	11,380	11,958	11,958
4	9,462	9,405	10,129
5	11,094	10,920	12,285
6	11,740	10,960	12,056
7	18,324	18,084	23,016
Mean	11,099	11,134	12,400

Both the direct count and the two indirect counts are given for comparison. The indirect smear count is somewhat higher than the other two, and is probably the more accurate.
From Chan and Yoffey [1960].

Stimulation of Basophil Production

Since the report by Levaditi [1902] on the production of a basophil leukocytosis in rabbits and guinea pigs by the injection of bacterial toxins, numerous observers have noted a relation between basophils, mast cells, and immune reactions. A quantitative study was done of the effect of foreign proteins on the marrow basophils, following daily injection of horse serum to four groups of guinea pigs. The first group received one injection, the second seven, the third 14, and the fourth 21.

In three animals whose marrow was examined 1 day after a single injection, the mean basophil count was 11,000 per μl; in another three animals examined 8 days after a single injection the count of the marrow basophils had risen to 33,500. At 15 days after a single injection the count was 18,000, and at 20 days 11,000. The response of marrow basophils to foreign proteins is thus slow in developing, and equally slow in returning to normal—perhaps even slightly below normal. The recent studies of Denburg et al [1981] on basophil production in liquid cultures suggest that the growth and differentiation of basophils is a slow process, taking place over a period of 7 days.

The gradual return of marrow basophils to normal and possibly even subnormal levels after a single injection of horse serum raised the obvious question of what would happen after repeated injections of horse serum. Accordingly, four animals were given seven daily injections of horse serum for 7 days, and the changes followed at 1, 8, 15, and 20 days after the last injection (Table IX.9). A further study was made of the changes in three groups of animals given 14 daily injections of horse serum, and examined at 1, 8, and 15 days after the last injection (Table IX.10). In these animals the

TABLE IX.9. Changes in Marrow Basophils After Seven Daily Injections of Horse Serum

Days after last injection	Basophils/μl				
	Animal 1	Animal 2	Animal 3	Animal 4	Mean
1	84,690	64,047	108,072		85,603
8	51,362	45,414	47,240	30,270	43,639
15	14,808	12,968	9,150		12,309
20	12,600	18,590	11,015		14,068

Three animals were used for the examination of marrow changes at 1, 15, and 20 days, and four animals at 8 days. The count is at its peak 1 day after the last injection and then gradually falls, being almost back to normal on day 15. The counts were made by the indirect smear method.
From Chan and Yoffey [1960].

basophil response is still marked. But in animals receiving 21 daily injections (Table IX.11) the response seems to have diminished.

Winquist [1960] also found that repeated injections of horse serum for a week or so gave rise to significant increase of basophils in the marrow.

Comparison of Marrow and Blood Basophils

From the data of Hudson [1958] for a total red marrow volume of 6.25 ml, and taking the basophils as 12,400 per μl, one may calculate that the total marrow population of basophils in the normal standard guinea pig is about 77 $\times$ 10^6, rising after repeated injections of horse serum to something like 500 $\times$ 10^6. The fall after a while in the numbers of marrow basophils could be due to disintegration in situ; but, if this is the case, it must be an extremely rapid process, since one rarely sees damaged basophils in marrow smears. The alternative explanation is that basophils are discharged into the bloodstream, like other granulocytes. The discharge of 500 $\times$ 10^6 basophils from the marrow would give rise to a count of about 20,000 basophils per μl of blood, but a basophil leukocytosis of this magnitude was never observed. In the experiments just cited, blood in four normal animals was found to contain a mean of four basophils per μl, whereas in two animals 8 days after a single injection of horse serum the blood basophils were 300 and 1,540 per μl respectively, and in another two examined 1 day after seven daily injections of serum the blood contained 480 and 1,060 basophils per μl. It is possible that one is dealing here with a masked leukocytosis such as was encountered with the neutrophils and eosinophils. Extravascular accumulation of basophils at the site of injection could be an essential part of the phenomenon [eg, Riley, 1959; Boseila, 1959; Osada and Ogawa, 1962, 1964]. But in addition to such local accumulation, some

TABLE IX.10. Changes in Marrow Basophils After 14 Daily Injections of Horse Serum

Days after last injection	Basophils/μl			
	Animal 1	Animal 2	Animal 3	Mean
1	122,012	75,091	84,459	93,854
8	17,376	13,293	18,291	16,320
15	8,540	10,388	7,840	8,923

The count is high 1 day after the last injection, but has fallen almost to normal by day 8, and is below normal by 15. Counts made by the indirect smear method. Three animals were used for each time interval.
From Chan and Yoffey [1960].

recent observations [Yoffey and Yaffe, 1982] raise the possibility of a more diffuse extravasation. In recent studies of murine peritoneal cells it was noted that, after a single subcutaneous injection of thioglycollate, mast cells began to appear in the peritoneum. Peritoneal fluid in the mouse, unlike that in the rat, does not normally contain mast cells. It has been repeatedly surmised that the peritoneal fluid is representative of the connective tissue in its cell populations, except that its cells are in a fluid medium. If this is the case, then it seems possible that in addition to the extravascular accumulation of basophils at the site of injection, there may be a generalized migration of these cells into the connective tissues.

Osada and Ogawa [1961] have reported the occurrence of basophilia in rabbits following repeated injections of egg albumen, which has a lower molecular weight than horse serum. They observed an associated eosinophilia which followed approximately the same time course [cf Osada and Ogawa, 1964]. Hudson [1963] noted a corresponding increase in the two cell types in the bone marrow.

The increase in the marrow basophils is due to their proliferation in situ. As already noted, in normal marrow the basophil population is almost static, 95.4% mature, 4.5% basophilic myelocytes, and 0.1% in mitosis. Compared with this normal distribution, 8 days after a single injection of horse serum 75% of the basophils were mature, 26.3% myelocytes, and 1.3% in mitosis. One day after seven daily injections of horse serum, 61.5% of the basophils were mature, 37.1% myelocytes, and 1.4% in mitosis. One day after 14 daily injections of horse serum, the basophil content was returning to its normal composition with 97.4% mature, 2.4% myelocytes, and 0.2% in mitosis. Evidently the basophils in normal marrow are proliferating very slowly, and even when stimulated by horse serum their proliferation is not

TABLE IX.11. Marrow Basophils After 21 Daily Injections of Horse Serum

Days after last injection	Basophils/μl					
	Animal 1	Animal 2	Animal 3	Animal 4	Animal 5	Mean
1	21,690	14,333	29,484	12,222	18,130	19,172
8	21,130	33,250				27,190
15	8,082	7,776				7,929

The marrow basophils are slightly raised up to day 8, after the last injection, but by day 15 they are below their normal level. Five animals used on day 1, and only two on days 8 and 15.
From Chan and Yoffey [1960].

very marked or long sustained when compared with erythroid cells or neutrophils.

It should be emphasized that the light microscope criteria of maturity are not as easy to observe in the case of the basophils as they are in other granulocytes, since the dense massing of the large granules may effectively hide most of the cytoplasmic and nuclear detail upon which a distinction may be based. Nuclear indentation is not usually as marked in the basophils as it is in the other granulocytes.

The quantitative study of basophil production is complicated by the fact that the cells may be formed elsewhere than in the bone marrow [Riley, 1959]. Considerations of this type also apply to the neutrophils in myeloid metaplasia, but in the case of the neutrophils, multiplication in the marrow occurs much more actively and on a very large scale, whereas with the basophils proliferation in the marrow may be so slight that even a moderate degree of formation elsewhere could well exceed it.

Basophils and Tissue Mast Cells

One of the recurring problems in the literature is the relationship between marrow basophils and tissue mast cells [Boseila, 1959; Riley, 1959]. Recent evidence [Hatanaka et al, 1979; Zucker-Franklin, 1980] suggests a myeloid origin for many if not all tissue mast cells. Zucker-Franklin [1980] raises the possibility that, in man, mast-cell precursors may migrate via the bloodstream to the tissues, and notes the occurrence of an intermediate cell, possessing the ultrastructural features typical of both basophils and mast cells. More recently Zucker-Franklin et al [1981] have reported the presence of mast-cell precursors in the bloodstream.

X.

Erythropoiesis

INTRODUCTION

In the erythrocyte production pathway there is a continuous process of differentiation from the stem cell via the proerythroblast to the mature red cell, with a number of cell divisions and intervening stages en route. At the stage of the orthochromatic erythroblast, cell division is virtually at an end, and mitoses are few and far between.

RETICULOCYTES

However, some degree of maturation occurs at the reticulocyte stage, even after nuclear extrusion. The reticulocytes are an integral part of the marrow erythroid population, and in some ways occupy the same position in the erythroid series as the segmented granulocytes in the myeloid. The rate at which reticulocytes are discharged from the marrow undergoes marked variation in response to functional needs. The use of reticulocyte grading brings out the fact that, when the demand for red cells is increased, reticulocytes are discharged from the marrow at an earlier stage of maturation than usual.

Substantia Granulofilamentosa

Reticulocytes contain a substance that stains with dyes such as Brilliant Cresyl Blue or New Methylene Blue. The substance which stains in this way has been termed the *substantia granulofilamentosa* (SGF). This name was given because the substance may occur in the form either of fine granules, or of filaments which, if present in sufficient amount, may form a network or *reticulum*. The term substantia granulofilamentosa is retained here as being more accurate than the "reticular substance," which has frequently been used. Dustin [1944] showed that the SGF disappeared after treatment with ribonuclease, thus indicating that it was composed predominantly of RNA.

Reticulocytes may readily be counted in marrow smears in relation to the nucleated red cells, or as a percentage of the nonnucleated red cells. This latter procedure makes it possible to confirm the observations of previous investigators [eg, Nizet, 1946; Seip, 1953] that, in the normal steady state, virtually all the reticulocytes in the marrow are situated extravascularly in the marrow parenchyma, from which they are then discharged into the bloodstream. This conclusion followed from a comparison of reticulocyte counts in marrow and blood, and a knowledge of the amount of blood contained in the marrow vessels. The latter, according to Osmond and Everett [1965], comprises about 6% of the total marrow volume. On this basis the blood contained in the marrow vessels would amount to about 300,000 erythrocytes per ml of marrow, and since the circulating blood contains 1–2% of reticulocytes, this would amount for 3,000–6,000 reticulocytes per ml, as against 200,000–300,000 reticulocytes usually found per ml of marrow. Hence, the contained blood would account for only a small proportion of the marrow reticulocytes, which must largely be extravascular unless a very large number can be stored in many stagnant sinusoids, for which there is no evidence.

Ultrastructural examination, which enables one to identify reticulocytes with ease, demonstrates clearly that virtually all the nonnucleated erythrocytes in the marrow are reticulocytes, in the vicinity of the erythroblastic islands [Ben-Ishay and Yoffey, 1971a, 1972] or close to the sinusoidal endothelium (Figs. X.1, 2), whereas in the normal steady state only an occasional reticulocyte is to be seen in a sinusoid. However, a powerful erythropoietic stimulus, such as bleeding, may stimulate a massive discharge of reticulocytes, in which case one can find sinusoids with many reticulocytes. Mature erythrocytes, once they have entered the circulation, do not appear to return to the marrow parenchyma [Nizet, 1946; Bond et al, 1964].

Grading of Reticulocytes

On the basis of the amount and distribution of SGF, Heilmeyer [1930] and Trachtenberg [1932] divided reticulocytes into four groups, according to their degree of maturity (group I being least and group IV most mature). In addition they observed SGF in nucleated erythroid cells, and these they termed group 0. Reticulocyte grading is of great value in making a more precise analysis than would otherwise be possible of the kinetics of reticulocyte formation in the marrow, and also of their discharge from the marrow and their subsequent changes in the bloodstream. In the marrow of the guinea pig, most reticulocytes are to be found in group III, and there are relatively few in group IV, the most mature. Groups III and IV are found in the blood in approximately equal numbers, so it might appear that most of the group IV reticulocytes are discharged from the marrow as soon as they are formed, whereas group III are discharged from the marrow in numbers that are appreciable, but not as great as in group IV. A complication is introduced by reticulocytes leaving the marrow at earlier stages and undergoing their final maturation in the blood stream, and similar consid-

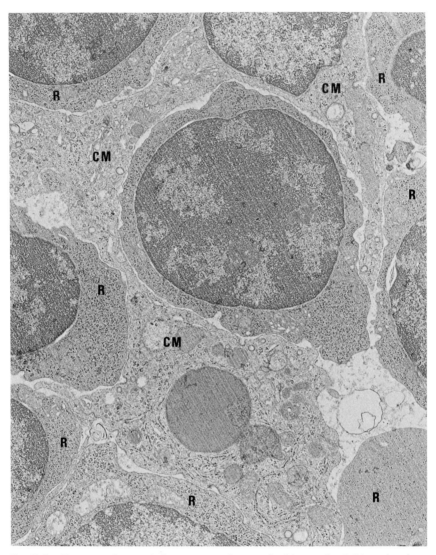

Fig. X.1. Tannic acid–treated thin section of an erythroblastic island. Note the sharp delineation of membranous structures, including cell membranes, by tannic acid. The figure is dominated by a central macrophage (CM) containing some secondary lysosomes and red cell debris. Note the extensive interdigitation with developing red cells (R); one of them is almost entirely embraced by process of the central macrophage. Note the coated vesicles in developing red cells, but coated vesicles are particularly frequent in the central macrophage (arrows). From Tavassoli and Shaklai [1979]. ×12,500.

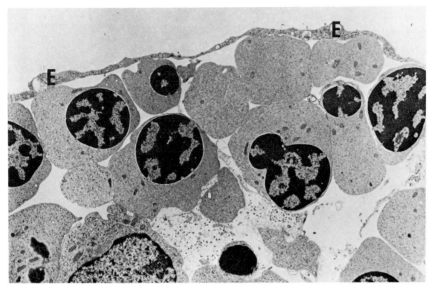

Fig. X.2. Reticulocytes and nucleated erythroblasts adjacent to the endothelium (E) of a sinusoid. From Tavassoli [1977]. ×6,500.

erations apply to the reticulocyte population of the marrow. But despite these difficulties, reticulocyte grading has made important contributions to an analysis of experimentally induced changes in erythropoiesis [see Griffiths et al, 1970, Fig. 1].

Seip [1953] studied the distribution of the different reticulocyte groups in human blood and marrow. In normal human blood, of 17 reticulocytes per 100 red cells, ten were in group IV, six in group III, one in group II, and virtually none in group I. In the bone marrow, the reticulocyte distribution was as follows: group I, 23%; group II, 40.5%; group III, 32.5%; group IV, 0%. Reticulocytes form 27.6% of the total marrow cells, of which the erythroid cells (including reticulocytes) are 43.5% and myeloid cells 47.18%. Hence, if one includes reticulocytes in the erythroid compartment, the M:E ratio is virtually 1.0. Seip also found that alterations in grading of blood reticulocytes were a very sensitive indicator of changes in the reticulocyte discharge from the marrow. After a person had breathed 10% oxygen for 15 min, there was an appreciable increase in the number of grade II reticulocytes in the blood stream.

MITOTIC AND OTHER CHANGES
Mitosis in the Erythropoietic Pathway

A number of attempts have been made to determine how many mitoses occur between the stage of the undifferentiated stem cell and the fully formed reticulocytes. The problem is complicated not only by the existence of species differences, but also by variation in any given species in accordance with functional needs. Alpen and Cranmore [1959] estimated that in the dog, in the normal steady state, only 2–3 mitoses were involved, and if the need for new red cells was great, one or more of these mitoses might be missed [cf Suit et al, 1957; Stohlman, 1961]. In the mouse, Hodgson [1967] inclined to the view that there were two mitoses between the undifferentiated stem cell and the mature red cell. Two mitoses are suggested in the rat also, by the data of McCool et al [1970], who made use of velocity sedimentation. They found that a large cell, with a sedimentation velocity of 6.6 mm/h, was the marrow cell most responsive to erythropoietin. "In the process of becoming hemoglobin-synthesizing cells it undergoes cell division and its sedimentation velocity decreases to 3.9 mm/h and then to 2.1 mm/h, the sedimentation velocity of mature red cells." In the guinea pig, Starling and Rosse [1976] concluded that in the normal steady state there were 2–4 divisions between the proerythroblast and the orthochromatic erythroblast.

Origin of Erythroid From Transitional Cells

The origin of the erythroid series from transitional cells has been established in several ways. In discussing transitional cell morphology, it was pointed out that at the light microscope level it was difficult to effect a clear-cut differentiation between basophilic transitional cells and blast cells. Cells with basophilic cytoplasm extending up to half-way round the nucleus were classified as transitional, whereas if the cytoplasm extended more than half-way round the nucleus, they were regarded as blast cells. Clearly this classification left much to be desired. At the ultrastructural level also there may be difficulty in deciding whether one is dealing with a transitional cell or a proerythroblast [Ben-Ishay and Yoffey, 1972].

Asynchronous Erythroblasts

Some interesting information at the light microscope level was obtained in cases of secondary hypoxia [Yoffey et al, 1965]. In one animal on day 4 of secondary hypoxia, and in three out of six animals on day 5, the marrow was seen to contain a number of atypical erythroblasts in which the differentiation of the cytoplasm was out of step with that of the nucleus, in comparison with which it seemed more advanced than usual. In one animal there were 19,000 of these cells per μl of marrow. Whereas the nucleus had the leptochromasia of a transitional or blast cell, the cytoplasm was already quite heavily hemoglobinized, corresponding from the point of hemoglobin content to the polychromatic and in some cases even to the orthochromatic erythroblast.

That these cells contained hemoglobin was first suggested by the eosinophilic staining of the cytoplasm. A positive Lepehne (benzidine) reaction supported this view, which was reinforced when the cells were examined in monochromatic light within the specific absorption of hemoglobin (wavelength 4,046 Å). The cytoplasm was dark, but the nucleus, which did not contain hemoglobin, was clear. In later studies Zucali et al [1974], and Rosse and his colleagues, provided conclusive evidence of the role of transitional cells as erythroblast precursors [Rosse, 1973, 1976; Rosse and Trotter, 1974a,b; Starling and Rosse, 1976; Rosse and Beaufait, 1978; Prothero et al, 1978].

Iron Incorporation

Zucali et al [1974] obtained enriched preparations of transitional cells from the marrow of rats in rebound by fractionating a suspension of marrow cells on a discontinuous bovine serum albumin density gradient. The various fractions were then cultured with erythropoietin and the heme synthesis was estimated. Analysis of the data pointed to the transitional cells as the population responding by heme synthesis to erythropoietin in vitro.

Rosse and Trotter [1974a] restimulated erythropoiesis in rebound guinea pigs by bleeding and hypoxia. Light microscope studies were made of ^{55}Fe incorporation in autoradiographs, while the presence of hemoglobin was also shown by the benzidine (Lepehne) reaction and the use of monochromatic light at 4,046 Å. The diaminobenzidine reaction facilitated the detection of hemoglobin on ultrastructural examination. In normal marrow, proerythroblasts were the earliest cells in which hemoglobin could be detected, but during the early phase of erythropoietin restimulation, "hemoglobin was demonstrated in transitional cells with all the methods employed."

Rosse and Beaufait [1978] made a study of the uptake of ^{55}Fe by transitional cells in vitro following stimulation by erythropoietin. They cultured cell fractions that were rich in transitional cells, but which contained no other cells calling for consideration as erythropoietin-responsive cells. Transitional cells were the only cells in which heme synthesis was dependent on erythropoietin.

Reference has already been made to the observations of De Gowin et al [1972], De Gowin and Gibson [1976], and Murphy et al [1971], who followed the development of transitional cells in the murine spleen. Further information about the erythropoietic role of transitional cells will be found in the reviews by Rosse [1976] and Yoffey [1980], and evidence of their pluripotential role is presented in a recent paper by Wolf and Rosse [1982].

HYPOXIA AND REBOUND

In discussing the transitional cell compartment (Chapter XIII) it is pointed out that in the normal steady state the compartment can cope adequately with its stem cell requirements, and in fact has a reserve of stem cells. When erythropoiesis is stimulated by hypoxia, the increased erythropoiesis is effected by the entry of additional stem cells into the erythropoietic pathway. This was first suggested by Yoffey [1957] on the basis of experiments at the Hochalpine Forschungsstation, Jungfraujoch, and was later confirmed by a number of workers [eg, Erslev, 1959; Alpen and Cranmore, 1959].

Hypoxia is believed to act by stimulating the secretion of erythropoietin, and in severe hypoxia the plasma erythropoietin can rise to 20–50 times above its normal level [Krantz and Jacobson, 1970]. Hypoxia can result either from alteration in the percentage of oxygen in the inspired air or from reduction of the pressure of air by means of a decompression chamber. The latter technique has been employed for the most part in the experiments described in the following pages, and the degree of hypoxia is expressed in terms of an equivalent altitude—eg, 3050, 4250, 5200, and 6100 m. The majority of the experiments have been performed on guinea pigs, but confirmating data were also obtained in the rat and mouse.

Since hypoxia gives rise to varying degrees of stress, it is important to recognize its limitations, which have been fully discussed elsewhere [Yoffey, 1974]. Campbell [1934] paid especial attention to the deleterious effects of hypoxia, and in the case of mice and rabbits he concluded that growth occurred normally until a stimulated altitude of 18,000 ft (12% oxygen) was reached. Above this, and certainly over 20,000 ft (10% oxygen) "animals cannot be acclimatized to live in health. . . . Growth ceases . . . and the animals die sooner or later with symptoms of chronic heart failure." The most informative experiments have been performed at 5200 m, but a few short-term experiments at 6100 m have yielded interesting results.

Though hypoxia acts essentially by stimulating erythropoiesis, there are associated changes in the other cell groups in the marrow, and these become more marked the more severe the hypoxia.

Primary Hypoxia, Rebound, and Secondary Hypoxia

When an animal in the normal steady state is subjected to hypoxia, we refer to this as *primary hypoxia* [Moffatt et al, 1964a], and the animal develops polycythemia as a result of the increased erythropoiesis. When such a polycythemic animal is then kept in ambient air, its oxygen-carrying capacity is greater than is needed, and the body reacts to this relative oxygen excess by a depression of erythropoiesis [Robertson, 1917; Boycott and Oakley, 1933]. The bone marrow in this phase of depressed erythropoiesis is known as in *rebound* [Moffatt et al, 1964a]. The term was used because in primary hypoxia both the lymphoid and myeloid cells fall, but they rebound to their normal or supernormal levels when polycythemic animals are kept in ambient air.

The term "rebound" is applied specifically to the marrow, and the rebound phase has proved to be of value in studying the changes in marrow lymphocytes and transitional cells, more especially since animals in rebound are entirely free from stress phenomena.

Assessing the Effects of Hypoxia

The effects of hypoxia can be assessed on the basis of changes in 1) marrow, 2) blood, and 3) other parts of the lymphomyeloid complex, notably the spleen. Moderate degrees of hypoxia give rise to changes mainly in marrow and blood, but in more severe degrees of hypoxia the spleen also becomes actively erythropoietic, and may undergo considerable enlargement.

Figure X.3 compares splenic weights in guinea pigs subjected to hypoxia at either 3050 or 6100 m. The difference between the two groups is also evident from the level of the blood reticulocytes (Fig. X.4). There is also a qualitative difference in the blood reticulocytes. Reticulocyte grading shows that at 6100 m many more grade III reticulocytes enter the bloodstream than at 3050 m [Yoffey et al, 1966].

Active and Passive Polycythemia

The polycythemia which develops when the animal's own red cell production is stimulated is known as *active polycythemia*, as opposed to *passive polycythemia*, induced by transfusion of red cells from another animal [Jacobson et al, 1960; Weitz-Hamburger et al, 1971]. In both types of polycythemia

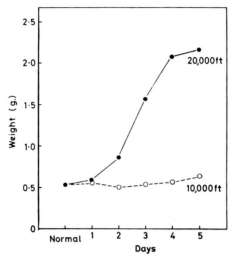

Fig. X.3. A comparison of splenic weights during hypoxia at 10,000 and 20,000 ft. At 10,000 ft the spleen undergoes virtually no change. At 20,000 ft, splenic hypertrophy is marked. Drawn from the data of Yoffey et al [1966]. Courtesy of Edward Arnold Ltd.

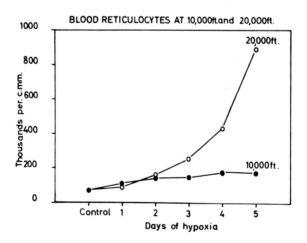

Fig. X.4. The difference between the blood reticulocytes at 10,000 and 20,000 ft. The difference becomes evident from day 3 onwards. From Yoffey et al [1966].

erythropoiesis is depressed, but with some significant differences. Passive polycythemia acts upon marrow in which red cell formation is proceeding at its normal steady pace, with just enough stem cells entering into the erythropoietic compartment to replace those undergoing maturation and differentiation. In the active polycythemia of rebound, the marrow is depressed at a time when greatly increased numbers of stem cells may be presumed to be entering the erythropoietic compartment.

There is another important difference between the two types of polycythemia. Passive polycythemia can be maintained indefinitely, by giving repeated red cell transfusions. The active polycythemia of rebound is self-terminating, for while hardly any new cells are being formed, the circulating red cells gradually diminish through normal wear and tear. As soon as they reach their normal level, erythropoiesis is resumed. This process takes about 12–14 days in the guinea pig subjected to 5200 m hypoxia for 7 days. After 12–14 days of rebound, erythropoiesis begins to return.

Quantitative Changes in Marrow Cells

A study of the marrow changes in moderate and severe hypoxia indicates that in both instances there is an increase in the nucleated erythroid cells, but on a very different scale in the two groups. At 6100 m the nucleated erythroid cells rise rapidly, from 520,000 per μl in the controls to 1,049,000 per μl on day 4 of hypoxia, whereas at 3050 m there is a more slowly rising trend, which in fact only becomes significant on day 5 of hypoxia, when they are 676,000 per μl [Yoffey et al, 1967]. Furthermore, the changes in the marrow reticulocytes also show a marked difference (Fig. X.5). In both groups the marrow reticulocytes fall during the first 2 days of hypoxia, but more so at 20,000 ft than at 10,000. Furthermore, the rise during the last 3 days of hypoxia is much greater at 20,000 than at 10,000 ft.

Interrelationships Between Main Cell Groups in Marrow

The experiments just cited bring out a fundamental fact that a significant change in one of the three main cell groups in the marrow usually involves changes in either or both of the remaining groups. Thus, at 3050 m marrow lymphocytes are virtually unchanged during 5 days of hypoxia, whereas at 6100 m they show a highly significant fall by day 5 (Fig. X.6). The myeloid cells, on the other hand, fell significantly both at 3050 and 6100 m, but much more so at 6100 than at 3050 m (Fig. X.7). In general, the more marked the change in one of the three main groups (ie, erythroid, myeloid, lymphoid), the greater the reciprocal change in the other two.

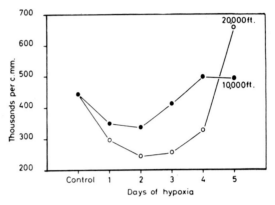

Fig. X.5. Marrow reticulocytes fall during the first 2 days of hypoxia, more so at 10,000 than at 20,000 ft. The rise during the last 3 days of hypoxia is much greater at 20,000 than at 10,000 ft. From Yoffey, Smith, and Wilson [1967].

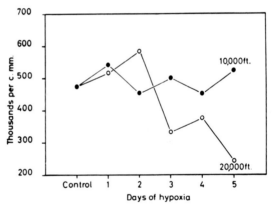

Fig. X.6. Marrow lymphocytes undergo little change at 10,000 ft, but at 20,000 ft show a highly significant fall after an initial rise. From Yoffey et al [1967].

Marrow and Blood Reticulocytes

Despite quite marked changes in erythrocyte production, the quantitative changes in the reticulocyte population of the marrow are relatively small compared to those in the blood reticulocytes. Figure X.8 depicts the total marrow and blood reticulocytes during primary hypoxia, rebound, and secondary hypoxia for 5 days at 4250 m. Blood reticulocytes rise strongly during 5 days of primary hypoxia, fall to below control level in

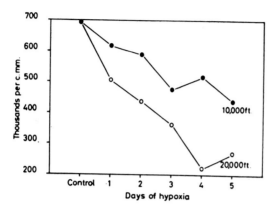

Fig. X.7. The myeloid cells of the marrow fell significantly both at 10,000 and 20,000 ft, but more markedly at 20,000. From Yoffey et al [1967].

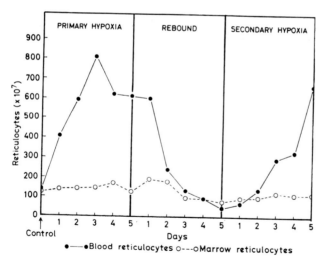

Fig. X.8. Total reticulocytes in blood and marrow during primary hypoxia (14,000 ft), rebound, and secondary hypoxia (14,000 ft). Marrow reticulocytes show only minor changes, but blood reticulocytes increase markedly both during primary and secondary hypoxia, whereas they fall to below control level during rebound. The blood reticulocytes increase more slowly in secondary than in primary hypoxia. Drawn from the data of Moffatt et al [1964a,b] and Yoffey et al [1965]. Courtesy of Edward Arnold Ltd.

rebound, and rise again in secondary hypoxia. Throughout this period, the marrow reticulocytes show comparatively minor numerical changes.

Immediate and Delayed Reticulocyte Response

The blood reticulocytes show a more rapid rise during primary than secondary hypoxia. In primary hypoxia the response is brisk, and is already quite marked after 1 day. In secondary hypoxia the response is much slower, the blood reticulocytes just reaching control levels after 2 days, and even by day 3 not reaching the level of the blood reticulocytes on day 1 of primary hypoxia. The delayed reticulocyte response in polycythemic animals has been repeatedly observed, and it also occurs in the polycythemic mice following erythropoietin [Gurney et al, 1961]. The explanation of the difference between the two responses must be sought in the bone marrow.

When erythropoiesis is stimulated at the end of rebound by secondary hypoxia, the initial level of the immediate reticulocyte precursors in the marrow—namely the late nucleated red cells—is a low one, and a rapid increase in the formation of reticulocytes to be discharged into the bloodstream is not possible. Before such an increase can occur, there must be an increase of the late nucleated erythroid cells from primitive precursors, and this takes 2–3 days, slower than in the normal marrow, which is geared to a higher level of red cell formation, and presumably has a more continuous rapid entry of stem cells ready to differentiate [cf Griffiths et al, 1970]. The data of Rosse et al [1970], in which erythropoiesis was stimulated in polycythemic rebound guinea pigs by bleeding, showed that the first significant increase in early erythroblasts occurred on day 3, though a slight and nonsignificant increase was observed after 36 hours. More recently, Aoki and Tavassoli [1981] have noted a biphasic reticulocyte response in rats after bleeding.

HYPOXIA AT 5200 METERS AND SUBSEQUENT REBOUND

In the studies of primary hypoxia, rebound, and secondary hypoxia at 4250 m, interesting changes were noted in lymphocytes and transitional cells [Yoffey, 1966, Fig. 3.7, p 54]. The small lymphocytes showed a slight fall in primary hypoxia, a slight rise in rebound, and a striking increase in secondary hypoxia. Their increase in secondary hypoxia ruled out stress as a cause of the fall in lymphocytes in primary hypoxia, since the animals were subjected to the same degree of stress in both primary and secondary hypoxia. Furthermore, the transitional cells, which had shown a slight rise during the first 2 days of primary hypoxia, showed a much sharper rise in secondary hypoxia [Yoffey et al, 1965]. Something seemed to be happening to the transitional cell compartment in rebound which led to greater activity in secondary hypoxia. The following represents the results of a series of experiments, mostly on guinea pigs subjected to 7 days hypoxia at 5200 m. These resulted in a greater degree of polycythemia than at 4250 m, and persisting through 7 days of rebound (Fig. X.9). Some confirmatory experiments were also performed in rats and mice.

Changes in the Bone Marrow

Reticulocytes. There are marked changes in the marrow reticulocytes (Fig. X.10). They fall during the first 2 days of hypoxia, while at the same time blood reticulocytes increase, both changes being significant by day 2. The fall in the marrow reticulocytes, while those in the blood are rising, suggests an accelerated discharge from the marrow, possibly due to erythropoietin [Krantz and Jacobson, 1970], though other reticulocyte release factors have been suggested [eg, Smith, 1962]. Fruhman and Fischer [1962] found young grade I reticulocytes in the blood of rats as early as 12 hours after the injection of erythropoietin. Gordon et al [1962], using the isolated perfused femur of the rat, noted a rapid stimulation of reticulocyte discharge from the marrow following the administration of erythropoietin. In the present experiments the highest level of marrow reticulocytes was found at

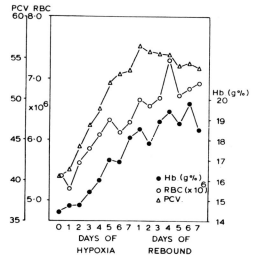

Fig. X.9. Changes in packed cell volume, hemoglobin, and red cell count during primary hypoxia at 5200 m and rebound. Polycythemia persists throughout the 7 days of rebound. From Yoffey et al [1968]. Courtesy of the New York Academy of Science.

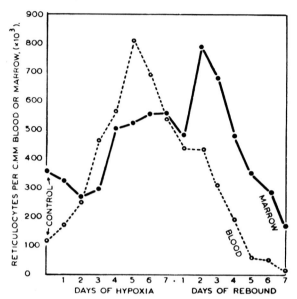

Fig. X.10.   Reticulocytes per μl of blood and marrow during primary hypoxia and rebound. The fall in the marrow reticulocytes during the first 2 days of hypoxia is associated with a very much greater increase in the blood reticulocytes. From Yoffey et al [1968]. Courtesy of the New York Academy of Science.

the beginning of rebound (Fig. X.10). The accumulation of reticulocytes in the marrow at a time when erythropoiesis is entering a phase of severe depression coincides presumably with the diminished formation of endogenous erythropoietin, and would therefore be in accord with the reticulocyte-discharging role of this substance.

Nucleated cells of marrow. The total nucleated cells of the marrow fluctuate for the first 4 days of hypoxia, fall significantly on day 5, and from then on continue to rise, with some fluctuation, until day 7 of rebound [Yoffey et al, 1968, Fig. 5]. Analysis of the three main cell groups—erythroid, myeloid, and lymphoid (Fig. X.11)—shows that both the lymphoid and the myeloid cells fall sharply during the first 5 days of hypoxia, whereas the nucleated erythroid cells rise rapidly during the first 4 days and then fall somewhat on day 5, though still above the control level. During rebound, the nucleated erythroid cells fall to a very low level, about one-fourth their number in the normal animal, but never disappear completely. The myeloid cells rebound to approximately their normal level. The lymphoid cells rise significantly during 7 days of rebound, at the end of which they are nearly

HYPOXIA (17,000 FEET) + REBOUND.
GUINEA-PIG BONE MARROW.

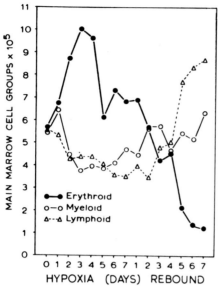

Fig. X.11. Changes (in absolute counts per µl marrow) of the main cell groups during hypoxia (5200 m) and rebound. The nucleated erythroid cells increase markedly during the first 4 days of hypoxia, level off for the next 3 days, and fall rapidly in rebound. Myeloid and lymphoid cells fall significantly during hypoxia, and return to normal or above normal in rebound. From Yoffey [1968]. Courtesy of the New York Academy of Science.

double their normal number. From the analysis of the change in the lymphoid cells, it is evident that the fall in these cells during hypoxia is primarily due to a diminution of the number of pachychromatic small lymphocytes, and not of transitional cells (Fig. X.12). In rebound, on the other hand, both the small lymphocytes and the transitional cells undergo a highly significant increase, and at the end of 7 days of rebound the transitional cells attain the remarkably high figure of 400,000/µl, compared wtih less than 100,000/µl in normal marrow. Rebound marrow is therefore an excellent source of transitional cells.

Erythroid cells. A comparison of Figures X.10 and X.11 brings out the fact that the increase in nucleated erythroid cells during the first 3 days of hypoxia precedes the increase in the marrow reticulocytes on day 4. This was to be expected, since the majority of nucleated erythroid cells are the late forms which are the immediate precursors of the reticulocytes. The fall in the marrow reticulocytes during the first 2 days of hypoxia (Fig. X.10) is

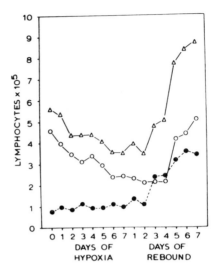

Fig. X.12. Changes in small lymphocytes (○) transitional (●) and total lymphoid (△) cells during hypoxia and rebound in the guinea-pig. In hypoxia the small lymphocytes show a marked fall whereas the transitional cells increase slightly. In rebound there is a highly significant increase in both groups. From Yoffey et al [1968].

due to the rapid maturation of late erythroid cells already in the erythropoietic pathway, and the accelerated discharge into the bloodstream of the newly formed reticulocytes. The large increase in marrow reticulocytes, evident on day 4, is due to the new wave of erythropoiesis induced by the hypoxia, starting ab initio by the differentiation of stem cells [cf Griffiths et al, 1970]. If this is the case, it would appear that the time taken from the stem cell to the mature erythrocyte is about 3 days [cf Starling and Rosse, 1976].

Lymphocytes and transitional cells. Although the transitional cells show only minor quantitative changes during the first 7 days of hypoxia, they are in fact actively proliferating, as shown by the evidence of thymidine labeling. However, despite this active proliferation, the number of transitional cells does not increase, presumably because for the most part they enter the erythropoietic pathway as soon as they are formed, and become proerythroblasts. Only a small number are available for granulocyte and lymphocyte formation, and the numbers of granulocytes and lymphocytes therefore diminish. But in rebound, when erythropoiesis is so greatly depressed, most of the transitional cells are no longer needed for erythropoiesis, so they are free to develop into lymphocytes or granulocytes. Hence the rapid increase of lymphoid and myeloid cells (Fig. X.11).

There appear to be many uncommitted cells in the transitional compartment capable of switching into either erythropoiesis or lymphocytopoiesis [Rosse, 1973]. Polycythemic guinea pigs in rebound were given injections of ^{3}H-thymidine, which labeled a large number of transitional cells. If no further stimulus was given, these labeled transitional cells gave rise to large numbers of labeled small lymphocytes. If, however, on day 7 of rebound, erythropoiesis was stimulated by bleeding, large numbers of nucleated erythroid cells were formed, and these were for the most part labeled. It is difficult to explain these results on any other basis than that many of the labeled transitional cells could undergo differentiation into either lymphocytes or erythrocytes.

The changes in rebound suggest the existence of some sort of control mechanism for transitional cell proliferation. If transitional cell proliferation continues during rebound at the same greatly increased rate as in hypoxia, more will be formed than are required for lymphocyte and granulocyte production, so the number of transitional cells will continue to rise, more especially as there is a lag of 4–5 days before the production of small lymphocytes begins to increase (Fig. X.12). The question then arises: How long can the increased proliferation of transitional cells continue? If it continued at the same rate for another few days, the marrow should come to consist largely of small lymphocytes and transitional cells.

Prolongation of Rebound

In order to see whether this was actually the case, in a further group of experiments, rebound was allowed to continue for 12 days instead of 7 [Jones et al, 1967]. Some of the results are illustrated in Figures X.13 and 14. When one examines the changing distribution of the three main cell groups, it will be seen that the lymphoid cells (ie, small lymphocytes and transitionals) continue to increase for another 2 days, reaching a peak on days 8 and 9 of rebound. At this point they constitute nearly three-fourths of the total nucleated cells of the marrow, which on superficial examination could well be regarded as leukemic. They then fall somewhat, though even on day 12 of rebound, the lymphoid cells still constitute about one-half of the total nucleated cells. Erythropoiesis remains at a low level throughout, though the erythroid cells appear to be rising slightly toward day 12.

The Secondary Myeloid Fall

During prolonged rebound the myeloid cells showed a surprising fall (Fig. X.13), which is difficult to explain. Two experimental situations have been encountered in which there is a fall in the myeloid cells. One is in hypoxia

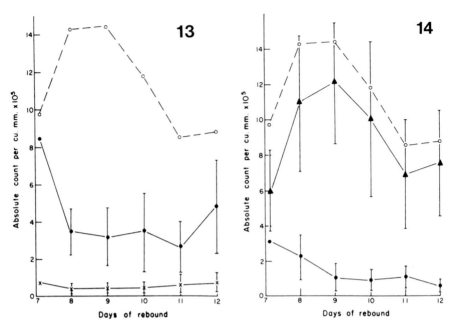

Fig. X.13.　Main cell groups in guinea pig marrow after 7 days hypoxia (5200 m) and 12 days rebound. On days 8 and 9 of rebound, lymphocytes rise sharply to almost 70% of the total nucleated cells. From Jones et al [1967]. X = erythroid; ● = myeloid; ○ = lymphoid.

Fig. X.14.　The rise in the marrow lymphoid cells in rebound is due to an increase in the pachychromatic small lymphocytes. Transitional cells show a significant fall. From Jones et al [1967]. ○ = total lymphoid; ▲ = small lymphocytes; ● = transitionals.

(Fig. X.11), the other in prolonged rebound (Fig. X.13). It seems unlikely that the same explanation for the fall is valid in both instances, for the attendant circumstances are quite different. The fall in myeloid cells during hypoxia one could readily attribute to stem cell competition, in that so many stem cells are being channeled into erythropoiesis that not enough are left for granulocyte or lymphocyte production. But the secondary fall in prolonged rebound is difficult to explain on these lines, for when the fall occurs, not only is erythropoiesis greatly depressed, but lymphocyte production is also beginning to fall.

Still more surprising than the secondary fall in the myeloid cells is that in prolonged rebound the transitional cells also ultimately fall to a very low level (Fig. X.14). This is a remarkable finding, since when the transitional cells fall (Fig. X.14) both red cell and granulocyte formation are at an abnormally low level, and even the small lymphocytes are beginning to fall.

A drop in transitional cells to the low level found on day 12 of rebound (Fig. X.14) cannot therefore be explained on the basis of an inordinate demand for stem cells. This is a situation where it may be worthwhile to look for factors inhibiting stem cell proliferation.

Erythropoietic Stimulation in Prolonged Rebound

The changes in the marrow during prolonged rebound suggested that it would be interesting to give these animals a powerful erythropoietic stimulus at a time of maximal erythropoietic depression coinciding with a falling trend in the transitional cell compartment. Day 9 of rebound (Figs. X.13, 14) was chosen because it has the additional advantage of being in the midst of a period when there was a sustained low level of blood reticulocytes (Fig. X.15) [Rosse et al, 1970]. In the unstimulated rebound animals, which served as controls, the first significant increase in the nucleated erythroid cells of the marrow occurred on day 14 of rebound. In the bled animals, there was a nonsignificant increase in the erythroid cells 1½ days after bleeding, but a highly significant increase by day 3 (Fig. X.16), 2 days earlier than the increase in the controls.

Erythroid Mitotic Index

Further information about the erythropoietic changes was obtained from a study of the mitotic index of the various cells in the erythropoietic

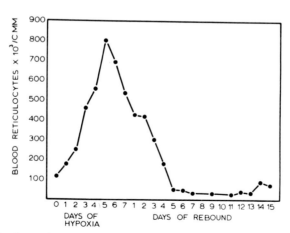

Fig. X.15. Blood reticulocytes in guinea pig during hypoxia for 7 days followed by 15 days of rebound. The first sign of the resumption of more active erythropoiesis is around days 13–14 of rebound. From Yoffey [1974]; drawn from unpublished data of Griffiths et al [1970]. Courtesy of the Chas. C. Thomas Company.

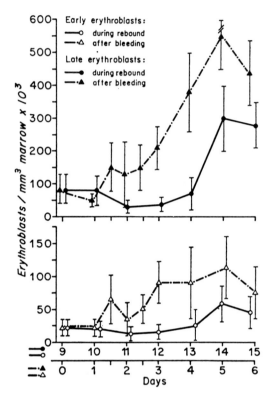

Fig. X.16. Numbers of early erythroblasts (proerythroblasts + basophilic erythroblasts) and late erythroblasts (polychromatic + orthochromatic) in the marrow of bled and unbled guinea pigs during rebound (mean values + SD). The increase in early erythroblasts, not quite significant after 1½ days, first becomes significant on day 3. From Rosse et al [1970]. Courtesy of S. Karger AG, Basel.

pathway. In the normal guinea pig, the mitotic index of early erythroblasts (proerythroblasts + basophilic erythroblasts) was found to be 4.25 ± 0.78%, and of the polychromatic erythroblasts 2.75 ± 0.93%. On day 9 of rebound the mitotic index was greatly reduced in both the early (1.5 ± 1.3%) and late (0.6 ± 0.3%) erythroblasts. In the bled animals the earliest change was a threefold increase in the mitotic index of early erythroblasts on day 2 after bleeding. On day 3 the index for early erythroblasts was 8.4 ± 2.2% (t-test done between day 9 of rebound and day 3 after bleeding gave a value of 15.6, P < 0.001). The first significant increase in the mitotic index of late erythroblasts was on day 4 (3.2 ± 2.3%). More recent studies of mitosis in the erythropoietic pathway have been made by Starling and Rosse [1976] and Rosse and Beaufait [1978].

Lymphoid Cells

As in the studies of Jones et al [1967], on day 9 of rebound the numbers of small lymphocytes and transitional cells were significantly above normal. Subsequently, small lymphocytes fell in both the bled and the unbled animals (Fig. X.17), though the fall began earlier and was greater in the former than the latter. In contrast, the transitional cells followed a significantly different course in the two groups. In the unbled animals, transitional cells declined steadily over a 6-day period, from days 9–15 of rebound. After bleeding, they decreased sharply for 24 hours, and after 2½ days rose

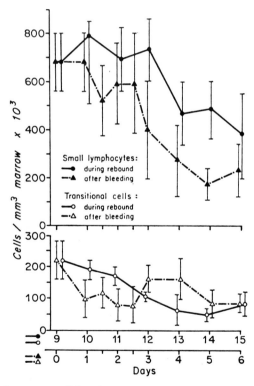

Fig. X.17. Pachychromatic small lymphocytes and transitional cells in rebound marrow of bled and unbled guinea pigs. In bled animals there is a significant increase in transitional cells after 3 or 4 days, whereas in unbled animals the transitional cells continue to fall. From Rosse et al [1970]. Courtesy of S. Karger AG, Basel.

sharply to a level significantly above the controls on days 3 and 4. This was followed by a peak rise of marrow erythroid cells on days 5 and 6 after bleeding.

In the context of all the other known facts concerning the relationship between transitional cells and erythropoiesis, the experiments on the stimulation of erythropoiesis during rebound are difficult to explain on any other basis than that the erythroblast precursors are to be found in the transitional cell compartment.

Hypoxia (5200 Meters) and Rebound in Rat

The studies of marrow changes in hypoxia and rebound have been performed mainly in guinea pigs. A small number of experiments have also been carried out in rats and mice. Transitional cells are a conspicuous element of rat marrow [Ramsell and Yoffey, 1961], where they form about 4% of the total nucleated cells. As in the guinea pig, they are an actively proliferating group. In guinea pig marrow the transitional cell compartment has an overall labeling index of about 35% in the normal steady state, whereas in the rat the index is aroundd 50% [Everett and Caffrey, 1967; Griffiths, 1969; Yoffey and Yaffe, 1980b]. Griffiths [1969] made a quantitative study of the lymphoid cells of rat bone marrow from day 5 to day 12 of rebound, following 7 days of hypoxia at 5200 m.

He found a highly significant rise in the total number of lymphocytes from the control value of $588 \pm 120 \times 10/\mu l$ to $1,143 \pm 2,043 \times 10^3/\mu l$ on day 5 of rebound, and to $1,515 \pm 100 \times 10^3/\mu l$ on day 6. The peak was reached at $1,603 \pm 132 \times 10^3/\mu l$ on day 9. From this peak they fell rapidly to $702 \pm 91 \times 10^3/\mu l$ on day 12. The transitional cells showed a significant increase on day 6, a little later than in the guinea pig, and not so marked [see Fig. 1, p 698, Griffiths, 1969].

In a recent study [Yoffey and Yaffe, 1980b], kinetic changes (^{3}H-thymidine and autoradiography) have been followed in rat bone marrow during 7 days of hypoxia at 5200 m and the subsequent 7 days of rebound. For the transitional cell compartment as a whole, the results are seen in Fig. X.18. The labeling index of over 50% in the controls fell to less than 40% on day 1 of hypoxia, but then rose sharply to nearly 70% on day 3. The great increase in the overall labeling index of the transitional compartment to its peak on day 3 was presumably related to the increased production of red cell precursors. The large transitionals, the most actively proliferating members of the compartment, had a labeling index of 80% by day 3 of hypoxia (Fig. X.19).

Hypoxia (5200 Meters) and Rebound in Mouse

After observing the changes in the transitional cell compartment in the guinea pig and rat, experiments were also performed on mice, in view of

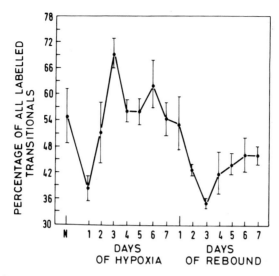

Fig. X.18. Rat bone marrow. Seven days hypoxia at 5200 m, and 7 days rebound. After an initial fall, the labeling index of the transitional compartment as a whole rises sharply to reach a peak on day 3, then falls to a low level on day 3 of rebound. From Yoffey and Yaffe [1980]. Courtesy of Journal of Anatomy.

their widespread use in experimental hematology. Figure X.20 presents some of the main quantitative changes in murine bone marrow during 5 days of hypoxia at 5200 m, and 9 days of rebound. The general pattern of lymphocytes, transitional cells, and nucleated erythroid cells is not essentially different from that found in the guinea pig, though there are minor differences both of degree and timing.

In both guinea pigs and mice, the small lymphocytes fall during hypoxia, though the fall is not evident on the first day. They then rise to well above control level during rebound, though in the case of the mouse, the secondary fall of small lymphocytes in late rebound did not become evident during the period in which the experiments were in progress. It remains to be established whether, had the experiments continued a few days longer, the same kind of secondary fall would have occurred as in the guinea pig.

The transitional cells fluctuated during hypoxia, but in rebound they reacted, like those of the guinea pig, by a sharp increase to levels well above normal. This raised level continued, with some minor changes, throughout the 9 days of rebound. Hurst et al [1969] made use of the spleen colony technique to observe the changes in CFU content of murine bone marrow during rebound (Fig. X.21). In their experiments, both the total lymphoid

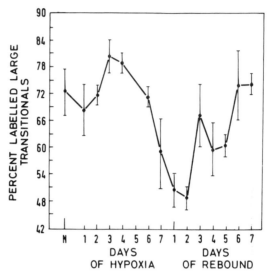

Fig. X.19. Rat bone marrow. Seven days hypoxia at 17,000 ft, and 7 days rebound. The highest labeling index is found in the large transitionals, reaching 80% on day 3 of hypoxia, and falling sharply to its lowest level on day of rebound. From Yoffey and Yaffe [1980].

cells (ie, transitional cells + small lymphocytes) and the CFU reached a peak on day 7 of rebound. In interpreting their results, Hurst et al [1969] kept open the possibility that some of the small lymphocytes might also be colony-forming units, though on the whole they concluded that "the number of transitional cells more closely correlates with colony-forming cell content than does the number of small lymphocytes." This view found support in the work of Mel and Schooley [1964], who employed a special technique for the fractionation of marrow cells, and did not find any correlation between the "small round mononuclear cell" (presumably small lymphocyte) content of murine marrow grafts and their spleen colony-forming ability. The recent studies of Thomas et al [1977], on the morphological identification of CFU-S, lend added force to this interpretation (cf Riches et al, 1976].

The literature contains a number of reports suggesting an increase in the CFU content of the marrow during rebound. Tribukait and Forssberg [1964] noted an improved survival time in mice irradiated after 2–3 days of rebound, as compared with normal mice. Okunewick et al [1969], following up these experiments, reported an increase in the numbers of CFU in the marrow of mice during rebound. Their experiments were performed on mice

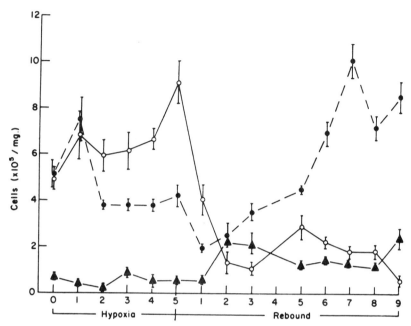

Fig. X.20. Quantitative changes in the F_1 mouse during hypoxia (5200 m) and rebound. The general pattern of the small lymphocyte and transitional cell changes is the same as in the guinea pig. During rebound, a marked increase in small lymphocytes and transitional cells accompanies diminished erythropoiesis. From Turner et al [1967]. ○ = erythroid cells; ● = small lymphocytes; ▲ = transitionals.

after 3 days of rebound following 3 weeks of hypoxia at 0.5 atm. Okunewick and Fulton [1970] noted that mice during rebound gave a greater response to erythropoietin than did normal mice.

LYMPHOID CELLS IN ERYTHROBLASTIC ISLANDS

Since all the experimental studies indicated that the erythropoietic stem cells are members of the transitional cell compartment, it seemed worth investigating the relation of transitional cells to the erythroblastic islands in which red cells are formed. An ultrastructural examination was made of erythroblastic islands in the marrow in different stages of activity: 1) in the normal steady state, 2) during 7 days of hypoxia at 5200 m [Ben-Ishay and Yoffey, 1971a], 3) during the subsequent 7 days of rebound [Ben-Ishay and Yoffey, 1971b], and 4) during the restimulation of erythropoiesis, after 7 days of rebound, by the withdrawal of blood [Ben-Ishay and Yoffey, 1972].

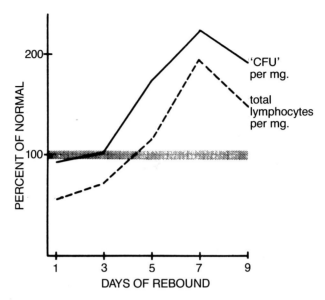

Fig. X.21. Colony-forming units (CFU-S) in murine bone marrow during rebound. From Turner et al [1967].

The Normal Steady State

In the normal steady state the structure of the islands conforms to the description given in Chapter IV. A typical island consists of a central macrophage, sometimes termed the "central reticular cell," surrounded by erythroblasts in various stages of maturation. The erythroblasts and the central macrophage cell are the two basic constituents. An occasional granulocyte or plasma cell may be found, but this is the exception rather than the rule. Fine processes of the central macrophage extend between the surrounding erythroblasts, with which they come into close contact.

The Influx of Lymphoid Cells in Hypoxia

Five hours after the start of hypoxia, pachychromatic small lymphocytes and an occasional medium or large transitional cell were seen either at the periphery or in the interior of erythroblastic islands [Ben-Ishay and Yoffey, 1971a, Fig. 1, p 950]. Small lymphocytes, close to the central macrophage, could often be seen at 12 hours.

Disappearance of Island Lymphocytes

By 24 hours, the lymphocytes seem to have disappeared from the islands. It is not known whether the entry of the lymphocytes into the islands is purely random, or whether any particular group of lymphocytes is concerned. The appearance of the occasional *transitional cell* seems to be more frequent after 12 hours of hypoxia [eg, Fig. 4, Ben-Ishay and Yoffey, 1971a]. At 24 hours one often sees the central macrophage surrounded by proerythroblasts [Fig. 6, Ben-Ishay and Yoffey, 1971a], which at a later stage can be seen in mitosis [Fig. 8, Ben-Ishay and Yoffey, 1971a].

The Erythroblastic Island in Rebound

For the first 2–3 days of rebound, the most obvious change in the islands is the replacement of immature by more mature erythroid forms. By day 3 of rebound, depression of erythropoiesis has been in progress long enough for most of the nucleated erythroid cells to have disappeared from the majority of the islands, although, however long rebound continues, they never disappear completely from all the islands. As already noted, there seems to be an irreducible minimum of erythropoiesis. In the depleted islands the processes of the central macrophages are retracted, so that the cells become more or less rounded. Instead of the nucleated erythroid cells, the central macrophages are now surrounded by small lymphocytes and an occasional transitional cell [Fig. 7, p 494, Ben-Ishay and Yoffey, 1971b].

Restimulation of Erythropoiesis

Even in islands in which erythropoiesis seems to have ceased entirely, the central reticular cells persist and are readily recognizable because of their characteristic inclusions. When erythropoiesis is reestablished, the first sign of regeneration is the appearance of a transitional cell or a proerythroblast in close contact with a central macrophage [Ben-Ishay and Yoffey, 1971b, Figs. 7, 8; 1972, Figs. 7, 8]. As soon as more erythroid cells appear, the processes of the macrophages begin to re-form, extending between the proliferating erythroid cells and coming into close contact with them [Ben-Ishay and Yoffey, 1972, Fig. 11]. La Pushin and Trentin [1977] have also emphasized the close contact between proerythroblasts and the central macrophages.

CONCLUDING COMMENTS

The stimulation of erythropoiesis, depending on its intensity, gives rise to a variety of changes not only in the erythroid cells, but also in granulocyte and lymphocyte production, associated with quantitative and kinetic changes in the transitional cell compartment. The transitional cell compartment is capable of a considerable degree of change in what can only be interpreted as adaptation to varying stem cell requirements. The modulation of the transitional cell compartment during the changing phases of erythropoiesis is meaningful only in the light of its stem cell role. Ultrastructural studies provide additional evidence in this direction.

In ultrastructural studies the only type of cell which can be envisaged as the proerythroblast precursor is a medium or large transitional cell. One sees no other cell in the erythroblastic island even remotely resembling a proerythroblast. It is true there are usually some small lymphocytes in erythroblastic islands, both in the early stages of hypoxia, where they appear transiently among the erythroid cells, and in rebound, where they are in fact more numerous than the transitional cells. But morphologically they are so very different from proerythroblasts that it is impossible to envisage the small lymphocytes as the *immediate* precursors of proerythroblasts, though one can conceive of a small number as more remote precursors after a suitable period of enlargement and transformation. This would apply especially to the "resting bone marrow lymphocytes" of Hoelzer et al [1975]. Although the role of small lymphocytes in erythroblastic islands awaits further investigation, transitional cells seem to be the only possible candidates for the role of the immediate proerythroblast precursors.

XI.

Platelet Production and Release

INTRODUCTION

Platelets are cytoplasmic fragments of megakaryocytes. Megakaryocytes develop in the bone marrow from their precursor cells, megakaryoblasts, which are in turn derived from stem cells. Substantial evidence now indicates that megakaryocytes share with myeloid and erythroid cells a common stem cell which is pluripotent. A progeny of this cell is committed to megakaryopoiesis [Ebbe and Stohlman, 1965]. Through a series of endomitosis, this cell develops into the megakaryocyte which, in the bone marrow, is located in the subendothelial region of marrow sinuses. In the course of maturation, megakaryocytes develop an elaborate membranous system known as the "demarcation membrane system." This system demarcates the megakaryocyte cytoplasm into platelet "zones" or "territories" each of which can then form a platelet, to be released into the circulation and leaving the megakaryocyte nuclei behind to be phagocytosed.

In this chapter only the cell biology of platelet formation and release will be treated. Numerous recent books and reviews obviate the necessity of giving consideration to kinetics, methodology, function, and pathophysiology of this process [Paulus, 1971; Baldini and Ebbe, 1974].

TERMINOLOGY AND PHYLOGENETIC CONSIDERATIONS

Platelets are nonnucleated cells and should be distinguished from the nucleated "thrombocytes" of lower vertebrates [Andrew, 1965; Jordan and Beans, 1929; Sugijama, 1926; Deckhuzyen, 1901]. However, in the literature pertaining to the mammalian system, the two terms are often interchangeably used, perhaps because Deckhuzyen [1901], who first described the functional equivalence of platelet and thrombocyte (and coined the latter term), overemphasized their similarities.

In the course of evolution, the megakaryocyte-platelet system is limited to mammals. In lower vertebrates (pisces, amphibia, reptiles, birds, and even some mammalia of lower orders), the functional equivalent of the platelet is the nucleated thrombocyte [Andrew, 1965; Jordan, 1929; Sugijama, 1926; Deckhuzyen, 1901]. They are derived through successive division of their precursor cells, "thromboblasts," in a manner similar to the derivation of red cells from erythroblasts. In invertebrates, a specific cell type is not endowed with the platelet function; the hemocyte, otherwise equivalent to the leukocyte, carries out this function (see Chapter II).

A simple computation indicates that the evolution of species has worked in an economic direction with regard to platelet formation: The majority of megakaryocytes have 8–16 nuclei with some even up to 64 [Penington et al, 1974; Odell et al, 1965; Garcia, 1964; Paulus, 1970; Paulus et al, 1971; Cronkite, 1958], and where nuclear division is associated with cytoplasmic division (as in thromboblast-thrombocyte system), at most 64 cells would have resulted, whereas a megakaryocyte, depending on its ploidy [Harker, 1968a,b, 1969] can produce an average of 4,000–8,000 platelets [Crosby, 1976; Becker and DeBruyn, 1976; Pedersen, 1978; Harker, 1968].

Phylogenetically, similarities exist between the platelet and the red cell. Both are nucleated cells in lower vertebrates and nonnucleated in mammalia. Both are produced intravascularly in lower vertebrates and extravascularly in mammalia. Both cell types are endowed with some transport function. Studies on the nucleated thrombocyte have contributed to the recognition of the significance of cell aggregation in thrombosis.

EVIDENCE FOR THE DERIVATION OF PLATELETS FROM MEGAKARYOCYTES

Derivation of platelets from megakaryocytes was first advocated by Wright [1906, 1910]. Wright's evidence was, however, strictly morphological, and his view only slowly penetrated the thinking in hematology; in fact, argument is advanced against it as late as 1976 [Leiter, 1976]. In addition to strong presumptive morphological evidence, the following findings indicate the presence of a megakaryocyte-platelet axis:

1) Experimentally induced thrombocytopenia is associated with compensatory increase in the size and the number of megakaryocytes [Harker 1968a,b, 1969; Ebbe et al, 1968; Odell et al, 1962, 1969; Rolovic et al, 1970; Matter et al, 1960; Craddock et al, 1955]. 2) Conversely, thrombocytosis results in suppression of megakaryocytopoiesis [Harker, 1968a,b; Pennington and Olsen, 1970; Odell et al, 1967; Paulus, 1967]. 3) Megakaryocytes and platelets share common antigens [Humphrey, 1955; Vazquez and Lewis, 1960; deLeval, 1967]. 4) There are also numerous similarities between the chemical composition of megakaryocytes and platelets [Zajicek, 1957; Jackson, 1973; Darzynkiewicz et al, 1967; Nagao and Angrist, 1968; Spicer et al, 1969; Rabellino et al, 1979]. 5) In the course of both phylogeny and ontogeny, temporal appearance of the megakaryocyte and the platelet is simultaneous [Andrew, 1965; Jordan and Beans, 1929; Sugijama, 1926; Deckhuzyen, 1901]. 6) When megakaryocytes are labeled, the label subsequently appears in platelets [Odell and McDonald, 1964; Evatt and Levin, 1969; Pennington, 1969; Najean and Ardaillou, 1969]. 7) Finally, derivation of platelets from megakaryocytes can directly be observed by microcinematography [Thiery and Bessis, 1956a,b; Albrecht, 1957; Hiraki et al, 1958; Izak et al, 1957; Kinosita and Ohno, 1958], the most convincing evidence yet in favor of Wright's theory.

MEGAKARYOCYTE MATURATION AND PLATELET FORMATION

In contrast to other hemopoietic cell lines, the megakaryocyte is a polyploid cell. It was once believed that the cytoplasmic maturation and nuclear divisions occur concurrently, as is the case with other hemopoietic cells. Hence, platelet formation should occur in the cell with high ploidy and in proportion to it. This is not the case, however. Before any evidence of cytoplasmic differentiation occurs, the cell synthesizes all the DNA that it ultimately will carry [Odell et al, 1965; Odell and Jackson, 1967; deLeval, 1964, 1966, 1968a,b; Paulus, 1968a,b, 1970]. During this period, the nuclear size increases without nuclear segmentation. Irrespective of the complement of DNA synthesized, the synthesis stops at the earliest sign of cytoplasmic differentiation. It has been postulated that the appearance in the cytoplasm of the contractile protein, thrombosthenin, may trigger a message to stop DNA synthesis [Paulus, 1967].

At any rate, the cytoplasmic maturation and nuclear segmentation of megakaryocytes proceed only after DNA synthesis has stopped, irrespective of ploidy. As a result, platelets are formed from megakaryocytes of different ploidy; yet simply because the ploidy number correlates positively with the cytoplasmic size, the numbers of platelets formed per megakaryocyte correspond to the degree of ploidy. Furthermore, there is some evidence that cells with different ploidy number may respond differently to various stimuli and may form platelets of different size [Paulus, 1970].

DEMARCATION MEMBRANE SYSTEM

The cytoplasmic maturation of the megakaryocyte is associated with the development of an extensive membranous system known as the "demarcation membrane system." It has been postulated that in the process of megakaryocyte development, the demarcation membrane system is the first organelle to appear [MacPherson, 1971, 1972]. This system demarcates platelet "zones" or "territories" by enclosing and defining parts of the megakaryocyte cytoplasm that would, in the end, be platelets. In this way, the demarcation membrane system appears as profiles of round, oval, or elongated vesicles where the membrane encloses an empty core or cisterna (Fig. XI.1). These profiles may show extensive budding, coalescing, and branching. The demarcation system is readily distinguished from the rough endoplasmic reticulum because, unlike the latter, its cytoplasmic surface is not studded by ribosomes, nor is a proteinaceous substance seen within the cisternae. The demarcation system can also be differentiated from the Golgi system by virtue of its distinctive morphology and by its localization in the intermediate rather than the perinuclear zone of the cell. In a well-developed megakaryocyte and in favorable sections, transverse sections of the demarcation system appear as circular vesicles that are arranged side by side, in a beadlike chain, thus forming the outline of a nascent platelet (platelet zone). In other areas, stacks of longitudinally sectioned profiles are seen to be oriented in parallel arrays. These have been called "dense compartment" by Behnke [1968, 1969], who suggested they were foci of membrane assembly and proliferation. Hence, observations on thin sections suggest that the demarcation system consists of cylindrical-tubular structures whose appearance depends on the plane of section. Intense proliferation of the demarcation system, inordinate with other aspects of cellular maturation, is seen in states of active megakaryocytosis, such as in experimental thrombocytopenia [Paulus, 1970] and in preleukemia [Maldonado and Pintado, 1974].

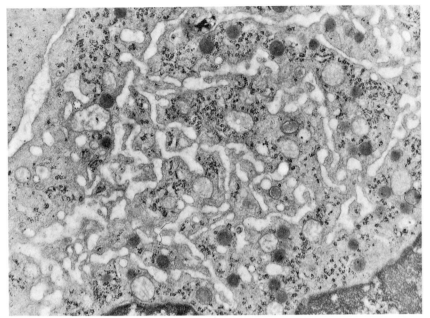

Fig. XI.1. Electron micrograph of a mature megakaryocyte in the rat. Portions of the nucleus are seen at the edge. Portion of the cell membrane is also seen. Note the round, oval, or elongated vesicles of the demarcation membrane system, distinguishable from the profiles of RER by the absence of ribsomes on the cytoplasmic surface. These vesicles form the outline of platelet zones or territories. (×42,500.)

Origin of the Demarcation Membrane System

The origin of the demarcation membrane system has variably been attributed to the megakaryocyte cell membrane [MacPherson, 1972; Behnke, 1969; Shaklai and Tavassoli, 1978a; Tavassoli, 1979a; Thiele et al, 1977], endoplasmic reticulum [Paulus, 1967; Berman and Fawcett, 1964; DeBruyn, 1964; Han and Baker, 1964; Schulz, 1968], Golgi system [Zucker-Franklin, 1970], and membranogenic areas of the cytoplasm [Yamada, 1957]. Current evidence indicates that none of the intracellular membrane systems are the origin of the demarcation system. However, there is abundant evidence to suggest that the demarcation membrane system is formed by invagination of the megakaryocyte cell membrane. This evidence is based on experiments with extracellular tracers that do not penetrate the intact biomembrane [Behnke, 1968; Shaklai and Tavassoli, 1978a; Geyer and Schaaf 1972; French, 1967; Behnke and Pedersen, 1974]. Ferritin, horseradish peroxidase, ruthenium red, thorotrast, and lanthanum nitrate have been used. In all cases the tracers have readily penetrated the cisternae of the demarcation system but not other cytoplasmic organelles, indicating communication of the demarcation system with the extracellular space and arguing for its origin from the megakaryocyte cell membrane. By contrast, the absence of tracers in the Golgi system and endoplasmic reticulum indicates the lack of communication with the demarcation system, and argues against its derivation from these intracellular membranous systems.

Other evidence in favor of the cell membrane derivation of the demarcation system is summarized here: 1) In murine leukemia, budding of viruses occurs not only on the cell surface but also on the cisternal surface of the demarcation system [DeHarven and Friend, 1960; Dalton et al, 1961], suggesting a unity. In other infected cells, budding occurs only on the cell membrane. 2) Freeze-fracture studies indicate an orderly progression, with respect to size and density of intramembranous particles, from the megakaryocyte cell membrane to the demarcation system to the platelet membrane [Shaklai and Tavassoli, 1978a], suggesting a direction in which the membrane differentiates. No such similarities are seen between the demarcation system and other intracellular membrane systems. 3) Acetylcholinesterase, a lipid-dependent enzyme, present on the outer layer of the red cell membrane and used as a marker [Martin, 1970], is also present in the megakaryocyte cell membrane in several species [Jackson, 1973; Darzynkiewicz et al, 1967]. Cytochemically, this enzyme has also been localized to the demarcation system [Lautenschlager et al, 1971]. 4) Platelets display a surface coat of acid mucosubstance that reacts with cationic dyes, ruthenium red, Alcian blue, lanthanum salts, and colloidal iron [Nagao and Angrist, 1968; Spicer et al, 1969; MacPherson, 1971; Behnke, 1968; Federenko and Levin, 1976]. This coat appears as a fuzz on the platelet surface. A coat with similar reactivity is also found in the megakaryocyte cell membrane and its demarcation system [Nagao and Angrist, 1968; Shaklai and Tavassoli, 1978a].

A Theoretical Dilemma

Although the consensus of opinion now favors the cells membrane origin of the demarcation system [Tavassoli, 1980a], until recently it was not clear how the process of platelet demarcation came about. For derivation of the demarcation system from the cell membrane, the latter must invaginate deeply into the cytoplasm. The invagination can give rise to the formation in the cytoplasm of cylindrical-tubular structures, the cisternae of which are in communication with the extracellular space. This view is consistent with observations on random sections and tracer experiments.

Here a theoretical dilemma exists: To enclose a part of the cytoplasm and to demarcate platelet zones, a flat sheet rather than tubular membrane is called for. It was MacPherson [1972] who appreciated the problem of transition from cylindrical-tubular membrane into a sheet of flat membrane capable of demarcating platelet zones. In search for a solution he advanced "the single site theory," which maintains that the initiation of the demarcation system formation occurs at a single localized linear area and proceeds by concentric infolding of the cell membrane. Thus, he attempts to resolve the theoretical problem by postulating that the system is a flat sheet from the beginning.

Because the random sections could not resolve the dilemma, this was left to the application of freeze-fracture technique [Shaklai and Tavassoli, 1978a; Tavassoli 1979a, 1980a; Thiele et al, 1977]. In contrast to sections, freeze-fracture technique permits, depending on the fracture path, a three-dimensional view of the inner parts of the cell and both its intracellular and cell membranes. In freeze-fracture, when the fracture line exposes the cell membrane, scattered invaginations are seen that are continuous with the demarcation system [Shaklai and Tavassoli, 1978a; Tavassoli, 1979a]. This does not support the single-site theory of MacPherson. When the system is fractured tangentially (Fig. XI.2), it appears as a fenestrated sheet, the fenestrations having a parallel alignment. When the fracture plane is transverse, however, it appears as a canal system, the basic element of which is membrane-wrapped tubules. These tubules may be cylindrical, like a pipe, or somewhat flattened, like an empty toothpaste tube. In favorable preparations, beadlike chains of these tubules, lying side by side (comparable to the profiles seen in thin sections), are seen connected by membranous bridges which, in oblique fracture planes, appear to be the result of focal fusion of membranes of two parallel tubules.

Fusion-Fission Reorganization of the Demarcation System

On the basis of these observations, it is now possible to reconstruct a developing membrane model whereby platelets are formed from megakaryocytes [Shaklai and Tavassoli, 1978a; Tavassoli, 1979a, 1980a]. This is shown schematically in Figure XI.3. Through the invagination of the cell membrane, tubules are formed within the cytoplasm (left upper part of Fig. XI.3). These tubules are membrane-wrapped, and their cisternae are in communication with extracellular space. When these structures are oriented parallel in their long axes, their membranes undergo point fusion in the direction "A." These point fusions become extensive, yet leaving unfused areas in between. These appear as fenestration in a tangentially fractured demarcation system. Separation or "fission" of these structures in direction "B" (perpendicular to "A") yields two sheets of scalloped membrane. Thus, the process of fusion-fission has reorganized the tubular membrane into two flat sheets. Upon the completion of fission, the two sheets of membrane form

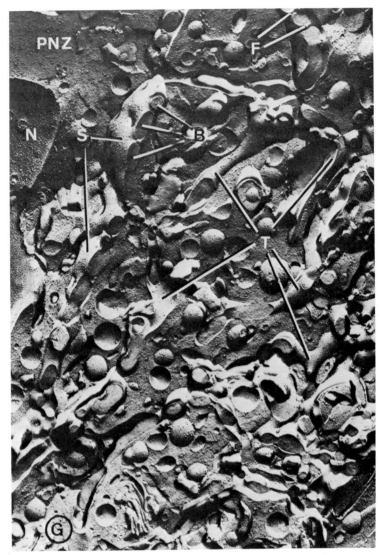

Fig. XI.2.   Freeze-fracture electron micrograph of the rat megakaryocyte. Transcytoplasmic fracture has revealed a portion of nucleus (N) and the perinuclear zone (PNZ). Note the Golgi system (G). Tangential fracture of the demarcation system has disclosed tubular structures (T) in some areas and fenestrated flat sheets elsewhere (S). Transverse fracture has revealed circular or oval spaces (B), which may be perceived as a chain of beads because they are linearly arranged. The continuity of the two fracture planes permits a three-dimensional view wherein the fenestrae (F) can be identified as the site of fusion of tubular structures. Demarcation of two nascent platelets can be perceived at the top of this figure. From Tavassoli [1979a]; courtesy of Springer-International. (×38,300.)

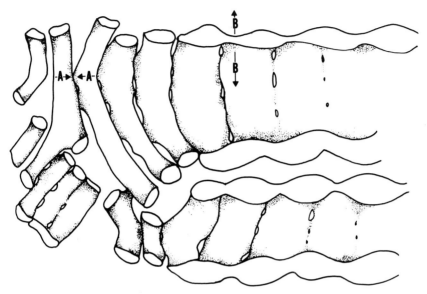

Fig. XI.3. Schematic reconstruction of the fusion-fission reorganization of the demarcation system. Tubular structures, resulting from the invagination of the megakaryocyte cell membrane, are aligned parallel (top left), undergoing point fusion in the direction "A." These point fusions extend, leaving fenestration in between. Fission of these structures (right) in the direction "B," perpendicular to direction "A," yields two sheets of scalloped membrane, thus forming the cell membranes of two adjacent platelets. From Tavassoli [1979a]; courtesy of Springer-International.

cell membranes of two adjacent nascent platelets. The open canalicular system of platelets may then be interpreted as unused demarcation membrane. The process is a dynamic asynchronous, and three-dimensional.

It is to be remembered that fusion-fission reorganization of membrane is not limited to the megakaryocyte-platelet system. It is one of the most ubiquitous events in cell biology, mediating such diverse biologic phenomena as fertilization, cytokinesis, neuromuscular transmission, endocytosis, exocytosis, formation of secondary lysosomes, and the release of enveloped viruses [Lucy, 1970; Shotton, 1978].

PLATELET RELEASE

In Wright-Giemsa–stained smears of aspirated marrow, mature megakaryocytes appear as if they were being fragmented into individual platelets. Indeed, this was the appearance that led Wright [1906, 1910] to formulate his concept of megakaryocyte-platelet axis. He postulated that cytoplasmic parts of the megakaryocyte projected through the neighboring vessel wall and were pinched off, as platelets, into the circulation. This concept still dominates the thinking of most practitioners of hematology. Moreover, Pisciotta et al [1953] studied megakaryocytes by phase-contrast microscopy, and reported that the cell membrane ruptured and platelets were extruded into the medium, but this observation has not been corroborated [Behnke, 1969]. As Crosby [1976] has pointed out, the appearance may be misleading, and the megakaryocyte in smears of marrow resembles the in vivo mega-karyocyte as a fried egg resembles the egg inside the hen. Platelet release should be studied in marrow megakaryocytes and with its anatomical relations intact.

Recent electron-microscopic studies using in situ–fixed marrow tissue [Shaklai and Tavassoli, 1979a], have indicated that megakaryocytes are located in the subendothelial region of vascular sinuses [Shaklai and Tavas-soli, 1978a, 1979; Tavassoli, 1979a; Tavassoli and Aoki, 1981]. Statistical analysis of Lichtman et al [1978] indicates that this arrangement is not a chance occurrence, and that it may be a determinant of platelet release [Tavassoli, 1979a; Lichtman et al, 1978].

In this subendothelial location, the cytoplasm of the megakaryocyte penetrates the endothelium to reach inside the lumen. This penetration is through the endothelium (transendothelial) and not between two endothe-lial cells (interendothelial) [Tavassoli and Aoki, 1981], a phenomenon that may have a regulatory function in platelet release [Becker and DeBruyn, 1976; Tavassoli, 1979]. In this manner, large segments of the cytoplasm enter the lumen. These are known as "proplatelets." Proplatelets are elongated structures of about 2.5×120 μm, and it has been computed that a mature megakaryocyte can produce about six proplatelets [Becker and DeBruyn, 1976]. Considering that a megakaryocyte might produce 8,000 platelets [Crosby, 1976], a proplatelet might be expected to give rise to some 1,200 platelets. It is not known if platelets are the immediate progeny of proplate-lets or if there are more intermediate steps. The concept of proplate-let may explain the size heterogeneity of circulating platelets, with younger forms being the larger ones [Karpatkin, 1969]. It is probably outside the marrow that proplatelets are further fragmented into platelets. This may occur within the general circulation or within the pulmonary circulation where proplatelets could be trapped. The finding that more platelets leave the lung than enter it (vide infra) supports the latter possibility.

Proplatelets were first observed in vitro by Bessis and his colleagues using microcinematography [Thiery and Bessis, 1956a,b]. They observed projections that became progressively elongated, giving the megakaryocytes an octopuslike appearance. Subsequent cinematographic and electron-microscopic studies have confirmed this observation [Becker and DeBruyn, 1976; Albrecht, 1957; Hiraki et al, 1958; Izak et al, 1957; Kinosita and Ohno, 1958; Behnke, 1969; French, 1967; Tavassoli and Aoki, 1981].

In vitro electron-microscopic studies of Radley and Scurfield [1980] have indicated the presence of microtubules in these proplatelets. The microtubules are oriented longitudinally along the axis of the long proplatelets and are concentrated at the sites of constriction where platelets are released. These constrictions bear structural similarities with the bridges separating midbody of cells in the terminal stages of cytokinesis. The presence of a centriole in these constriction sites has also been demonstrated, suggesting the possibility that the process of platelet release from proplatelets is a special form of cytokinesis. In this context, it may be pertinent to mention that the enucleation of red cells is also considered a special form of cytokinesis in which the cytoplasmic division occurs without nuclear division [Tavassoli, 1978a]. It is of interest that the exposure to microtubule depolymerizing agents results in the retraction of the proplatelets and reformation of "megakaryocytes" [Radley and Haller, 1982]. This observation not only provides evidence for the involvement of microtubules in the process of platelet release, but also indicates that the process can be reversible.

The Fate of Megakaryocyte Nuclei

After the megakaryocyte is depleted of its platelet content, its nuclei remain in the extravascular compartment of the bone marrow, surrounded by a thin layer of cytoplasm and a membrane. Electron-microscopic studies of Radley and Haller [1983] suggest that such cellular remnants undergo a process known as "apoptosis" [Kerr et al, 1972; Willie et al, 1980]. This degenerative process involves the formation of protrusions from the surface which later separate to form membrane-bound apoptotic bodies. Nonlysosomal endonucleases are activated to excise nucleosomes. Chromatin undergoes condensation. Bundles of microfilaments appear in the nucleus, and the cellular remnant may then undergo phagocytosis.

EXTRAMEDULLARY DISTRIBUTION OF MEGAKARYOCYTES

Not only the cytoplasmic pieces of megakaryocytes, the proplatelets, but also the whole cell can pass the marrow-blood barrier and move into the circulation [Tavassoli and Aoki, 1981]. This passage has actually been documented in the elegant studies of Kinosita and Ohno [1958]. During their study on the living microscopy of the rabbit bone marrow, these authors produced a microcinematographic film. In one sequence, a mega-karyocyte is shown attached to the wall of a sinus. Within a few seconds, the cell tumbles into the sinus and off the screen, carried away by the bloodstream. They suggested that if these megakaryocytes do not complete further development in the marrow or within the circulation, they may be trapped in the pulmonary circulation, completing their development in alveolar capillaries.

Moreover, the presence of megakaryocytes in the circulation has been amply documented [Hansen and Pedersen, 1978; Efrati and Rozenszajn, 1960; Herbeuval et al, 1961, 1962a; Melamed et al, 1966; Minot, 1922; Scheinin and Korvuneimi, 1962, 1963; Breslow et al, 1968; Whitby, 1948], and the contention that these cells may reflect a serious disorder of the marrow [Minot, 1922; Whitby, 1948] has not been validated. It is now evident that megakaryocytes are normal constituents of blood and that they are derived from the marrow [Kaufman et al, 1965a]. Their reported concen-tration varies, depending on the technique [Efrati and Rozenszajn, 1960; Herbeuval et al, 1961, 1962a; Melamed et al, 1966] and on the state of health or disease [Scheinin and Korvuneimi, 1963; Breslow et al, 1968; Whitby, 1948; Hume et al, 1964; Herbenval et al, 1962b]. It may be said that in healthy adult humans, ten megakaryocytes per milliliter of peripheral blood is a reliable figure. Their concentration is increased after surgery and in cancer and inflammatory diseases. In cancer, they can be misinterpreted as circulating cancer cells. Cytochemistry [Jackson, 1962] and differential lysis of cancer cells [Scheinin and Korvuneimi, 1963] have been helpful in differentiating them from circulating cancer cells.

Megakaryocytes are also found in other tissues, including the lung, spleen, kidney, liver, and heart [Smith and Butcher, 1952; Rothermel, 1930]. Here again, their number is increased and their distribution is wider in disease states than in health [Smith and Butcher, 1952], and this has been considered a sign of "stress" [Minot, 1922].

Pulmonary Megakaryocytes

Megakaryocytes are particularly abundant in the lung and the pulmo-nary circulation [Pedersen 1974, 1978; Scheinin and Korvuneimi, 1963; Kaufman et al, 1965a,b; Jordan 1940; Aschoff, 1893; Maniatis, 1969]. As-choff [1893], who first observed intravascular pulmonary megakaryocytes, proposed that they originated from the marrow and were embolized into the lung. Kaufman et al [1965a] rearranged the pulmonary vessels in dogs so that blood from the right side of the heart perfused first the right lung and then went through the left lung. Many megakaryocytes were seen in the right lung but few in the left lung, suggesting that circulating mega-karyocytes are filtered out by the lung. This is in complete agreement with the postulate of Aschoff [1893] and of Kinosita and Ohno [1958] as de-scribed above. It has also been demonstrated that the platelet count is higher in the pulmonary vein than in the pulmonary artery [Melamed et al, 1966; Scheinin and Korvuneimi, 1963; Pedersen, 1974; Maniatis, 1969; Howell and Donahue, 1937], inevitably suggesting that pulmonary mega-karyocytes contribute to the platelet production.

It is now generally accepted that these pulmonary megakaryocytes origi-nate from the marrow, and because of their size, most are trapped in the pulmonary circulation where they release platelets. It has been estimated that 40,000 megakaryocytes are delivered in this manner to the lung every minute [Pedersen, 1978]. Agreement is lacking, however, on the extent of their contribution to the total platelet production. Values as varied as 7% [Kaufman et al, 1965a,b] to almost 100% [Crosby, 1976; Pedersen, 1978] have been reported. These values are invariably derived at by computations based on either differential platelet counts in pulmonary artery and vein or the estimation of the number of megakaryocytes that may reach the lung and the number of platelets that each can produce. The data base is subject to too wide a variation to permit reliable information. Labeling kinetic studies may help to clarify this point.

MEGAKARYOCYTE-ENDOTHELIAL RELATION

Localization of megakaryocytes in the subendothelial region of marrow sinuses has been implicated as a determinant of platelet release [Lichtman et al, 1978]. The arrangement may be of more functional significance. In this location, megakaryocytes subserve an adventitial function, since adven-titial cells are absent where megakaryocytes are present [Shaklai and Tavas-soli, 1979a]. They may also serve as a component of the marrow-blood barrier, so that the cell traffic takes a transmegakaryocytic route to enter the circulation [Tavassoli, 1981b]. In this respect, they are similar to marrow fat cells, also located in the subendothelial region [Tavassoli, 1976]. Fat cells, however, are believed to derive from adventitial cells [Tavassoli, 1976; Weiss, 1965], whereas megakaryocytes are not.

Moreover, in this location, megakaryocytes project multiple small pro-cesses through the endothelium into the lumen [Tavassoli and Aoki, 1981]. These processes may contain cytoplasmic organelles, similar to those of platelets, and their luminal penetration may be a part of proplatelet formation and platelet release [Becker and DeBruyn, 1976; Weiss, 1965]. Often, however, they are remarkably free of organelles [Tavassoli, 1976b, 1979a] and their endothelial penetration may simply serve as an anchoring mechanism, giving the cell some stability in this location. A similar arrangement is reported in the spleen, where cordal macrophages "anchor" into the endothelium of splenic sinuses and presumably screen the cells passing by [Tavassoli and Weiss, 1973].

This arrangement may also serve as a mechanism to "monitor" the circulation and to receive information as to the requirement of the body for platelet formation [Tavassoli, 1979a]. A similar arrangement has been reported for perisinal macrophages in the rabbit marrow where macrophages penetrate the endothelium, reaching the lumen and phagocytizing red cells [Tavassoli, 1977b]. The nature of the regulatory information that may be so received by the megakaryocyte is not clear, although it is believed that the oxygen tension may have a regulatory function, either directly or through thrombopoietin, on platelet formation and release [Pulvertaft, 1958; McDonald et al, 1970]. Information is scant in these areas, which deserve further exploration.

XII.

Lymphocyte Production

INTRODUCTION

Osmond and Everett [1964] provided the first positive evidence that small lymphocytes are produced actively and in very large numbers in the bone marrow itself. This was first shown in the guinea pig [Osmond and Everett, 1964; Harris and Kugler, 1965; Osmond, 1967], and subsequently confirmed in the rat [Craddock, 1965; Everett and Caffrey, 1967]. At the outset it should be emphasized that the occurrence of extensive lymphocytopoiesis in the marrow does not rule out the entry of some lymphocytes into the marrow from the bloodstream, as has been shown in rats [Everett et al, 1960], dogs [Keiser et al, 1967], and guinea pigs [Rosse, 1972a]. The earlier studies were on lymphocytes as morphological entities, without distinction of the type of lymphocyte concerned. More recent studies differentiate between B cells, null cells, T-cell precursors, and natural killer (NK) cells, which are also closely related to the marrow lymphocyte population. Recent surveys by Osmond [1975, 1980], Rosse [1976], and Cooper [1981] provide evidence of the rapid progress in this field.

FORMATION OF LYMPHOCYTES FROM TRANSITIONAL CELLS

Osmond and Everett [1964] first observed the labeling sequence in lymphocytes and transitional cells in the marrow after a single intraperitoneal injection of tritiated thymidine, and they confirmed the early labeling of transitional cells, which reached a peak at 24 hours. The number of labeled transitionals then fell rapidly, while at the same time the number of labeled small lymphocytes increased, reaching a peak at 3 days, following which they too rapidly diminished (Fig. XII.1).

Osmond and Everett [1964] followed up this observation by two further experiments. In one experiment, the circulation was occluded in one hind limb for 20 min, while tritiated thymidine was injected into the femoral vein of the other limb. The occlusion was maintained until there was no more free thymidine in the circulation. The marrows of the occluded and the unoccluded limbs were examined 72 hours later.

In the unoccluded marrow 39.7% of the small lymphocytes were labeled, and in the occluded marrow only 1.7%. Assuming that the temporary occlusion does not damage the marrow, a point investigated by Osmond [1967], the inference seems clear that large numbers of marrow lymphocytes are formed in situ, and are therefore not hematogenous in origin.

In a further experiment, humeral bone marrow was taken 1–2½ hours after the IP injection of tritiated thymidine and cultured in a diffusion chamber in the peritoneum of an unlabeled animal. Whereas there were no

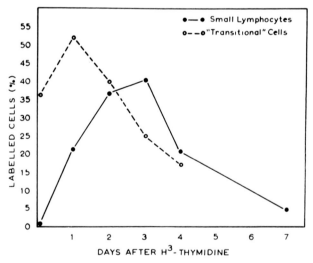

Fig. XII.1. Labeling of transitional cells and small lymphocytes in guinea pig bone marrow after a single IP injection of tritiated thymidine. Note that the peak of labeled transitional cells occurs about 2 days before that of the pachychromatic small lymphocytes. From Osmond and Everett [1964].

labeled small lymphocytes at the outset, their number "showed a marked and progressive increase with culture times" [Osmond and Everett, 1964]. Harris and Kugler [1965] performed a similar experiment, except that it was a free suspension of labeled marrow cells that was injected into the peritoneum of an irridiated recipient, and removed 7½ hours later.

On the basis of their observations, Osmond and Everett [1964] concluded not only that there was active production of lymphocytes in the marrow, but also that "analysis of the labeling curves and grain counts indicates that the population of marrow lymphocytes is maintained in a dynamic steady state with an average turnover time of 3 days or less." Following these studies, Craddock [1965] reported the extensive formation of lymphocytes in the bone marrow of the rat, as did Everett and Caffrey [1967].

Osmond et al [1973], in a further study of guinea pig bone marrow, concluded that "the observed rate of cell production by proliferating lymphoid cells" (ie, transitional cells) "considerably exceeded the requirements for renewal of small lymphocytes." The proliferation over and above what is needed for small lymphocyte production is presumably required for differentiation into other blood cells. In the case of the mouse, Miller and Osmond [1974, 1975] confirmed the high proliferative activity of the transitional cell compartment, and also drew attention to the fall in this activity in older animals.

Quantitative Data

The scale of lymphocyte production in the bone marrow is readily appreciated if a comparison is made with the thoracic duct lymphocyte output, and the number of lymphocytes in the circulation. Table XII.1 presents these data for the standard guinea pig. For every lymphocyte

TABLE XII.1. Comparative Data on Lymphocytes in Bone Marrow, Blood, and Thoracic Duct Lymph (400 g Guinea Pig)

Thoracic duct lymphocyte output in 24 h[a]	373×10^6
Total blood lymphocytes[b]	131×10^6
Total marrow lymphocytes[c]	$2,670 \times 10^6$

[a]Based on the findings of Yoffey et al [1958].
[b]Yoffey [1966].
[c]Based on the data of Hudson et al [1963] and Hudson [1958].

present in the blood, three are daily entering the bloodstream via the thoracic duct, and 20 are present in the marrow. Allowances must of course be made for species' differences, which have been discussed elsewhere [Yoffey and Courtice, 1970]. The data of Osmond and Everett [1964] indicate a turnover time for marrow lymphocytes of about 3 days, which means that the daily production is about six times the normal blood lymphocyte population. There is no evidence to indicate lymphocyte destruction in the marrow to any marked extent, so that large numbers must constantly be discharged into the bloodstream.

The Short Production Pathway

From a consideration of the size spectrum in the transitional cell compartment [Patinkin et al, 1979] it is clear that, at the most, there are only three mitoses in the course of marrow lymphocyte production. This is on the assumption that lymphocyte production starts with the large transitional cell, as has been suggested for B lymphocytes on immunological grounds [eg, Owen et al, 1977]. There would then be three mitoses, as compared with the long production pathway of 6–8 mitoses in thymus or lymph node [Yoffey and Courtice, 1970]. The existence of the short production pathway for marrow lymphocytes should result in less dilution of label, and therefore heavier labeling, in autoradiographic studies of marrow lymphocytes when compared with thymocytes. Everett and Caffrey [1967] emphasized that bone marrow lymphocytes labeled more heavily than thymocytes, and for this reason they thought it unlikely that there was extensive migration of thymocytes to the marrow. However, a certain amount of migration of thymocytes to the marrow does occur, and may subserve important functions [cf Rosse, 1972a].

Lymphocyte Populations With Different Turnover Times

Though the majority of marrow lymphocytes are a rapidly renewing population, this does not apply to all. There are differences in turnover times, as has been emphasized by Rosse [1971b], who performed two main groups of experiments.

In one group, a daily injection of ^{3}H-thymidine was given to guinea pigs for 10 days. This procedure labels rapidly proliferating cells, as well as a smaller proportion of cells with a slow rate of turnover. After the injections have been completed, the concentration of ^{3}H-thymidine undergoes progressive reduction with each division of the proliferating cells, until finally it is too weak to be detected by autoradiography. Provided isotope reutilization can be excluded, labeled cells must have been formed during the period of thymidine administration and persisted until the time of sampling.

In another group of experiments, ^{3}H-thymidine was injected every 4 hours for periods up to 4 days. This injection schedule should label all cells entering into DNA synthesis during the injection period, and afforded an interesting contrast to the first group. In the marrow of the guinea pigs receiving daily injections for 14 days, the only unlabeled cells were reticular, endothelial and plasma cells, some damaged cells, and 14.1% of small lymphocytes. Six weeks after receiving the injections, 7% of marrow lymphocytes remained labeled. Conversely, in guinea pigs injected four times hourly for 4 days, 14.4% of small lymphocytes remained unlabeled.

Rosse [1971b] therefore concluded that in the bone marrow of the guinea pig 86% of the lymphocytes have a short life-span and rapid turnover, whereas 14% turn over more slowly, and 7% have a life-span exceeding 4 weeks. The same general conclusion was reached by Haas et al [1971], working with rats. They used an injection schedule [Fliedner et al, 1968] which started with the pregnant mother, so that growing fetal cells were labeled in utero, while in addition the administration of ^{3}H-thymidine was continued for 26 days after birth, at which time the thymidine administration was discontinued. Four weeks later, a small number of marrow lymphocytes were still labeled. Both in these experiments and in those of Rosse [1971b] an unknown number of the labeled lymphocytes may have been hematogenous, belonging to the recirculating lymphocyte pool. But whatever the numbers of these latter, the evidence seems clear that most of the marrow lymphocytes turn over rapidly and are derived from transitional cells.

Labeling of Lymphocytes In Situ

Everett and Caffrey [1967] showed that transitional cells, and subsequently small lymphocytes, could be labeled in situ by the direct injection of ^{3}H-thymidine into the marrow whose circulation had been temporarily occluded. When the occlusion was released, the labeled cells left the marrow, and 48 hours later were identified in autoradiographs of blood, spleen, and unoccluded marrow. Brahim and Osmond [1970] noted that lymphocytes, thus labeled in the occluded marrow, were subsequently found, for the most part, in the blood, mesenteric lymph node, and spleen. A small number of labeled lymphocytes (1:5,000) were also seen in thoracic duct lymph.

In the case of the rat, later experiments [Howard, 1972; Howard et al, 1972] seemed to indicate that some B (marrow-derived) lymphocytes join the long-lived recirculating cells found in thoracic duct lymph. During prolonged thoracic duct drainage, it is possible that a considerably greater number of marrow lymphocytes than usual may find their way into thoracic duct lymph, for the marrow lymphocytes then fall quite sharply (rat: Yoffey et al [1964]; guinea pig: Dineen and Adams [1970]), though the transitional cells do not. In fact, in the rat experiments the transitional cells in the marrow actually increased during the period of thoracic duct drainage.

UPTAKE OF CELLS BY THE MARROW

The experiments of Osmond and Everett [1964], in which the circulation to one limb was occluded, while ^{3}H-thymidine had free access to the other, showed that when the occlusion was released, a small but definite number of labeled lymphocytes found their way from the bloodstream into the previously occluded marrow. In ultrastructural studies of guinea pig marrow, Hudson and Yoffey [1966] discussed ways in which the entry of lymphocytes into the marrow might occur. The passage of lymphocytes from the blood into the marrow presumably would be most likely to occur in temporarily stagnant sinusoids [Branemark, 1959, 1961]. The observations of Keiser et al [1964, 1967] indicated that in the dog a larger number of lymphocytes than in the guinea pig might be entering the marrow from the bloodstream.

Rosse [1972a] demonstrated the uptake of lymphocytes by the marrow by the technique of parabiosis:

> Guinea pigs in which cells with long lifespan were selectively labeled were joined in parabiosis to non-labeled syngeneic litter-mates at a time when label reutilization detectable by autoradi-ograph could be excluded. Of all cells with a slow rate of turnover and long life span, only small lymphocytes entered the circula-tion and crossed the anastomosis in detectable numbers. . . . The presence of a minor population of lymphocytes with a long lifespan was confirmed in the marrow. Ten to 30 times as many lymphocytes migrated into the bone marrow of initially unla-beled animals as were found in an equal volume of blood. The majority, if not all long-lived lymphocytes migrate to the marrow from the blood and they also reenter the blood.

Ropke and Everett [1947a] performed parabiotic experiments in mice, and here too they demonstrated the entry of lymphocytes into the marrow from the bloodstream. Ropke et al [1975] found long-lived T and B lympho-cytes in murine bone marrow, as well as part of the recirculating pool.

The entry of T lymphocytes into the marrow may have hematological significance in view of recent studies. Goodman and her associates have repeatedly emphasized the role of thymic cells in hemopoiesis, and bone marrow growth [Goodman and Shinpock, 1968; Goodman et al, 1979, 1979]. Shinpock and Goodman [1978] assigned to thymic lymphocytes the ability to influence the kinetics of colony-forming units in radiation chimeras. These experiments have acquired added interest in view of studies of erythroid colony formation in vitro, involving T cells in the process [Nathan et al, 1978; Reid et al, 1981; Sawada and Adler, 1981]. An association of small lymphocytes with erythropoiesis was reported by Ben-Ishay and Yoffey [1971a,b], when studying the changes in erythroblastic islands during hypoxia. During the first few hours of hypoxia some lymphocytes were to be found close to or in the erythroblastic islands. But it was not possible to ascertain whether this was a random movement, or whether any specific type of lymphocyte was involved.

B-LYMPHOCYTE FORMATION

A full account of the formation of B lymphocytes in the marrow from transitional cells is beyond the scope of this volume. In the immunological literature B lymphocytes are frequently described as originating in "B-cell precursors," another of the many synonyms for transitional cells.

The formation of small lymphocytes in the marrow is not in itself evidence of B-cell formation, for which one needs to demonstrate the presence of immunoglobulins. Unanue et al [1971] first drew attention to the bone marrow as a source of B cells in mice that had been thymectomized, lethally irradiated, and transfused with a suspension of marrow cells.

Basten et al [1972a,b] separated transitional cells from B cells by passage through a specially designed column. They thus obtained enrichment of the precursor cells, which appeared to be colony-forming units—ie, transitional cells—which could give rise to B lymphocytes. Lafleur et al [1972] removed B cells from a marrow suspension by velocity sedimentation, and then injected the remainder of the suspension, containing the larger and lighter precursor cells, into irradiated animals. The precursor cells began to produce detectable numbers of B cells within 3 days after transplantation. B-cell activity then increased with a doubling time of 24 hours, again pointing to the transitional cells as the precursors, since there are no other cells in the marrow that can meet this situation.

The formation of the B lymphocytes involved changes in two directions. The first is a reduction in size, the result of one or two divisions. The second is the development of various surface receptors, including IgM [reviewed eg by Osmond, 1975, 1980; Ryser and Vassalli, 1974; Rosse, 1976; Cooper,

1981]. These changes can take several days, and the final maturation may occur outside the marrow, notably in the spleen [Rosse et al, 1978]. Osmond and Nossal [1974a,b] and Ryser and Vassalli [1974] showed that cells with surface IgM (sIgM+) were derived from sIgM− cells in the marrow and fetal liver. Raff et al [1976] postulated the appearance of heavy chains in the cytoplasm before the B-cell precursors became sIgM+. The initial formation of heavy chains in the cytoplasm was subsequently emphasized by Burrows et al [1979] and by Levitt and Cooper [1980].

On the question of size changes, Owen et al [1977] described, in murine marrow, a pool of large, rapidly proliferating cIgM+ cells which gave rise to smaller cIgM+ cells, and these in turn expressed surface IgM (sIgM+). Gathings et al [1977] reported the presence of pre–B cells in the marrow of 13-week-old fetuses, a stage when transitional cells are conspicuously present [Yoffey et al, 1961]. They noted further that the pre–B cells could be either large or small, and that the larger pre–B cells divided at a very rapid rate, with a labeling index as high as 90%. This recalls the finding by Miller et al [1978], in murine marrow, of a labeling index approaching 100% in the larger transitional ("lymphoid") cells. Okos and Gathings [1977] comment on the marked size spectrum in the transitional ("pre-B") cell compartment. Lau et al [1979] also emphasize the size variations in adult "pre-B" cells in the marrow. All these observations point to the transitional cells as the only possible B-cell precursors, since there are no other cells in the marrow with these size and kinetic properties.

T-LYMPHOCYTE PRECURSORS

Several lines of evidence [reviewed by Yoffey, 1981] indicate that the marrow supplies stem cells which migrate to the thymus and in the thymic environment undergo their specific differentiation [Jordan and Robinson, 1981]. Kaplan and Brown [1952] showed that marrow shielding in mice during systemic irradiation not only conferred hemopoietic protection, but also promoted regeneration of thymus and lymph nodes. In guinea pigs, Osmond et al [1966] also reported a beneficial effect on thymic regeneration of thigh-shielding during sublethal irradiation. That migrating cells were involved was demonstrated by the use of chromosome markers, when it was shown that grafted thymuses soon became repopulated with host cells [Metcalf and Wakonig-Vaartaja, 1964; Dukor et al, 1965; Koller et al, 1967]. Schlesinger and Hurvitz [1968] arrived at the same conclusion on the basis of immunological differences between host and donor. Komuro et al [1975] followed up these immunological observations by showing that a suspension of splenic cells—hemopoietic in the mouse—could also repopulate the thymus.

Another line of approach has been to show that bone marrow cells can develop T-cell antigens in vitro [eg, Komuro and Boyse, 1973; Cohen and Patterson, 1975], though it must be noted that even pluripotential stem cells express thy-1 antigen [Hunt, 1979; Goldschneider et al, 1980]. Rosse and Press [1978] reviewed the earlier work, and summarized their own experiments, from which they concluded that T cells develop from uncommitted transitional cells. This fits in with various observations that the T-cell precursors are larger and less dense than the mature T cells, which are pachychromatic small lymphocytes.

We do not have quantitative data on the production of T-cell precursors, but it is probable that the number is not large since on reaching the thymus they enter into the long production pathway of eight mitoses [Yoffey and Courtice, 1970]. On this basis one precursor cell should give rise to over 200 mature T cells. Micklem et al [1975] endeavored to give a more precise assessment of the number of marrow-derived precursors required by the thymus. In a study of the repopulation of the thymus in irradiated mice, Kadish and Basch [1975] have reemphasized the small number of progenitors required to effect this repopulation.

NATURAL KILLER CELLS: "LARGE GRANULAR LYMPHOCYTES"

The existence in the bone marrow of a hitherto unrecognized cell type, with what appears to be a fundamentally important biological role, is one of the intriguing hematological discoveries of recent years. The cell has been described as a "large granular lymphocyte" containing azarophilic granules (LGL) [reviewed by Herberman, 1981]. The work of Bennett [1973] pointed to the presence of such cells in the marrow by making use of the uptake of ^{89}Sr, which destroys the marrow cells, while the immunohemopoietic cells of the spleen still function. Since these mice were unable to reject marrow allografts, it was concluded that a distinctive group of marrow cells was responsible for the rejection.

Haller and Wigzell [1977] confirmed and extended this finding, again making use of the bone-seeking properties of ^{89}Sr and the associated marrow destruction. They arrived at the same basic conclusion, that natural killer (NK) cells were distinguished from other killer cells by their selective sensitivity to ^{89}Sr, indicating that a functioning bone marrow was needed for their generation and maintenance.

Timonen et al [1981] devised a technique for obtaining highly enriched (over 90%) populations of large granular lymphocytes, thereby greatly facilitating their study. According to Herberman [1981], NK cells are 2.5% of human and rat peripheral blood leukocytes, and they have been found in the blood of most other species. Morphologically, LGL often seem to have marked nuclear indentations, and to be monocytoid in appearance [Timonen et al, 1979]. The presence of azurophilic granules in some lymphocytes was described as far back as 1902 by Michaelis and Wolff. Because of the association of these granules with NK cells they have become the subject of more detailed study. Grossi et al [1982] identify the granules as primary lysosomes, and emphasize that LGL in some ways resemble monocytes. However, they are not phagocytic.

Miller [1982] has recently reported the results of kinetic studies in the mouse. Repeated administration of hydroxyurea eliminated newly formed lymphoid cells in spleen and marrow. After the first hydroxyurea injection, the NK activity of femoral marrow was not affected for 10.5 hours, the time taken, presumably, for the DNA-synthesizing precursor to become an NK cell. "This was followed by an exponential decline with $T_{1/2}$ pf 7.9 hours, indicative of rapid exponential renewal of NK cells in the marrow." Thus, though the NK cells themselves are not in cell cycle, they appear to be the product of rapidly dividing precursors in the marrow. Although these rapidly renewing NK precursor cells have not yet been identified, the transitional cell compartment would appear to be their most likely source. According to Miller [1982], NK cells leave the marrow randomly, and an unknown number enter the spleen, from which they also depart after a short time ($T_{1/2} = 24.8$ h). Their subsequent life history is obscure.

NULL CELLS

The so-called "null" cells are a heterogeneous group. Almost half the small lymphocytes in murine bone marrow do not possess surface markers that would identify them as B or T cells [Osmond and Nossal, 1974a], though many of these are newly formed immature B lymphocytes which sooner or later develop surface IgM [Osmond and Nossal, 1974b; Ryser and Vassalli, 1974]. However, there appears to be a residue of null cells whose identity is still in doubt.

One possibility to be borne in mind is that some of these null cells are the small nonproliferating stem cells which, as already noted, are much less leptochromatic than the typical transitional cell, and come close in morphology to the pachychromatic small lymphocyte. This interpretation is in agreement with the view put forward by Hoelzer et al [1975], who suggested that "the nonproliferating dormant form" (of the stem cell) "can have the morphological appearance of small lymphocytes, which enlarge to become transitional cells capable of self-replication."

XIII.

Transitional (Stem) Cell Compartment

INTRODUCTION

From the evidence that has been steadily accumulating during the past two decades, it is clear that the transitional cells (TC) constitute the stem cell compartment not only of bone marrow, but ultimately of the lympho-myeloid complex as a whole. As new facts have emerged concerning the kinetic and other properties of transitional cells, they have been the subject of continuous review and reappraisal [Yoffey, 1957; Osmond and Everett, 1964; Yoffey and Courtice, 1970; Rosse and Yoffey, 1967a,b; Harris, 1956; Harris et al, 1963; Osmond et al, 1973; Thomas et al, 1977; Osmond, 1975; Rosse, 1976].

Transitional cells are a heterogeneous group of cells whose primary habitat is the bone marrow, where most of them are to be found. In smaller laboratory animals such as the mouse, transitional cells are present in the spleen, though it is possible that these may be of secondary importance in relation to similar cells in the marrow [Kretchmar and Conover,

1970; Silini et al, 1976]. Transitional cells are to be found in varying numbers in the bloodstream, and throughout the lymphomyeloid complex, including the serous cavities and connective tissues. The problem of migrating stem cells is discussed in Chapter VIII.

Some of the basic properties of transitional cells were first described by Osmond and Everett [1964], who were the first to demonstrate the active production of lymphocytes in the bone marrow [cf Harris and Kugler, 1965]. Three recent reviews [Rosse, 1976; Osmond, 1980; Yoffey, 1980] have dealt in detail with various aspects of the structure and properties of the transitional cell compartment. The present account will therefore deal briefly with some of its more salient features. The recognition of the stem cell role of the transitional cell compartment has been greatly aided by the fact that other classical contenders for the role of stem cell, notably the ill-defined reticulum cell, possessed neither the kinetics nor the migratory properties we now know stem cells to possess.

Our understanding of the transitional cell compartment has been greatly hindered by a number of factors, one of which has been confused terminology. The very name "transitional," though it now turns out to be singularly appropriate, was in fact originally given in error by Yoffey [1957]. Transitional cells were at first thought to be intermediate stages in the formation of blast cells from small lymphocytes entering the marrow from the bloodstream, and because of this they were for some time referred to as "transitional lymphocytes." Despite this initial error the name has been retained, since the compartment contains an inordinately large number of transitions linking together an apparently heterogeneous cell population which, by virtue of these transitions, functions as an integrated cell group. The most obvious transitions are in size, nuclear structure, DNA synthesis, and cytoplasmic basophilia.

Of the many other names given to transitional cells, the commonest is "lymphoid." This is a term that is sometimes useful in describing transitional cells and lymphocytes together in contradistinction to myeloid and erythroid cells. But it should be used with caution, since "lymphoid" cells are found throughout the lymphomyeloid complex, in situations where there are few or no transitional cells. The position is further complicated by the fact that some of the smallest transitional cells, in a kinetically resting state, are prone to be confused with lymphocytes [Rosse, 1972b; Haas et al, 1973; Hoelzer et al, 1975].

MORPHOLOGY OF TRANSITIONAL CELLS
High N:C Ratio

One feature common to all transitional cells is the high ratio of nucleus (N) to cytoplasm (C). In air-dried, Romanowsky-stained smears this high

N:C ratio tends to be accentuated, and the cytoplasmic shrinkage may give the cytoplasm the appearance of a tuft at one pole of the cell. This polar cytoplasm is not as a rule seen in ultramicroscopic preparations, where there is much less shrinkage, so that even though the N:C ratio is still high, there is usually a complete rim of cytoplasm surrounding the nucleus (Fig. XIII.1).

Size Spectrum

Transitional cells show a spectrum of sizes, ranging from the small transitional, around 7–8 μm in diameter, to the larger transitional cells 12 μm in diameter. In earlier studies, most of the measurements were made in smears, and although measurements of cell or nuclear size in smears can only be approximate, they have proved extremely useful in autoradiographic studies with the light microscope [Yoffey et al, 1965; Rosse and Yoffey, 1967; Osmond, 1967; Moffatt et al, 1967; Keiser et al, 1967; Rosse, 1973]. More recently large numbers of transitional cells—together with small lympho-cytes—have been measured in a coulter counter [Yoffey et al, 1978; Patinkin et al, 1979]. For this purpose it was necessary to obtain populations of these cells in as pure a state as possible, free from contamination by other cells. As the starting point, guinea pigs were used between 7 and 10 days of rebound (Chapter X), after 7 days of hypoxia at 0.5 atm. The marrow in these animals contains not only greatly increased numbers of transitional cells and lymphocytes, but also markedly diminished numbers of nucleated erythroid cells, and a trend toward diminished production of myeloid cells. Passage of rebound marrow through Ficoll and albumin density gradients reduces to two or three the number of components to be measured in each fraction, in which the size distribution can then be easily analyzed.

Four peaks were obtained in all. Peak 1 was a population of small cells (volume 53–59 fl) composed mainly of pachychromatic small lymphocytes with a few slightly larger cells. Peak 2 was a population of somewhat larger cells (volume 154–160 fl), consisting of small transitional cells with little or no cytoplasm. Peak 3 was a population of still larger cells (volume 200–218 fl), consisting entirely of medium to large transitional cells with a large leptochromatic nucleus, and clearly visible pale to basophilic cytoplasm. These cells were found exclusively in the lighter-density fractions of 17% and 19% albumin. Peak 4 was a population of very large transitional cells (volume 350–400 fl) with a large leptochromatic nucleus, and relatively more, and usually much more, basophilic cytoplasm. These cells were somewhat inconstant, and their numbers were smaller than those in the other peaks. From these measurements it appears that there are three main size groups in the TC compartment (Fig. XIII.2), so that presumably two

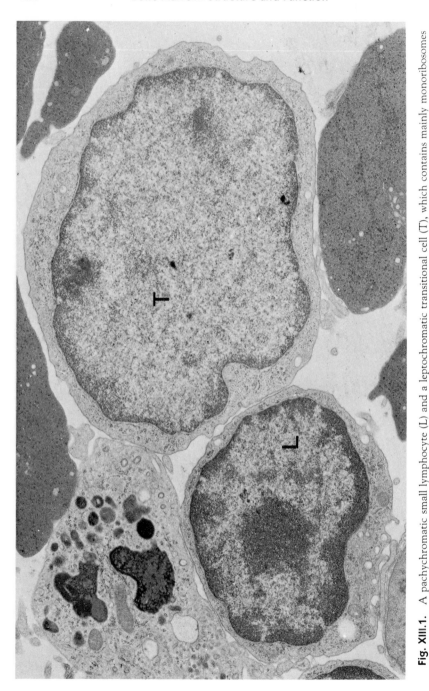

Fig. XIII.1. A pachychromatic small lymphocyte (L) and a leptochromatic transitional cell (T), which contains mainly monoribosomes and corresponds to the pale transitional cell of light microscopy. Some transitionals contain mainly polyribosomes, and these are the basophilic cells. The small lymphocyte has a characteristic condensation of chromatin at the nuclear membrane. [Adapted from Yoffey and Weinberg, 1976.] ×7,500.

proliferative cycles are possible, namely between small and medium, and between medium and large transitional cells.

The cycle between the small and medium transitional cells would increase the number of cells at the smaller end of the compartment, whereas that between the medium and large cells would increase the larger cells. The cycling between small, medium, and large transitional cells results in a continuous spectrum of cell sizes. In guinea pig marrow, Yoffey et al [1965] have illustrated the continuous size spectrum both of unlabeled transitional cells [Figs. 1–13, Yoffey et al, 1965] and of cells labeled with tritiated thymidine [Fig. 25, Yoffey et al, 1965], as have also Osmond [1967] and Osmond et al [1973]. Illustrations in color have been published by Harris and Kugler [1963], Rosse and Yoffey [1967], and Rosse [1970b]. Everett and Caffrey [1967] illustrated TC in rat marrow [cf Morrison, 1967], and Sharp et al [1976] and Riches et al [1976] have illustrated TC in murine marrow. Electron micrographs (TEM) are also available: guinea pigs [Bainton and Yoffey, 1970], rats [Ben-Ishay and Yoffey, 1972], mice [Yoffey and Weinberg, 1976], and mouse, monkey, and man [Dicke et al, 1973].

Nuclear Structure

The nuclei of transitional cells show varying degrees of leptochromasia, most marked in the larger cells, least so in the smaller cells. The leptochromatic TC nucleus is in sharp contrast to the pachychromatic nucleus of the small lymphocyte (Fig. XIII.1). The nuclear membrane of the transitional cell is thin, contrasting with the juxtamembranous condensation of chromatin in the small lymphocyte. The interior of the TC nucleus is less dense than that of the small lymphocyte, and has a higher proportion of parachromatin. The one or two nucleoli in the TC are usually pale, without the thick coating of nucleolar-associated DNA found in the lymphocyte. TC

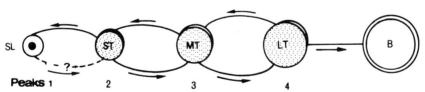

Fig. XIII.2. There are three basic groups in the transitional cell compartment—large (LT), medium (MT), and small (ST) transitionals. Self-maintenance can be effected by cycling by small and medium, or medium and large transitionals. (--?--) indicates the possible reentry of a small subgroup of uncommitted small lymphocytes (SL) into the transitional cell compartment. Lymphocyte production occurs through the short production pathway, involving two or three mitoses. [Modified from Yoffey et al, 1978.]

nuclei frequently posess deep indentations. The significance of these indentations is unknown, though one may speculate that as they increase the
surface of the nuclear membrane, they may perhaps be an indication of
increased nuclear and cellular activities. Rosse [1971b] observed that, in
cultures of bone marrow, the nucleus of the living transitional cells was
"very active, even in stationary cells, showing a marked streaming of nuclear
material and deep invaginations of the nuclear membrane."

Cytoplasmic Basophilia

By light microscopy after the customary hematological stains the cytoplasm of transitional cells shows varying degrees of basophilia, ranging from
pale to intensely basophilic [Yoffey et al, 1965; Rosse and Yoffey, 1967b;
Jones et al, 1967; Osmond et al, 1973]. In TEM one sees varying numbers
of monoribosomes and polyribosomes. Cells containing predominantly
monoribosomes would no doubt be the pale cells of light microscopy, whereas those with many polyribosomes would correspond to the basophilic cells.
There seems to be some degree of correlation between basophilia and cell
size, since as a rule there appear to be more pale cells among the small, and
more basophilic cells among the large ones.

Apart from the degree of basophilia, there appears to be relatively more
cytoplasm in the pale than in the basophilic cells, so that even in air-dried
smears the pale TC may have a complete rim of cytoplasm. Though many
of the pale transitionals are in Go [Rosse, 1970a], they are nonetheless
capable of some proliferation [Moffatt et al, 1967; Miller and Osmond,
1973].

The basophilic transitionals merge through a continuous series of intermediate stages with the various blast cells, the most numerous of which are
the proerythroblasts and myeloblasts. Whereas some transitionals have only
a small tuft of basophilic cytoplasm, one also finds a whole series of cells
with progressively increasing amounts of cytoplasm, and at the stage when
there is enough basophilic cytoplasm to surround the nucleus, the cell is
regarded as a fully formed blast cell; but the classification of the stages
between the basophilic transitional and the fully formed blast cell presents
a problem on both light and electron microscopy. For purposes of light
microscopy classification, cells have been arbitrarily regarded as transitional
if the cytoplasm extends up to half-way round the nucleus, and as blast cells
if it extends more than half-way. Though this classification is not precise, it
has been found to be of some use in assessing marrow reactions.

The more intensely basophilic transitionals tend to be more numerous
among the larger members of the group. Thus in the 10-μm + size group in

normal guinea pig marrow, over 50% were recorded as basophilic, whereas about 20% were intermediate and 25% were pale [Moffatt et al, 1967; Jones et al, 1967].

The Proliferation Gradient: DNA Synthesis

The kinetics of the TC compartment are complex. One of the most striking features is the *proliferation gradient*, by which is meant the gradual increase in the labeling index from the small to the large transitionals (Fig. XIII.3). The gradient is a fundamental property of the compartment. It seems to involve at least three known factors—cytoplasmic basophilia, nuclear size, and length of the S phase. As to nuclear diameter, in general

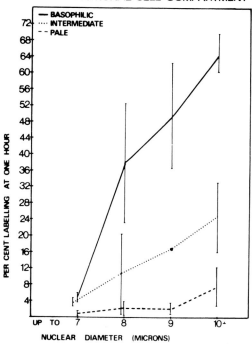

Fig. XIII.3. The cells of the transitional cell compartment (guinea pig) exhibit a characteristic proliferation gradient 1 hour after in vivo labeling of bone marrow cells with tritiated thymidine. The highest labeling index is to be found in the basophilic transitionals, the lowest in the pale cells. The cells with intermediate degrees of basophilia are between these two groups. In all three groups, the larger cells have a considerably higher labeling index than the small ones. [Redrawn from the data of Moffatt et al, 1967.]

the larger the cell, the higher the labeling index. The difference is most marked in the basophilic group, in which the figures for the labeling percentages are $\leqslant 7$ μm, 4.9%; $\leqslant 8$ μm 38.2%; $\leqslant 9$ μm, 49.5%; $\leqslant 10$ μm+, 65.4%. In the pale group the index was very much lower: $\leqslant 7$ μm, 1.4%; $\leqslant 8\mu$m, 2.4%; $\leqslant 9$ μm, 2.2%; $\leqslant 10$ μm+, 7.7%. For the group with intermediate degrees of basophilia the figures were $\leqslant 7$ μm, 3.6%; $\leqslant 8$ μm, 10.9%; $\leqslant 9$ μm, 17.5%; $\leqslant 10$ μm+, 25.2% [Moffatt et al, 1967]. Another noteworthy feature in the transitional cell compartment is the variation in the duration of the S phase, which according to Miller and Osmond [1973] is 3.5 hours in the largest transitionals with a cell cycle of 6.4 hours, whereas in the smaller transitionals S phase is 10.9 hours. The pale transitionals could be regarded as the resting phase of the stem cell population, and this view seems to be supported by the work of Rosse [1970a], who noted that many pale transitionals could be out of cycle for several days [cf Osmond et al, 1973]. This observation fits in well with the view emerging from CFU-S studies, that an appreciable number of pluripotential stem cells are in a resting, nonproliferative state. But it must be borne in mind that similar considerations could also apply to the small basophilic transitionals, since they too have a low labeling index. Whichever resting cells are concerned, whether pale or basophilic, the entry of a small number of nonproliferating stem cells into a highly proliferative state could provide an obvious amplifying mechanism if increased numbers of stem cells are required. From a consideration of the proliferation gradient, it would appear that the change from the nonproliferating to the proliferating state must be accompanied by cell enlargement and an increase in the labeling index. Both these changes occur in conditions of increased marrow activity.

In view of the fundamental importance of the cells forming the stem cell compartment, repeated efforts have been made to develop techniques for their more precise analysis, and among these we may briefly note the following. A physical technique to separate the large from the small cells is the *velocity-sedimentation test* [Peterson and Evans, 1967; Miller and Phillips, 1969]. This technique depends on the simple fact that large cells sediment more rapidly than small ones, from which it follows that changes in the sedimentation velocity indicate changes in cell size. Furthermore, by separating small cells from large one can compare their kinetic and other properties. Another test depends on killing cells in DNA synthesis, leaving behind the cells that are not in S phase. This can be done by exposing the cells to high-specific-activity thymidine, which is incorporated into the duplicating DNA (the so-called thymidine suicide test) or by substances such as hydroxyurea. Selective destruction of cells in DNA synthesis would obviously result in the death of many more large than small cells, leaving an enriched population of small cells.

An important adjunct to separation techniques has been the discontinuous albumin density gradient technique [eg, Murphy et al, 1971; Dicke et al, 1973]. The last-named authors described, following the use of this technique, a "new and dominant cell type" which is in fact a typical transitional cell. More recently the fluorescence-activated cell sorter has been used to obtain greatly enriched populations of pluripotent hemopoietic stem cells [Goldschneider et al, 1980], and these too appear to be transitional cells. Their Figure 7a, p 427, is an electron micrograph of a transitional cell with many monoribosomes and a few mitochondria. Immunological techniques have also been employed to an increasing extent, since Golub [1972] noted that hemopoietic stem cells and brain tissue shared a common antigen.

TRANSITIONAL CELLS AND COLONY-FORMING UNITS

In the earlier studies on colony-forming units, investigators paid little or no attention to the morphology of the cells. Various stem cell models were devised, starting usually with an unknown stem cell "not known to possess characteristic morphological features." However, a number of workers have since tried to identify the colony-forming units, notably CFU-S and CFU-GM, and have found them to possess typical transitional cell morphology.

The earlier studies were performed mainly in the mouse, by means of the spleen-colony technique. Following the work of Turner et al [1967] and Hurst et al [1969], Murphy et al [1971] further investigated changes in murine bone marrow during rebound. After 3 days of rebound, marrows were treated by density gradient centrifugation. They found that 80–95% of a light-density fraction was composed of mononuclear cells that had a typical transitional cell structure. A suspension of these cells was injected directly into the spleen of mice that had received a lethal dose of irradiation 48 hours previously. The animals were killed at times ranging from 15 min to 8 days later. The injected cells developed into typical spleen colonies, containing varying numbers of erythrocytes, granulocytes, and megakaryocytes.

De Gowin et al [1972] and De Gowin and Gibson [1976] performed some interesting experiments in which they used the endocolonization technique. Except for one leg, which was shielded, mice were given whole-body irradiation (850 rads). Three hours later the shielded leg was also irradiated with 850 rads. During these 3 hours a number of stem cells migrated from the shielded marrow to the spleen, in which their subsequent development could be followed. Over the next 3–4 days, while the migrating stem cells proliferated and differentiated in the spleen, tritiated thymidine was injected intravenously and the spleen was examined in two stages. One hour after the thymidine injection, a portion of the spleen was removed and was found to contain heavily labeled mononuclear cells resembling "medium to large leptochromatic lymphocytes." These "leptochromatic lymphocytes" exhibited all the characteristics of transitional cells, including the size spectrum, leptochromatic nucleus, and high labeling properties. When the remainder of the spleen was removed 24–48 hours later, it was found to contain lightly labeled erythroblasts and myeloid cells. Still more labeled erythroblasts and myeloid cells were found on days 5 and 6, as were "lymphoid" cells. Grain counts suggested that about four divisions occurred during the formation of erythrocytes from transitional cells, and 2–3 during granulocyte formation.

Another approach to identifying the relationship between transitional cells and colony-forming units was employed by Riches et al [1976a,b] and Thomas et al [1977]. They administered mustine hydrochloride to mice, folowing which the nucleated cell content of the marrow fell to 20% of control values, whereas the CFU-S at first were depressed to 10% of control values and rose sharply to 60% on day 4. From day 5 onward there was evidence of varying degrees of marrow regeneration. The marrow on day 4, greatly enriched in transitional cells, also contained a correspondingly greater number of CFU-S. The transitional cells are sometimes referred to as such, sometimes as "leptochromatic mononuclear cells." The illustrations, including the autoradiographs, are of typical transitional cells.

Transitional Cell Enrichment

The experiments just cited are but some of many examples of transitional cell enrichment. A variety of techniques to obtain greatly enriched populations of transitional cells have made it possible to investigate their stem cell role with much greater ease and certainty than when they are only a small fraction of a large population. The experiments of Thomas et al [1977] are an excellent example of enrichment in vivo, contrasting with many experiments in which enrichment has been obtained in vitro. Rebound marrow is an excellent starting point for enrichment techniques, since it already contains an appreciably higher percentage of transitional cells than does normal marrow.

Moore et al [1972] employed buoyant density gradient separation of rhesus monkey bone marrow, and obtained a light-density distribution profile of cells capable of forming colonies in agar culture (CFU-GM). High-resolution density gradient separation performed on a light-density fraction of bone marrow produced on average a 100-fold enrichment of the in vitro CFU-GM. The most enriched fractions contained the majority of the CFU-GM population present in the original marrow, and fractions were routinely obtained in which up to 23% of cells formed colonies. The thymidine suicide technique, combined with autoradiography and morphological studies, showed that the in vitro CFU-GM was a transitional cell—in their terminology, a "transitional lymphocyte," as illustrated in their Figure 4, p 290. They concluded that single cells could finally give rise to colonies containing both granulocytes and macrophages.

Dexter et al [1977] devised a technique in which they obtained the proliferation of both CFU-S and CFU-GM in vitro. Under the conditions prevailing in their culture system no lymphocytes developed. Their description in the text [p 40, Dexter et al, 1977] fits transitional cells. Daniels [1980], Tavassoli and Takahashi [1982], and subsequently others performed TEM studies of the cells in the same type of culture. Daniels's Figure 3, from a 7-day culture, shows a typical transitional cell with what appear to be monoribosomes.

In addition to these and other attempts to identify the colony-forming units morphologically, one frequently encounters kinetic changes in the colony-forming units which can only be accounted for on the basis of the identity of these units and transitional cells. A number of these changes are discussed in Chapter XIV. It must be emphasized, however, that though colony-forming units possess transitional cell morphology and have the kinetic properties of transitional cells, the reverse is not necessarily the case. Not all transitional cells are colony-forming units. A large number are already fully committed to specific lines of differentiation.

Rosse [1972b] made observations on living transitional cells from guinea pig marrow. He noted that some of the transitional cells divided into daughter cells, which then enlarged as transitional cells. This was in fact the first direct demonstration that the TC compartment was self-maintaining. He further noted that in many instances the daughter cells resulting from the division of the smaller transitionals gradually underwent a process of shrinkage and condensation over a period of 5–6 hours and then acquired the characteristic morphology of small lymphocytes [cf Osmond et al, 1973]. Rosse further tried to determine the cell cycle time of transitional cells by observing the distribution of labeled mitoses after a pulse label in vivo. Though there was some variation, for most cells the duration of the cell cycle in vitro was thought to be around 15 hours (G1, 5–6 h; S, 7–8 h; G2, ~ 1 h).

Kinetic Data

In view of the fundamental importance of the TC compartment, it would obviously be desirable to have full quantitative kinetic data both on the compartment as a whole and on the different types of cell, committed and uncommitted, which it contains. Unfortunately, the available data do not give us this information, though they do give a clear indication of great proliferative activity.

In the guinea pig, about 35% of transitional cells are in DNA synthesis in the normal steady state [Osmond and Everett, 1964]; in the rat, the figure is around 50% [Everett and Caffrey, 1967]. However, when increased numbers of stem cells are required, the labeling index of the compartment in the rat can rise from 50% to 70% [Yoffey and Yaffe, 1980]. In the mouse, Miller et al [1974] reported a labeling index of 60% of "lymphoid" (ie, transitional) cells at 4 weeks, 42% at 8 weeks, and 36% at 16 weeks. It is therefore clear that even in the normal steady state, transitional cells are a very actively proliferating group in all the species studies so far.

In addition to the age variation noted by Miller and Osmond [1974], there are considerable variations for which we cannot account. Thus, to take the 400-g guinea pig, Table IX.2 gives a count of around 50,000/μl TC in the normal animal. Moffatt et al [1967] give a different figure of 90,000, and Griffiths and Rieke [1960] report a count of 122,000/μl. The figure in Table IX.2 is the lowest TC count in an extensive series of investigations, and about 100,000 TC/μl of marrow is probably a more representative figure. Taking Osmond and Everett's [1964] figure of 35% for the labeling index of the compartment as a whole, and a generation time of around 12 hours, the TC compartment would come close to doubling every day provided no cells left the compartment. But as cells are continually differentiating and leaving the compartment, it does not double but just about meets its normal requirements, remaining more or less constant.

Obviously, if the smaller cells grow in size and move to the large end of the proliferation gradient, the TC compartment could increase much more rapidly. With an S period of 3½ hours [Osmond et al, 1973] and a cell cycle time of 12–15 hours [Rosse, 1971b], the TC population could markedly increase its rate of growth. In hypoxia, the labeling index of the large transitionals in rats rises to 80% [Yoffey and Yaffe, 1980].

The Transitional Cell Compartment as a Whole

There are two opposing processes at work in the transitional cell compartment (Fig. XIII.4). One process is the constant proliferation of the cells without any other change—ie, a process of self-maintenance which in itself would merely result in their continued increase. The other is the differentiation of its cells into lymphocytes and the various blast cells, a process which would have the opposite effect and diminish the number of cells in the compartment. The actual size of the compartment at any time reflects the dynamic equilibrium between these two processes. The factors that control the extent of transitional cell proliferation are not well understood.

Self-replication is at first sight an apparently simple process, in which large transitionals give rise to smaller ones, and these in turn enlarge. There appear in fact to be two possible proliferative cycles—between small and medium, and between medium and large transitionals. The speed with which the smaller cells enlarge, and the larger transitionals divide, determines the rate at which new stem cells are formed, and this rate can undergo considerable variation. Differentiation occurs in a number of directions, but in quantitative terms the three main pathways of differentiation are into proerythroblasts, myeloblasts, and lymphocytes. In the normal steady state it seems to be the larger transitionals that follow the erythropoietic or granulopoietic lines of development, via the stage of the basophilic blast cell. But in some experimental situations the transitionals may apparently undergo differentiation without going through the blast cell stage.

Increased Stem Cell Demands

In the normal steady state the transitional cell compartment can cope adequately with all stem cell requirements, and in fact there is a stem cell reserve, in the form of resting cells which can be stimulated to proliferate when there are increased stem cell demands. But this drawing on reserves

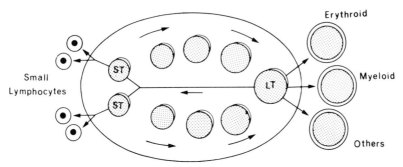

Fig. XIII.4. A scheme of the transitional compartment in bone marrow. The compartment is capable of self-maintenance and of differentiation, giving rise to the various groups of blood cells—mainly small lymphocytes, erythrocytes, and granulocytes. There is a spectrum of cell sizes in the compartment. Small lymphocytes, predominantly B cells, are formed by the division of small transitional cells. [From Yoffey, 1977.]

can keep pace with the demand only up to a point, beyond which the supply of stem cells ceases to be adequate for all requirements, and the production of one or more cell groups falls accordingly (Chapter VIII). This type of change can readily be investigated by means of varying degrees of hypoxia. As more and more stem cells are induced by the stimulus to differentiate along the erythropoietic pathway, not enough are left for granulocyte or lymphocyte production, both of which undergo diminution.

Heavy Fetal Demand for Stem Cells

The bone marrow of the human fetus is an interesting example of a marrow in which there is a physiologically high demand for stem cells. Transitional cells appear to be present in the bone marrow from the outset, and have been illustrated in photomicrographs [Yoffey et al, 1961, Fig. 1] from which it is evident that the size spectrum is clearly present in the bone marrow of a 15-week fetus. Lymphocytes and transitional cells average around 25% of the cells in fetal marrow (range 10–45%), and of these the transitionals constitute about 15%. These large numbers of TC are found during a period of several months when there is a sustained high demand for stem cells. One must attribute this primarily to the needs of red cell production. Between weeks 12 and 25 of gestation, the erythrocyte content per unit volume of blood is more than doubled, and the body weight increases 17-fold [Thomas and Yoffey, 1962]. If the increase in blood volume during this period of development is of the same order, then the circulating erythrocyte population will increase more than 30-fold.

This must be a conservative estimate, since it does not take into account the replacement of effete red cells, and in addition there is suggestive evidence that the mean red cell life is shorter during the early stages of development than in the adult [Mollison, 1947]. In the third trimester there is a further rapid increase in the number of erythrocytes per cubic millimeter of blood [Thomas and Yoffey, 1962]. From the data of Hudson [1965] it is clear that the available volume of bone marrow in relation to body weight is substantially less in the fetus than in the adult, and this must be a limiting factor in the capacity of the bone marrow to meet the great demand for red cells. The erythropoietic role of the liver is therefore essential during the fetal period to compensate for the temporary inadequacy of the marrow. But even with this hepatic assistance, the maximal level of red cell production is still required from the bone marrow, especially during the later stages of pregnancy, when hepatic hemopoiesis is being phased out in preparation for its postnatal metabolic activities. It is doubtless the high rate of erythropoiesis in the marrow which necessitates a large number of transitional cells to function as stem cells. This may apply to some extent also in the early postnatal period, when transitional cells constitute about 2% of the total nucleated cells for the first few months [Rosse et al, 1977]. The early postnatal period imposes on the bone marrow the added burden of increased B-lymphocyte and granulocyte production, when the infant is exposed to an external environment full of immunological stimuli.

Transitional cells constitute a mean of 4% of the nucleated cells in fetal marrow, and in some instances rise to nearly 7%. This is a high concentration of stem cells compared with adult marrow, and fetal marrow should therefore be a valuable source of these cells for transplantation purposes. A recent report indicates that this is in fact the case. Kelemen et al [1982] confirmed the earlier data of Yoffey et al [1961] on the high lymphoid cell content of fetal marrow, in which they identified both lymphocytes and "lymphocytelike" cells—ie, transitional cells. On the basis of histochemical studies they concluded that these "lymphocytelike" cells were not T cells. A successful transplant, in a case of aplastic anemia, consisted of 2.5 $\times$ 10^6 fetal marrow cells per kg body weight.

Once the adult stage is reached, so that in the normal steady state new red cells are required only to replace normal wear and tear, the need for stem cells becomes minimal, and because of their small numbers their identity has frequently been a matter of controversy. The enrichment technique of Dicke et al [1973] enabled them to identify a stem cell that was a typical transitional cell. Kempgens et al [1973] made a careful study of the transitional ("lymphoid") cells in the marrow of eight healthy adults, where they found them, though few, to resemble the transitional cells in the marrow from laboratory animals. In man they constituted 0.85% of the total marrow cells, and their overall labeling index with thymidine was 32.5%. They also noted that whereas the pale transitionals possessed only the diploid number of chromosomes, the basophilic had a range from diploid to tetraploid (see their Abb 2, p 438). In a later paper [Kempgens et al, 1976] they reported that in seven cases of renal anemia the transitional cell content of the marrow increased, ranging from 1.4% to 6.4% of the nucleated cells. Though the transitional cells were proliferating more slowly than in normal subjects, their numbers nevertheless increased, presumably because they were not differentiating into red cells.

This type of condition, in which there is an element of maturation arrest, is one in which transitional cells are particularly prone to accumulate. In drug-induced agranulocytosis [Pisciotta et al, 1964] there is a marked increase in transitional cells in the period during which they are not differentiating into granulocytes, but their numbers fall sharply during the recovery stage, when they begin to differentiate into granulocytes once more. Some cases of aplastic anemia, especially those of the hyperplastic type, may also have an element of maturation arrest. Rhoads and Miller [1938] compared the marrow, in those cases of aplastic anemia they considered to be due to maturation arrest, with the marrow in cases of agranulocytosis, and concluded that the two conditions had much in common. Boggs and Boggs [1976] interpret the pathogenesis of aplastic anemia in terms of a defective pluripotential stem cell and a disturbance of the normal dynamic equilibrium between self-replication and differentiation. Transitional cells ("Q cells" [Davidson et al, 1943]) also accumulate in the marrow in some types of refractory anemia [cf Tillman et al, 1976].

In general, it appears that the transitional cell content of human marrow, high in the fetus, is at its lowest in the healthy adult in the normal steady state, when it is also appreciably lower than the figures usually obtained in the small laboratory animals.

TERMINOLOGY

In view of the fundamental importance now attached to transitional cells, it has become increasingly desirable to resolve the growing confusion in terminology. No other cells in the marrow have been given so many different names. No other cells in the marrow have so often been rediscovered, redescribed, reillustrated, and renamed. Although, as already noted, the term "transitional" was originally introduced on the basis of a mistaken hypothesis, it still seems to have more in its favor than any other name, since it suggests both the morphological and kinetic attributes of a very distinctive cell group.

There is no doubt, when one surveys the hematological literature, that from the early days of hematology transitional cells have been repeatedly observed. But attention was usually focused on one or another cell type in the compartment, which consequently was not recognized as a whole, although some observers came near to doing so. Had these observers had at their disposal the more sophisticated techniques now employed for kinetic studies, the true state of affairs would long since have been understood. The problem was complicated not only by the great confusion in terminology, but also by the difficulty experienced in abandoning widely held but erroneous stem cell concepts, such as the origin of stem cells from reticulum cells or endothelium.

Naegeli's [1900, 1931] preoccupation with the myeloblast is a case in point. He could not find an origin for the myeloblast from mesenchymal cells, even in the embryo, where the myeloblast seemed to appear all of a sudden, in both blood and tissues, without any obvious precursor. His "micromyeloblast" [1931, Abb 67, cells 2 and 3] is a typical small transitional cell, which he would almost certainly have identified as the precursor of either small lymphocytes or larger myeloblasts, had tritiated thymidine been at his disposal. He automatically ruled out the formation of lymphocytes in the marrow since, following Ehrlich, he believed that lymphocytes had nothing to do with the marrow tissue proper, but were "extraparenchymatous"—a view adopted by the majority of hematologists for many years. All this is now hard to believe, just as it is equally difficult to believe that for many years the vast majority of hematologists considered the small lymphocyte to be quite incapable of growth.

Pappenheim [1907], in his description of large and small hematogones, also seems to have been dealing with transitional cells. At a later date [Pappenheim and Ferrata, 1910, and subsequent publications] the terminology was changed to "lymphoid cells" and "lymphoidocytes." Here, too, the concern was obviously with transitional cells, since the 1910 paper was based to a large extent on the bone marrow of guinea pigs, in which transitional cells are conspicuous. The "primitive" cells of Cunningham et al [1925] are also typical transitional cells, but like Naegeli they too refused to recognize lymphocytes as an integral part of the marrow. In addition, they derived the "primitive" cells from a somewhat ill-defined reticulum cell. Of the many other names given to transitional cells one may note: "Q" cells in the bone marrow of patients with refractory anemia [Davidson et al, 1943]; "lymphocytelike" cells [Burke and Harris, 1959; Harris, 1961; Cudkowicz et al, 1964b; Bennett and Cudkowicz, 1967]; "lymphoid" [Thomas et al, 1965; Osmond et al, 1973; Kempgens et al, 1973, 1976]; resting bone marrow lymphocyte [Hoelzer et al, 1975]; hematopoietic precursor cell [Murphy et al, 1971]; hemopoietic stem cell [Dicke et al, 1973]; "X" cell [Simar et al, 1968]; presumptive hematopoietic stem cell [Rubinstein and Trobaugh, 1973]; leptochromatic lymphocyte [De Gowin and Gibson, 1976]; leptochromatic mononuclear cell [Sharp et al, 1976; Riches et al, 1976]. Kincade [1981, Fig. 3] has illustrated a group of monoclonally selected "B-cell precursors" which are typical transitional cells with the characteristic size spectrum.

In recent ultramicroscopic studies, Morris et al [1975] described a transitional cell in cord blood as a "blastlike" cell [cf Faulk et al, 1973], Korbling et al [1979] illustrate a "canine hemopoietic blood stem cell" which has the morphology of a typical transitional cell with an indented nucleus and monoribosomes, and Meer et al [1979] illustrate a "monoblast" closely resembling a transitional cell with polyribosomes. The "inactive lympho-cyte" of Zucker-Franklin [1969, Figs. 1, 2] seems to have typical transitional cell morphology. It would be interesting to know more about its distribution and properties.

ADDITIONAL OBSERVATIONS

It is interesting to compare what is known about transitional cells with some of the properties of "morphologically unrecognizable" stem cells which have emerged from a large number of experimental studies, and which may be summarized in a series of stem cell postulates. 1) Stem cells must be present in adequate numbers for normal steady-state requirements, and also be capable of rapid proliferation when demands for them are increased. 2) Stem cells must exist in two forms, proliferating and nonproliferating. 3) Within the stem cell compartment the proportion of proliferating to non-proliferating cells can vary in accordance with stem cell requirements. 4) Stem cells must be capable of varying degrees of mobilization and migration into and out of the hemopoietic tissues.

In considering the stem cell role of transitional cells, it is important to bear in mind that there is no other cell group in the marrow that has the postulated stem cell properties. The autoradiographic studies of Caffrey et al [1966] and the continuous labeling studies of Fliedner et al [1968] and Haas et al [1973] effectively rule out all the classical contenders for the role of stem cell, notably reticulum cells or endothelium.

But transitional cells still present many problems. They are a heterogene-ous population, both functionally and morphologically. The present posi-tion with regard to the heterogeneous transitional cell compartment resem-bles in some ways that which prevailed in relation to small lymphocytes before new techniques made it possible to sort out the lymphocytes into their different groups.

XIV.

Stem Cell Considerations

INTRODUCTION

In several of the preceding chapters, the evidence presented points to the postnatal location of the hemopoietic stem cells in the transitional cell compartment. These cells are outstandingly prominent in the fetus, in which, however, they are preceded by cells in the yolk sac and liver and possibly the primitive mesenchyme.

On the question of definition, a stem cell is here broadly defined as a cell that does not exhibit any obvious signs of differentiation but which is nevertheless capable, if appropriately stimulated, of undergoing differentiation. The present chapter deals with only a few aspects of the stem cell problem. More comprehensive treatment will be found in a number of monographs and reviews [eg, Metcalf and Moore, 1971; Metcalf, 1977].

FETAL HEMOPOIESIS

Four main hemopoietic sites have been described in the fetus—the yolk sac, the liver, the primitive mesenchyme, and the bone marrow (see Chapter III). To a lesser extent, other constituents of the lymphomyeloid complex also call for consideration.

Yolk Sac

An account of earlier work on the yolk sac, as studied by light microscopy, has been given by Bloom [1938]. Subsequently, ultrastructural studies were performed by Sorensen [1961], Fukuda [1974], and others. In company with most observers, Bloom [1938] followed Maximow [1927] in attributing a mesenchymal origin to the vitelline stem cells, though a derivation from endoderm has also been suggested [Gladstone and Hamilton, 1941]. Whatever their origin, the cells are quite distinctive, being large and basophilic, bearing no resemblance to transitional cells. This is a point to be emphasized, since Moore and Metcalf [1970] and others have maintained that the yolk sac in the mouse, and presumably in other mammals, is the primary source of all hemopoietic stem cells, which were thought to migrate subsequently to the liver, bone marrow, and the remainder of the lymphomyeloid complex. This view was greatly reinforced by studies of the avian yolk sac, a much more substantial source of cells than the vestigial yolk sac of mammals. If the cells of the mammalian yolk sac are indeed the ultimate source of all the transitional cells in the organism, they must be capable of a remarkable degree of proliferation and they must also undergo a striking change in morphology, for neither in the liver nor in the bone marrow do they occur in the form in which they are found in the yolk sac. In a recent study, Symann et al [1978] conclude that in birds, amphibia, and mice "the experimental evidence . . . questions the dependence of intraembryonic hemopoiesis on a migration stream of hemopoietic cells which would develop ab initio in the yolk sac."

Liver

Hepatic hemopoiesis in mammals, to which Von Kolliker first drew attention in 1853, is much more extensive than in the yolk sac. But as in the case of the yolk sac, here too most observers seem to have accepted Maximow's [1927] view that the hemocytoblasts that appear in such large numbers are mesenchymal derivatives. Schridde [1907] was unable to find in fetal liver the wandering primitive mesenchymal cells described by Maximow, and Thomas and Yoffey [1964] were unable to see them in most of the liver parenchyma, though a few cells which might be regarded as such could be observed in the vicinity of the larger blood vessels. Maximow's [1927] evidence for the mesenchymal origin of the hepatic blood cells is not very convincing, though for many years the weight of his authority gained widespread acceptance of his views.

In human fetal liver, Thomas and Yoffey [1964] thought that the hemocytoblasts were derived from the undifferentiated cells of the liver and would therefore be endodermal in origin, a view first put forward over a century ago by Toldt and Zuckerkandel [1875]. The developing erythroid cells were an integral part of the hepatic cords, in which here and there one could see cells resembling the neighboring hepatic cells but beginning to develop basophilia. Cells with the morphology of yolk sac erythroblasts were never seen in the hepatic cords, a finding subsequently confirmed by Rifkind et al [1969]. Some transitional cells are present in the liver [Thomas, 1973; Hoyes et al, 1973; Fukuda, 1974], but these appear to be relatively few in number.

Hemopoiesis in the liver is predominantly erythropoietic, and fetal liver contains very few granulocytes or lymphocytes [Thomas and Yoffey, 1964; Rosenberg, 1969]. This is presumably due to the local environment, since transfusion of fetal liver cells into lethally irradiated animals gives rise to a normal bone marrow [Thomas, 1973], though Micklem and Loutit [1966] drew attention to the not infrequent occurrence of lymphoid tissue hypoplasia in syngeneic fetal liver chimeras. Kincade et al [1975] found that B lymphocytes could develop in ^{89}Sr-treated fetal mice in which virtually all bone marrow had been eliminated. Johnson and Metcalf [1978] noted that, despite the absence of granulopoiesis in the fetal liver in vivo, the in vitro culture of fetal liver resulted in the development of typical granulocyte-macrophage colonies. They also made the interesting observation that fetal liver CFU-GM were much larger cells than those in bone marrow (in the normal steady state), with sedimentation velocity (SV) peaks of 9.4 mm/h and 7.7 mm/h as against 4.5 mm/h for bone marrow. Williams and Moore [1973] had previously found that liver CFU-GM were larger than those in the marrow, and were homogeneous in volume, "indicative of a single non-cycling population with no evidence of an S or G_2 component." Nicola et al [1981], by the FACS technique, identified the erythropoietic stem cells in mouse fetal liver as cells of 13–17 μm in diameter, appreciably larger than the cells of the TC component.

Since suspensions of fetal liver cells can effectively repopulate the remainder of the lymphomyeloid complex, it seems to be tacitly assumed that from the intact fetal liver in vivo stem cells are continually migrating into the blood stream. However, in sections of fetal liver, Thomas and Yoffey [1964] could find no evidence of cells becoming detached from the hepatic cords to enter the bloodstream.

Primitive Mesenchyme

Maximow [1927—an extensive review summarizing all his earlier studies] was the foremost advocate of the concept that primitive mesenchymal cells are capable of developing into hemopoietic stem cells, the basophilic hemocytoblasts. His illustrations to show this [1927—Abb 90-93] are not very convincing. He seems to have been impressed by the occasional presence of hemopoietic foci in the embryonic connective tissues, but those which he describes, as he himself points out, are neither very extensive nor particularly active. He emphasized that granulocytes are seen only in pairs, but he also noted that the occasional small group of erythroblasts consisted typically of cells that were all at the same stage of development [Abb 92, 93, Maximow, 1927]. Although this appearance might conceivably be due to the proliferation of a hemocytoblast resulting from the transformation of a primitive connective tissue cell—a transformation, incidentally, which he does not illustrate—it could equally well be due to a circulating stem cell that had migrated out of the bloodstream into the connective tissues. From what we now know about the cellular migration streams through the connective tissues even in postnatal life, and of the greatly increased numbers of stem cells in the fetal circulation, this seems at least as likely an explanation of Maximow's findings as that which he advanced.

Bone Marrow

Hammar [1901] described the earliest stages of the bone marrow as "primary" marrow, consisting of loose connective tissue between dilated, thin-walled vessels. This is quickly followed by infiltration with lymphoid cells, and the subsequent formation of the definitive bone marrow. The origin of the cells appearing in Hammar's "lymphoid" marrow is unknown, whether autochthonous or immigrant. Maximow [1927] ascribed the initial formation of marrow to invasion by mesenchymal hemocytoblasts, which he believed to be present in the deeper layers of the periosteum, from which they presumably made their way into the marrow cavity. But Naegeli [1900, 1931], in formulating his views on the myeloblast, was unable to find any evidence in developing marrow for the origin of blast cells from mesenchyme.

Yoffey et al [1961] studied the marrow in a series of 50 human fetuses, ranging in age from 8 to 28 weeks. Femoral marrow was first clearly in evidence at 12 weeks. The marrow was first studied in smears, and later in sections [Yoffey and Thomas, 1964]. The appearances seen in the sections confirmed the findings of Hammar [1901]. In none of the many sections examined were hemocytoblasts seen in the periosteum. Soon after the appearance of the lymphoid marrow, all the main cell groups became evident, in proportions which did not vary greatly throughout pregnancy. The lymphoid cells form about 25% of the total nucleated cells of the marrow in the fetus (range 10–45%). They are diffusely scattered, never forming aggregates or nodules. Transitional cells are a striking feature of the marrow throughout fetal life. It is noteworthy that the characteristic size spectrum is present from the outset [Yoffey et al, 1961] and that, at 15% of the lymphoid cells, transitional cells form on the average 4% of the total nucleated cells of fetal marrow, rising at times to 7%. There are therefore proportionately more transitional cells in the marrow of the fetus than at any other time throughout life. Kelemenen et al [1982] have recently confirmed the high percentage of lymphocytes and "lymphocytelike" (ie, transitional) cells in human fetal marrow. From what we now know of the transitional cell compartment, it is clear that fetal marrow should be an excellent source of transplant material, as was found in the case reported by Kelemenen et al [1982].

MIGRATION OF HEMOPOIETIC CELLS

The general concept of "Cellular Migration Streams" [Yoffey et al, 1959] includes the migration through the bloodstream of hemopoietic stem cells. The idea that stem cells might be present in the bloodstream goes back to the early days of hematology. Neumann [1890] suggested it as a possibility in discussing the formation of bone marrow in calcified laryngeal cartilages. But the experimental study of the problem dates from the pioneer experiments of Jacobson et al [1949], who found that shielding the spleen protected animals against otherwise lethal irradiation. The irradiated bone marrow underwent complete regeneration, and it was soon established that the protection was essentially due to recolonization of the damaged tissue by stem cells migrating through the bloodstream. The same conclusion followed from experiments such as those of Kaplan and Brown [1952], in which thigh shielding during otherwise lethal irradiation also conferred hemopoietic protection, and promoted the regeneration of the entire lymphomyeloid complex, including lymph nodes and thymus. Transfusion of marrow cell suspensions also conferred protection, in accordance with the numbers given, but with a maximum upper limit. Furthermore, young donors were more effective than old [Jacobson et al, 1954], a finding which correlates well with the greater number of transitional cells in the former than the latter.

Hemopoietic Stem Cells in Blood

Though an obvious corollary of stem cell migration is the presence of stem cells in the bloodstream, some time elapsed before their presence was clearly demonstrated by the protective capacity of blood leukocyte suspensions in the mouse [Popp, 1960; Goodman and Hodgson, 1962], dog [Cavins et al, 1964; Korbling et al, 1979], and guinea pig [Malinin et al, 1965]. The development of the in vitro colony technique [Pluznik and Sachs, 1965; Bradley and Metcalf, 1966] was soon followed by the growth of a variety of colonies from human blood cells as well as marrow [Robinson and Pike, 1970; Chervenick and Boggs, 1971a; Kurnick and Robinson, 1971; Fauser and Messner, 1978; Barr et al, 1975; Liu et al, 1979; Lipton et al, 1981]. The earlier work on stem cell migration was performed mainly in mice, and was largely directed to migration between marrow and spleen.

Quantitation of Stem Cells

In the mouse, a number of studies have been directed to quantitating the CFU-S. Trobaugh and Lewis [1964] concluded that in the adult mouse, the blood contains 1/100th the number of CFU-S present in the marrow. Barnes and Loutit [1967c] estimated that there are 50,000 CFU-S in adult mouse marrow as against 1,000 in the spleen and 20 in blood. Hodgson et al [1968] estimated the CFU-S content of the spleen to be 1/10th that of the marrow. Hellman and Grate [1968] gave estimates of the same order, but in the case of the marrow drew a distinction between a smaller group of CFU-S that could be easily mobilized so as to obtain ready access to the bloodstream, and a much larger group which was relatively static and could only be mobilized at a slow rate. Metcalf and Moore [1971] give the total CFU-S content of adult murine marrow as 44,000, compared with 7,000 in the spleen and 20 in the blood, the latter comparing with 80 in the blood of the neonate. The blood of the fetal mouse, according to Barnes et al [1964], contains 100 times as many stem cells as that of the adult—about 2,000 CFU-S. In human fetal blood transitional cells are encountered frequently [Winter et al, 1965] and have been illustrated [Yoffey, 1971]. At birth, it was noted that 14% of the blood lymphocytes possessed leptochromatic nuclei; and 2% of the blood lymphocytes, typical transitional cells, showed spontaneous DNA synthesis as opposed to 0.2% in the adult. Faulk et al [1973] found corresponding figures of 2.05% and 0.08%.

It is evident from the literature that transitional cells, though not named as such, have been recognized on purely morphological grounds in fetal and neonatal blood. Efrati et al [1961] described them as "atypical mononuclear cells" in cord blood. Rind [1967] noted their presence in fetal blood, and warned against regarding these atypical cells as leukemic.

Methods of Studying Migration

An early approach to the study of CFU-S migration (in mice) was to shield a limited portion of the marrow, usually the femur, while irradiating the rest of the animal, including the spleen. Stem cells migrating from the shielded marrow then formed colonies in the spleen [Wolf and Rosse, 1982]. Hanks [1964], using this technique, arrested the migration of stem cells from marrow to spleen by lethally irradiating the shielded thigh at times ranging from 2 to 7 hours after the first irradiation. By this and other procedures he made estimates of the number of CFU-S leaving the marrow, and arrived at a figure of 250 CFU-S per day from a shielded femur, with a calculated total of about 5,000 CFU-S per day going into the bloodstream from what was considered to be the "total hemopoietic tissue." Croizat et al [1980] estimated a migration rate from leg marrow to spleen of 8 CFU-S/h, and 80 CFU-S/h for the whole marrow. Croizat et al [1976] calculated a total migration of 100 CFU-S/h to the exteriorized spleen, irradiated while the rest of the mouse was shielded. These figures give a relatively short life in the blood for the CFU-S migrating through the bloodstream. Maloney and Patt [1976], also using the autorepopulation technique, estimated the life of CFU-S in the blood to be 2.5–6 hours, an appreciably longer life than that estimated by Hodgson et al [1968], who induced anemia in mice by phenylhydrazine. During the course of the anemia an increased number of CFU-S appeared in the bloodstream and also in the spleen. They concluded that these cells passed quite rapidly through the blood, in which they were calculated to have a half-life of only 6 min.

Maloney and Patt [1978] emphasized that the uptake of cells by the irradiated spleen might be very different from the uptake by the unirradiated spleen. Furthermore, the use of the spleen as a target organ for estimating the number of migrating cells could be misleading for another reason, namely that an unknown and variable number of stem cells may be leaving the bloodstream for destinations other than the spleen. In addition, the position with regard to the murine spleen is very different from that of larger animals and man. In the normal human spleen, for example, Freedman and Saunders [1981] could find neither CFU-E nor CFU-GM.

Stem Cell Migration to Bone Marrow

Thus far we have considered stem cells as being formed in the marrow and there undergoing differentiation, or leaving the marrow to enter the bloodstream. Another possibility is the entry of stem cells into the marrow from the bloodstream (see also Chapter VI). Congdon et al [1952] showed in an early study that intravenously transfused marrow cells migrate readily into marrow that has previously been depleted by irradiation. But the uptake of stem cells by normal marrow is a different matter.

Micklem et al [1968] transfused marrow cells from normal male CBA-T6T6 mice into the normal male CBA recipients. Donor cells were found in the bone marrow, and also in the spleen, thymus, and lymph nodes. Since there was no prior irradiation, one might expect these experiments to approximate to the pattern of cell migration found in the normal animal, though it is still possible to raise the objection that the transfused marrow might introduce into the circulation a larger number of stem cells than would usually be present in the bloodstream.

Parabiosis

Difficulties of this nature can presumably be avoided by the use of parabiotic animals, in which one parabiont is labeled with ^{3}H-thymidine while the circulation between the two animals is temporarily occluded. When the occlusion is subsequently released, labeled cells from one animal can migrate via the bloodstream and be identified in the other.

Tyler and Everett [1966] performed parabiotic experiments with rats, in which the hind limbs of one rat were shielded while the animals were irradiated with 100 rads. A "monocytoid" cell was the major cell type which crossed from the shielded to the nonshielded marrow, and from their description it seems probable that these were in fact transitional cells with indented nuclei. Rosse [1972a] performed parabiotic experiments on guinea pigs with somewhat different design from those performed by Tyler and Everett [1966]. In these experiments there was no irradiation. Repeated injections of ^{3}H-thymidine were administered to one animal in order to label lymphocytes with a long life-span; these animals were then joined in parabiosis to nonlabeled littermates. It was found that only small lymphocytes entered the circulation and crossed the anastomosis in appreciable numbers. Although these experiments avoided the damaging effects of irradiation, Rosse [1972a] brings out one point of note: Parabiosis appears to give rise to considerable stress, which is presumably the cause of an appreciable fall in marrow lymphocytes in both parabionts. It would appear that caution is needed in applying to normal animals findings on cell migration based on the examination of parabionts. Harris et al [1964] joined in parabiosis two pairs of mice of different chromosomal constitution (CBA, CBA/T6T6) and observed the changes in bone marrow after 4 and 5 weeks. Parabiosis was effected when the mice (of the same sex) were 4 weeks old. After 4 weeks of union, the CBA marrow contained 5% of T6T6 cells, and the CBA/T6T6 marrow had 3% of CBA cells. In the experiment of 5 weeks' duration, the marrow of the CBA mouse had 4% of T6T6 cells, and the CBA/T6T6 mouse had 3% of CBA cells. Barnes and Loutit [1967b] referred to work on six additional parabiotic pairs, killed at intervals of up to 30 weeks. "Bone marrow equilibration appeared to take place with 5 to 10% of partner's cells," and was attained between 4 and 8 weeks.

Ford et al [1966] performed experiments which in some respects were similar in principle to those involving parabiosis, even though only one animal was used. The experiments had the great advantage of avoiding parabiotic stress. After lethal irradiation of the lower extremities, animals were given a transfusion of chromosomally marked marrow cells, which "promptly and permanently recolonized the irradiated portion of the recipient's bone marrow, which however also contained a substantial minority of host cells which had previously migrated from the shielded part of the body." In these experiments, once the animals had recovered from the effects of the experimental procedures, it seems reasonable to suppose that cell migration was as near normal as possible. The experiments confirmed that the irradiated marrows took up many more cells than those that were not irradiated [cf Congdon et al, 1952]. They seem to indicate further that though some stem cells do migrate via the bloodstream, this migration may not be very extensive in the normal animal. In fact, it would appear from these experiments that the majority of the stem cells are a relatively static population in the normal mouse and tend to remain confined largely to their own marrow, despite their undoubted mobility when hemopoietic needs appear to warrant it [cf Hellman and Grate, 1968].

STEM CELL MIGRATION TO NONMYELOID SITES

Stem cells of different varieties can migrate to a number of sites other than the bone marrow. Among these sites one may note the thymus and other constituents of the lymphomyeloid complex, including the connective tissues.

Apart from the various committed stem cells in the blood, there are also present some CFU-S, and it is these which confer protection against lethal irradiation. Micklem et al [1975] have suggested that many—though not all—of the CFU-S in the circulation are the victims of clonal senescence and have been "expelled as waste products from the bone marrow." This concept of stem cell rejection is based on the observation that there are marked differences between blood and marrow stem cells in their capacity for self-renewal and in the size of the descendant populations which they produce under identical conditions. This view has been supported recently by Chertkov et al [1982], who also found that circulating CFU-S have a lower self-maintenance than the "resident CFU-S" in the marrow, though they agreed that there were some "high-maintenance" CFU-S even in the circulation.

Vos et al [1981] present some interesting data on the relative potency of CFU-S from different sources. They found that the number of CFU-S required to prevent 50% mortality of irradiated mice was about three for fetal liver, 7–10 for bone marrow, 20 for normal blood, and 80 for the spleen of normal mice. The data show the same general trend as those of Duplan et al [1979], though they differ somewhat in regard to splenic CFU-S [cf Rencricca et al, 1976].

Stem Cells and the Thymus

The migration of stem cells to the thymus has been reviewed recently [Yoffey, 1981], and will be dealt with here only briefly. In the case of the fetal thymus, it has been suggested that there is a thymopetal migration stream from the yolk sac [Moore and Owen, 1967; Moore and Metcalf, 1980], though this view has been queried [Le Douarin et al, 1975; Dieterlen-Lievre et al, 1976; Le Douarin, 1978; Symann et al, 1978].

In postnatal life, Kaplan and Brown [1952] observed that thigh-shielding during systemic irradiation not only conferred hemopoietic protection, but also promoted regeneration of lymph nodes and thymus [cf Osmond et al, 1960]. The fact that the thymus continually receives immigrant stem cells was shown by a study of thymic grafts. Metcalf and Wakonig-Vaartaja [1964] grafted thymus glands of AKR mice into normal (AKR × T6) F1 mice. The central part of the graft undergoes necrosis, but the peripheral rim, in contact with blood vessels, survives and for a time is the site of active proliferation of donor lymphocytes. However, as shown by chromosome analysis, from day 10 onwards the donor lymphocytes fall sharply and become completely replaced by host type cells [cf Dukor et al, 1965; Koller et al, 1967]. Schlesinger and Hurvitz [1968] analyzed thymus grafts on the basis of immunological differences between host and donor. The donor thymus contained TL+ cells, whereas the host thymocytes were TL−.

They observed that the invading host cells acquired TL antigenicity after residing in the thymus graft for 3–4 days, a change they attributed to the surviving reticuloepithelial cells of the graft "guiding and directing the differentiation of the invading host cells." Following these studies, Komuro and Boyse [1973] noted that cells from bone marrow, spleen, or fetal liver of nu/nu mice could be induced in vitro to express TL antigen. Komuro et al [1975] concluded that a prothymocyte normally migrates from the hemopoietic tissues to the thymus, where it is induced by thymopoietin to express the phenotype of an early T cell.

Several subsequent immunological studies were in accord with this concept. Press and Rosse [1977] demonstrated that null lymphocytes in murine bone marrow acquired T-cell surface antigens during the course of the blastogenic response to PHA [cf Cohen and Patterson, 1975]. Press and Rosse [1977] were able to show that even in nude mice there were T-cell precursors in the bone marrow that responded to PHA in the same way as in normal mice. Rosse and Press [1978] reviewed earlier work and summarized their own experiments, from which it appeared that both B-cell and T-cell precursors in bone marrow developed from transitional cells.

In addition to prothymocytes as T-cell precursors, CFU-S should be given consideration. They are present in the fetal thymus in considerable numbers [Barg et al, 1978], though hardly any are present in the neonate [Micklem and Loutit, 1966; Micklem et al, 1976]. At the times when they are present in the thymus, CFU-S should presumably be capable of acting as thymocyte precursors. It is interesting to note that, as indicated by velocity sedimentation, buoyant density, and cell surface charge, thymocyte precursors have the same characteristics as CFU-S [Boersma et al, 1981].

Stem Cells and Connective Tissue

The connective tissues of the body contain hemopoietic stem cells concerning whose life history we are largely in ignorance. The serous cavities, notably the peritoneum, are generally regarded as possessing the same kind of cell population as connective tissues elsewhere, but with a fluid matrix. Goodman [1963] and Cole [1963] showed that among the cells of the peritoneal cavity there were hemopoietic stem cells that were able to confer protection against otherwise lethal irradiation. The number of these peritoneal stem cells was relatively small, since Goodman [1963] noted that marrow was about 250 times as effective as peritoneal cells in conferring protection. A number of typical transitional cells are present in the peritoneum [Yaffe and Yoffey, 1982].

In the case of the connective tissues generally, Tyler et al [1972] examined the subcutaneous inflammatory exudates formed in mice 18 hours after the implantation of coverslips. They found that the cells of these exudates were capable of promoting erythropoietic recovery when transfused into lethally irradiated recipients, as measured by ^{59}Fe incorporation into the spleen. The exudate cells were at least twice as effective in their repopulating ability as an equal number of blood leukocytes, and one-tenth as effective as bone marrow cells. They were impressed by the fact that the erythropoietic cells seemed to be closely associated with a population of monocytes, macrophages, and cells termed "monocytoid." At a later date Scuderi et al [1977] noted that the exudates contained cells with both monocyte and transitional cell morphology. Sokol et al [1982] have recently illustrated cells with typical transitional cell morphology in skin window preparations from normal subjects.

The peritoneal cavity in the mouse contains not only CFU-S, but also atypical CFU-GM, as shown by Lin and Stewart [1973]. Lin [1980] noted further that the number of CFU-GM could greatly increase after the intraperitoneal injection of thioglycollate. Here too, as in the case of the CFU-S, the evidence indicates that the CFU-GM are members of the transitional cell compartment [cf Moore et al, 1972]. Under the culture conditions of Moore et al [1972], CFU-GM could develop into both macrophages and granulocytes, but it would appear that it is only the macrophage line of development which usually occurs in the peritoneal cavity.

The presence of CFU-GM and CFU-S in the peritoneum, and of either CFU-S or BFU-E in the other connective tissues, raises a number of questions we are unable to answer. Granulocytopoiesis does not normally occur in the peritoneum, nor erythropoiesis in connective tissues elsewhere. But whether in the peritoneum or in the subcutaneous connective tissues, the stem cells always seem to be associated—as emphasized by Tyler et al [1972] in the case of subcutaneous exudates—with monocytes and macrophages. One possibility therefore to be considered is that these cells, unable because of the local microenvironment to develop into either granulocytes or erythrocytes, are continually differentiating into macrophages.

SIZE HETEROGENEITY IN STEM CELLS

From the proliferation gradient (Fig. XIII.3) and the data on the main size groups in the transitional cell compartment (Fig. XIII.2), several conclusions follow for the properties of stem cells: 1) The existence of three main size groups in the transitional cell compartment suggests that stem cells may exist in one, two, or three sizes. 2) The smaller the size of the stem cells, the lower the percentage of cells in DNA synthesis. 3) Since the percentage of cells in DNA synthesis is higher in the larger cells, one is able, by means of mitotic poisons—eg, high specific activity thymidine or hydroxyurea—to effect selective killing of the larger cells and leave intact a greater proportion of small cells. 4) Velocity sedimentation enables one to separate cells on the basis of size. Data thus obtained can be correlated with those on DNA synthesis. 5) When increased production of stem cells is required, this can be effected by the more rapid and extensive enlargement of the smaller transitional cells, feeding into the more actively proliferating and larger cells of the stem cell compartment. In terms of the standard velocity sedimentation curve, this is a shift to the right, and will be referred to as such in this context.

Stem Cells in Different Sizes

The existence of stem cells in two or three sizes has been noted by a number of observers. One of the early observations, by Worton et al [1969], was directed toward differentiating CFU-S from CFU-GM. They noted that the former sedimented at 3.9 mm/h, the latter at 4.9 mm/h and they therefore concluded that CFU-S and CFU-GM are not identical. A number of observations of size heterogeneity have since been published, not only for CFU-S, but also for granulocytic and erythrocytic precursors.

The work of Monette et al [1974] suggested that CFU-S exist in three sizes. In the normal steady state, most of the CFU-S are at the small end of the stem cell spectrum, and are not in cycle; their SV is 4.2 mm/h. But hydroxyurea (HU), which kills most of the cells in cycle—ie, the larger cells—triggers off the proliferation of most of the smaller resting CFU-S [cf Necas, 1981], which then enlarge. Twelve hours after HU, the CFU-S show three peaks, sedimenting at 4.2, 5.3, and 7.0 mm/h. Furthermore, whereas in normal marrow they found 16% of the CFU-S in cycle, after HU the percentage in cycle rose to 43%. Necas [1981] gives an even higher figure than Monette et al [1974] for CFU-S in cycle—65%, 12 hours after HU.

Heath et al [1976], in an analysis of the action of erythropoietin on stem cells, found that they sedimented in two peaks which differed in their erythropoietin response. Cells in one peak, sedimenting at 5.7–7.0 mm/h, responded rapidly to a low dose of erythropoietin, and formed colonies of hemoglobin-synthesizing cells which reached their highest number in 2 days, ending up as small colonies (up to 65 cells) of nonnucleated cells. These rapidly responding cells were termed CFU-E. By contrast, in cultures treated with a high dose of erythropoietin, with which they were continually fed, crops of new colonies appeared after about 6 days and were termed "bursts," the stem cells that gave rise to them being known as BFU-E. BFU-

E and CFU-E differed in size. BFU-E sedimented at 3.7–4.1 mm/h, whereas the CFU-E sedimented at 5.7–7.0 mm/h.

Iscove and Sieber [1974], in methyl cellulose cultures of murine bone marrow, found that the BFU-E sedimented at 3.9 mm/h, with a thymidine suicide rate of 25%, whereas the larger CFU-E sedimented at 5.5 mm/h and had a suicide rate of 70%. Gregory and Eaves [1978] subdivided the BFU-E into early and late forms, and so obtained three erythropoietin progenitor cells: 1) BFU-E with bursts at 8 days, 2) BFU-E with bursts at 3 days, and 3) CFU-E which develop into erythroid cells very rapidly. The most primitive cells were the 8-day BFU-E (SV 3.8 mm/h, thymidine suicide rate 21.7%), whereas the 3-day BFU-E (SV 4.4 mm/h, thymidine suicide rate 51.5%) were intermediate in maturity, and the CFU-E (SV 7.0 mm/h, thymidine suicide rate 70.1%) were the most mature. In these and other examples, the relation between cell size and DNA synthetic activity corresponds to a similar relationship in the transitional cell compartment. There are no other cells in the marrow that can account for the observed facts.

Transfusion polycythemia caused a significant fall in marrow CFU-E, but not in the 3-day or 8-day BFU-E, which if anything rose slightly. This raises the possibility that some of the increased numbers of transitional cells that appear in the bone marrow during rebound could in fact be BFU-E.

Ogawa et al [1977] described three types of erythroid colonies in human marrow: small, peaking on day 4–5; medium, peaking on day 8; and large, peaking on day 11.

The general trend of the size data is in accord with the results of other workers. In murine marrow, Hara and Ogawa [1978] also described three types of erythropoietic colony-forming cells: 1) CFU-mix—ie, cells giving rise to colonies of erythroid cells mixed with macrophages and other cells, including megakaryocytes (SV 3.4 mm/h, virtually none in S); 2) BFU-E (SV 3.9 mm/h, 36% in S); and 3) CFU-E (SV 6.4 mm/h, 74% in S). Peschle et al [1981] also identified three classes of erythroid progenitors in human fetal liver, cord blood, and adult marrow, but the lack of sedimentation velocity data makes it dificult to compare their results with those cited.

The circulating erythroid progenitors in postnatal life seem to be entirely BFU-E [Lipton et al, 1981]. Clarke et al [1979] thought that these circulating BFU-E were programmed to produce fetal, not adult, hemoglobin, though Papayannopoulou et al [1978] had suggested that the switch to fetal Hb production might be the result of the culture conditions.

The CFU-GM also have been the subject of extensive kinetic studies, which have demonstrated size heterogeneity. The earlier literature has been extensively reviewed by Metcalf and Moore [1971]. It was concerned largely with animal studies. In the same year, Chervenick and Boggs [1971a] and Kurnick and Robinson [1971] reported the presence of CFU-GM in human blood, since which time there have been numerous studies. There is considerable variation in the numbers of colonies reported, as noted and discussed by Kreutzmann and Fliedner [1979], Barrett et al [1979], and Grilli et al [1980].

Initially, only one variety of CFU-GM appears to have been recognized. Miller et al [1978] described in human marrow two types of CFU-GM: rapidly sedimenting cells, SV 7.0–8.0 mm/h, forming colonies after 7 days; and more slowly sedimenting cells, SV 6.5 mm/h, forming colonies after 11 days. But the heterogeneity of CFU-GM had been appreciated in animal marrows several years previously [Metcalf and Moore, 1971]. Metcalf and MacDonald [1975] separated colony-forming and cluster-forming cells in murine bone marrow. Colony formers sedimented at a single peak (4.4 mm/h), whereas cluster formers sedimented at two peaks, mostly at 5.7 mm/h, and were considered to be the progeny of the colony-forming cells. Niskanen et al [1979] described two varieties of stem cell in human blood: One variety, which they termed the CFU-DG—more frequently CFU-D— grew in plasma clots in diffusion chambers; the other formed granulocyte colonies in vitro in agar. The CFU-D were considered to be the more primitive and to give rise to the CFU-GM. Jacobsen et al [1978] obtained cells from normal human bone marrow, and separated them into three groups by velocity sedimentation: 1) CFU-D, SV 5.0 mm/h, 7% in S; 2) rapidly sedimenting CFU-GM (SV 7.3 mm/h, 48% in S) forming clusters of 3–50 cells after 7 days; and 3) slowly sedimenting CFU-GM (SV 6.0 mm/h, 21% in S) forming clusters at 14 days. Bol et al [1979] and Bol and Williams [1980] have also described three types of macrophage-granulocyte progenitors in murine bone marrow, but the size differences between the three types seem to be comparatively small.

In the preceding pages we have given a few representative examples of heterogeneity in size and kinetic status of CFU-S, and of erythrocyte and granulocyte-macrophage progenitors. It is only the transitional compartment that contains cells of the same range of size and kinetic qualities.

SIZE CHANGES IN STIMULATED MARROW

In discussing the proliferation gradient (Fig. XIII.3), it was suggested that one of the most obvious ways to increase cell production was by the enlargement of a greater number of the small nonproliferating cells, which would then become capable of DNA synthesis and division. In terms of the proliferation gradient this sounds eminently reasonable, but does it in fact occur? There are a number of experimental situations in which it appears to do so.

If one takes the thymidine-labeling index as a guide to cell size (Fig. XIII.3), then the experiments of Becker et al [1965] show evidence of CFU-S enlargement when more stem cells are needed. They studied inter alia the kinetic state of regenerating marrow, in which cell proliferation is very active, and they observed that instead of the usual 10% of CFU-S in DNA synthesis, the figure rose to 40–65%.

Sublethal irradiation is another situation in which greatly increased proliferation of stem cells is needed, to give rise to new erythroid and other cells to replace those destroyed. A major contribution was made by Harris [1956], who subjected guinea pigs to whole-body irradiation (150 rads) and then, by a quantitative technique, followed the changes in the bone marrow for 36 days. An initial abrupt fall in all the radiosensitive nucleated cells— the most sensitive being the transitionals [Harris, 1960]—was succeeded by a series of changes. Regeneration began with the transitional cells and lymphocytes, which multiplied rapidly from day 4 onwards, until by day 16 they were about twice their control value. Recovery of the nucleated erythroid cells was slow at first, but became more marked from days 14–20, with a slight overshoot above control values. Myeloid regeneration started around day 16, and rose to 50% above control values. From days 16 to 20, when the combined erythroid and myeloid regeneration were reaching the peak of their activity, transitional cells and lymphocytes fell abruptly to less than half their control level. The striking increase in transitional cells, preceding the great spurt in erythropoietic and granulopoietic regeneration, is what one would expect from the stem cell role of the TC compartment. Blackett et al [1964] studied the marrow changes after sublethal irradiation in the rat, and also found a great increase in "lymphoid" (obviously transitional) cells in the marrow following irradiation.

Data about size changes after sublethal irradiation, as measured by the sedimentation velocity, came from Metcalf et al [1977], working with mice. They found that 2 days after 250 rads, the sedimentation velocity of the CFU-GM had risen sharply from 4.3 to 7.8 mm/h. The shift from small to large CFU-GM, was associated with an equally sharp increase in the thymidine suicide rate, from 39% in the normal to 70% in the animals recovering from irradiation.

In regenerating marrow following transplantation, there is increased proliferation not only of CFU-S, as already noted, but also of CFU-GM.

Cudkowicz et al [1964b] described the active proliferation of "lymphocyte-like" cells in regenerating murine bone marrow after transplantation. Sutherland et al [1971] observed that, in regenerating marrow 6 days after transplantation, CFU-GM were sedimenting at 7.3 mm/h, as against the usual peak value of 5 mm/h. Another interesting example of size change was reported by Metcalf and Wilson [1976]. They noted that, 2 days after the injection of endotoxin, the CFU-GM in murine bone marrow showed a marked increase in sedimentation velocity, from 4.5 mm/h to 5.5–6.5 mm/h, the cluster-forming cells sedimenting at 7.6–8.0 mm/h.

Gerhartz and Fliedner [1980] performed leukapheresis in dogs for 24 hours, and found that larger than normal CFU-GM began to appear in the bone marrow. The enlargement is nicely shown in their Figures 6a and 6b, a typical "shift to the right." Together with the enlargement there was a rise in the thymidine suicide rate from 26.5% before the leukapheresis to 49.5% after the leukapheresis had been in progress for 24 hours. Keiser et al [1967] have shown that canine bone marrow contains a typical transitional cell compartment, with the characteristic size spectrum. They also noted that, in the early recovery phase after irradiation, the labeling index of the large transitional ("lymphoid") cells rose to 70%.

CFU-GM in blood appear to be null cells, lacking surface receptors for immunoglobulin, sheep erythrocytes, and complement [Richman et al, 1978]. Barr et al [1975], who obtained mixed cultures from blood leukocytes, were also dealing with null cells.

CIRCULATING STEM CELLS: CHANGES WITH AGE

There are a number of differences in the circulating stem cells in the prenatal, perinatal, and postnatal periods. In terms of CFU-S, reference has already been made to the findings by Barnes et al [1964] that there are 100 times as many stem cells in the blood of fetal as in adult mice. In terms of transitional cells, Winter et al [1965] and Yoffey [1971] drew attention to the large numbers of transitional cells in fetal blood, though actual counts were not made. In the neonate 14.4% of the circulating lymphoid cells had leptochromatic nuclei, and about half of them were typical transitionals. Faulk et al [1973] noted the presence in cord blood of a number of cells which were neither typical transitional cells nor typical small lymphocytes, and they provisionally termed them "intermediate." In the adult, Winter et al [1965] found that about 6% of blood lymphocytes were leptochromatic, though very few could be regarded as typical transitional cells. As far then as transitional cells in human blood are concerned, a high content in fetal blood contrasts with a low content in the blood of the adult. In man, the blood of the adult contains relatively few pluripotential stem cells, though they are definitely present [Messner and Fauser, 1980], and concentration techniques have made it possible to obtain them in increased numbers [Lasky et al, 1982]. In the case of stem cells in blood, as in marrow, whenever attempts are made to identify them morphologically they show transitional cell characteristics—eg, the "large lymphocytes" of Barr et al [1975]. According to Monette and Stockel [1980], CFU-S in murine blood are immunologically different from those in other tissues.

In fetal blood, attention seems to have been largely directed to the erythropoietic and granulopoietic stem cells. Ogawa et al [1976] examined the erythropoietic precursors in cord blood, which contained per ml 2,084 ± 454 BFU-E, and 169 ± 58 CFU-E. Beuzard et al [1979] investigated the content of BFU-E and CFU-E in fetal, cord, and adult blood. In the blood of a 32-week fetus they found 720 BFU-E per 10^6 plated cells, in cord blood at full term 400 per 10^6, and in 15 normal adults $75/10^6$. In agreement with many other observers, CFU-E were not found in adult blood, but were present in cord blood, 292 per 10^6 plated cells in 7-day cultures.

Darbre et al [1981] compared erythroid bursts (BFU-E) in fetal, neonatal, and adult blood. The fetal blood was obtained during fetoscopy for antenatal diagnosis of spina bifida. In normal adult blood the plating efficiency ranged from three to 40 colonies per 10^5 cells plated. Colony numbers in fetal blood ranged from 100 to 200 per 10^5 nucleated cells, and nonerythroid colony growth was very dense if adherent cells were not removed. In cord blood the maximal colony numbers ranged from 20 to 70 per 10^5 nucleated cells plated, and here too nonerythroid colony growth was quite marked. A noteworthy feature was that the erythroid bursts began to develop significantly earlier in fetal than in cord or adult blood, being first visible by day 4, compared with cord blood at day 5, and adult blood at 8–9 days.

Hassan et al [1979] investigated erythroid colony growth in adult and cord blood and in fetal liver. Cells were incubated for 14 days in plasma clot cultures with erythropoietin. Adult blood gave no early colonies (CFU-E), but only late colonies (BFU-E) on day 14—100 colonies per 0.1 ml. Fetal liver produced many early colonies by day 7 (over 1,500/0.1 ml), whereas cord blood cultures contained both early and late colonies—200/0.1 ml on day 7, and 125/0.1 ml by day 12.

CFU-GM in cord blood fall rapidly after birth. Knudtzon [1974] found that cord blood gave a mean CFU-GM count of 122 per 2×10^5 cells plated (range 17–385 colonies) compared with a mean of 3 per 2×10^5 cells in adult blood (range 0–11). Prindull et al [1978] reported at birth one CFU-

GM in 1,678 cells, falling rapidly during the first 10 days, to virtually none in adult blood. Ueno et al [1981] observed in cord blood 93.5 CFU-GM per 10^5 mononuclear cells, falling to $29.8/10^5$ cells at 3 days, $7.0/10^5$ at 7 days, and $1.1/10$ in the adult. Prindull et al [1981] found high levels of CFU-GM in the blood of preterm infants.

In addition to granulocyte and erythrocyte precursors, other colony-forming cells have been found in both fetal and adult blood. Vainchenker et al [1979] succeeded in growing megakaryocyte colonies from fetal, neonatal, and adult peripheral blood cells. Barr et al [1975] had previously observed the occasional appearance of megakaryocytes in cultures of adult human peripheral blood cells. Presumably the CFU-M found in cultures of murine bone marrow and spleen [Metcalf et al, 1975; Nakeff and Daniels-McQueen, 1976] are present in the blood also. Kirshner and Goldberg [1980] emphasized the presence of eosinophil colonies in cord blood, and Ijima et al [1982] thought that as many as 80% of the colony-forming cells in cord blood gave rise to macrophages.

Petrakis et al [1961] cultured normal human leukocytes in subcutaneously implanted diffusion chambers in autologous and homologous subjects, for periods up to 6 weeks. The development of macrophages from monocytes was to be expected, but in addition there appeared fibroblasts even occasionally fat cells. Fibroblast colony-forming cells (CFU-F) (see also Chapter IV) have been studied in human bone marrow [Castro-Malaspina et al, 1980], where they were shown to have a modal sedimentation velocity of 4.95 ± 0.15 mm/h, as against 3.4 mm/h for small lymphocytes. Some of the CFU-F were large, sedimenting at 10 mm/h. The size range could mean that the CFU-F are transitional cells, but if so they are unusual as they were not in S, not being killed by thymidine suicide.

Mast cell precursors are in all probability present in human peripheral blood [Zucker-Franklin, 1980], where they have been thought to be present in "lymphocyte" fractions. In the case of rat blood, Zucker-Franklin [1981] obtained numerous mast cell colonies from "mononuclear" cell fractions, cultured in soft agar.

Enhanced Reactivity of Fetal Cells

The finding by Darbre et al [1981] that colony-forming cells in the fetus, and up to the time of birth, reacted more rapidly than adult cells finds a parallel in the response of fetal lymphocytes. Papiernik [1971] examined lymphocytes from fetuses aged 15–39 weeks. Until week 32 of pregnancy they showed a high spontaneous rate of transformation. He also noted that fetal blood lymphocytes showed a higher rate of transformation in response to PHA than did those of infants from 3 days to 16 years. Yoffey et al [1978] compared the response to PHA and Con A of lymphocytes from cord blood with those of adults. At varying intervals ranging from 20 to 48 hours after the start of the cultures, the percentage of lymphoid cells in DNA synthesis was measured by the uptake of tritiated thymidine and autoradiography. In both the PHA and the Con A cultures, the increase in the percentage of labeled cells occurred significantly earlier in cord than in adult blood.

The question arises whether the greater reactivity is a general property of fetal as opposed to adult cells, or whether the lymphocytes are a special group in this respect, for immunological reasons. Stites et al [1972] inclined to the view that "fetal lymphocytes are already partially stimulated in vivo." Weber et al [1973] appear to have thought along similar lines when they suggested that "the fast response of fetal lymphocytes to exogenous stimulation may reflect a state of readiness for immunological defence." Melchers and Abramzuk [1980] have emphasized the presence of "precursor B cells" (ie, transitional cells) in mouse fetal blood.

THE ROLE OF CIRCULATING STEM CELLS

The life history and role of the circulating stem cells are not understood. A small percentage, the T-cell precursors or prothymocytes, en route from bone marrow to thymus, serve an obvious purpose. But the thymus, at least in the adult, requires a relatively small number of stem cells, since the prothymocytes are believed to undergo something like eight mitoses in the course of the thymocyte production pathway [Yoffey, 1981]. It is true that occasionally a small amount of granulocyte or erythrocyte production takes place in the thymus, but this is by no means a regular occurrence, and when it does occur it is on a relatively minor scale. The thymus cannot be considered as a major target organ for circulating erythrocyte or granulocyte precursors; nor, except possibly for very small animals, can the spleen be regarded as the major destination of migrating stem cells.

It may be that the stem cells in the bloodstream are a spillover from the bone marrow, in which case the more stem cells there are in the bone marrow, the greater the number likely to be present in the bloodstream. This, conceivably, could be one factor responsible for the higher stem cell content of fetal blood. However, even in the normal steady state in the adult there always seem to be some stem cells in the bloodstream.

Stimulation of erythropoiesis is also at times associated with an increased number of stem cells in the blood. Hodgson et al [1968] noted in mice an increased number of CFU-S in the bloodstream during phenylhydrazine anemia, a finding confirmed by Rencricca et al [1970], who suggested that in severe anemia stem cells migrated from marrow to spleen. Harris and Kugler [1971] observed the presence of unusual mononuclear cells in the peripheral blood of guinea pigs during phenylhydrazine anemia. Forty percent of the atypical cells were transitionals, mainly large and basophilic, of which one-third were in DNA synthesis. The atypical cells reached a peak of 50/ml on day 5, and 70/ml on day 15. These may not appear to be large numbers, but if the atypical cells in the guinea pig—or at least the transitionals among them—are the counterpart of the murine CFU-S, then according to Hodgson et al [1968] they pass rapidly through the bloodstream, in which it was calculated that they had a half-life of 6 min. On this basis even a small number of stem cells in the blood would be compatible with a considerable degree of production.

Whereas in the smaller laboratory animals the presence of stem cells in the bloodstream may be attributed to their migration from bone marrow to spleen, this explanation does not seem so readily applicable to man. Cooper and Firkin [1964] reported the presence of increased numbers of DNA-synthesizing cells, flash labeling with thymidine, in the blood of patients with refractory anemia. In the normal adult, virtually no blood leukocytes label with tritiated thymidine [Bond et al, 1958]. This was confirmed by Cooper and Firkin [1964], who found no labeling cells in the blood of two normal individuals, and 0.02% in a third [cf Winter et al, 1965; Faulk et al, 1973]. On the other hand, in three cases of aplastic anemia, 0.3%, 0.5%, and 0.6% of cells were found to take up the label. In a case of hemolytic anemia, 1.1% of blood leukocytes became labeled, as did 0.8% in a case of paroxysmal nocturnal hemoglobinuria. The labeled cells were described as "young lymphocytes," and from comments in the text it seems evident that they must have been transitional cells. In fact it seems to be generally the case that where investigators try to identify the circulating stem cells, the most apt description seems to be "lymphocyte," large rather than small [cf Barr et al, 1975]. Liu et al [1979] identified circulating CFU-GM in man as "lymphocytes," and noted further that 26% of the colony-forming cells, and 14% of the cluster-forming cells, took up thymidine. This finding clearly rules out small lymphocytes, which do not label with thymidine.

Whether they originate in hyperactive or normal marrow, some stem cells always seem to be present in the bloodstream. Whether some of the circulating stem cells find their way back to the marrow, and if so in what numbers, has yet to be established. Those that do not return to the marrow may, as already noted, enter the various constituents of the lymphomyeloid complex, and the connective tissues. But in all these situations their subsequent fate is obscure, and may vary with their microenvironment. For example, the CFU-S known to be present in the peritoneum do not, in that situation, seem to give rise to red cells or granulocytes, though they are quite capable of doing so when they reach the bone marrow of irradiated animals, presumably because the marrow provides the appropriate microenvironment. A somewhat atypical CFU-GM, which gives rise only to macrophages, and then only rather slowly, has been described by Lin [1980] in the peritoneal cavity also. Volkmann [1966], who transfused intravenously a suspension of labeled marrow cells in rats, found subsequently in the peritoneum both labeled macrophages and labeled "lymphocytelike"—presumably transitional—cells. It is conceivable that some of the CFU-GM in the bloodstream are escaping continually into the connective tissues and replenishing the macrophage population. Other possible stem cell migrants into the connective tissues are fibroblast and mast-cell precursors, in addition, of course, to the usual drift of mature granulocytes, small lymphocytes, and monocytes.

In our ignorance of the fate of stem cells in the circulation, one is tempted to speculate that there is constant reinforcement of the senescent cells of the connective tissues by the continued influx of primitive cells from the bloodstream. If this speculation should turn out to be correct, then the bone marrow would be one of the major factors in maintaining the integrity of the connective tissues.

References

Abercrombie M (1967): In DeReuck AVS, Knight J (eds): "Cell Differentiation." Boston: Little, Brown.
Abramson S, Miller RG, Phillips RA (1977): J Exp Med 145:1567.
Akai H, Sato S (1971): J Invest Physiol 17:1665.
Albrecht M (1957): Acta Haematol 17:160.
Alpen EJ, Cranmore D (1959): In Stohlman F (ed): "The Kinetics of Cellular Proliferation." New York: Grune and Stratton, p 290.
Amsel S, Maniatis A, Tavassoli M, Crosby WH (1969): Anat Rec 164:101.
Andrew W (1965): "Comparative Hematology." New York: Grune and Stratton.
Aoki M, Tavassoli M (1981a): J Ultrastruct Res 74:255.
Aoki M, Tavassoli M (1981b): Br J Haematol 49:337.
Aoki M, Tavassoli M (1981c): Exp Hematol 9:231.
Archer RK (1963): "The Eosinophil Leukocytes." Oxford: Blackwell.
Archer RK (1970): In Gordon AS (ed): "Regulation of Hematopoiesis," vol. 2. New York: Appleton-Century-Crofts, p 917.
Arndt R (1881): Virchows Arch 83:15.
Aschoff L (1893): Arch Pathol Anat Physiol 134:11.
Askanazy M (1911): Virchows Arch 205:346.
Askanazy M (1918): Zentralbl Allg Pathol 29:409.
Askanazy M (1927): In Heneke F, Lubrasch O (eds): "Handbuch der speziellen pathogischen Anatomie und Histologie." Berlin: Springer.
Aye MT (1977): J Cell Physiol 91:69.
Bailkow A (1870): Zentralbl Med Wissensch 24:371.
Bainton DF, Yoffey JM (1970): In Yoffey JM, Courtice FC: "Lymphatics, Lymph and the Lymphomyeloid Complex." New York: Academic Press, p 648.
Baker JE, Keenan MA, Raphals L (1969): J Cell Physiol 74:51.
Baldini MG, Ebbe S (1974): "Platelets." New York: Grune and Stratton.
Bankston PW, DeBruyn PPH (1974): Am J Anat 141:281.
Barcroft J, Binger CH, Bock AV, Doggart JH, Forbes HS, Harrop G, Meakins JC, Redfield AC (1923): Phil Trans R Soc Lond (SB) 211:351.

Barg M, Mandel TE, Johnson GR (1978): Aust J Biol Med Sci 56:195.
Bargmann W (1930): Z Zellforsch 11:1.
Barnes DWH, Ford CE, Loutit JF (1964): Lancet 1:1395.
Barnes DWH, Loutit JF (1967a): Lancet 2:1138.
Barnes DWH, Loutit JF (1967b): Haematol Latina 10:1.
Barnes DWH, Loutit JF (1967c): Nature 213:1142.
Barr RD, Watt J (1978): Acta Haematol 60:29.
Barr RD, Whang-Peng J, Perry S (1975): Science 190:284.
Barrett AJ, Faille A, Ketels F (1979): Br J Haematol 42:337.
Basten A, Beeson PB (1970): J Exp Med 131:1228.
Basten A, Miller JFAP, Sprent J, Pye J (1972a): J Exp Med 135:610.
Basten A, Warner NC, Mandel T (1972b): J Exp Med 135:627.
Bateman AE, Cole RJ (1971): J Embryol Exp Morphol 26:475.
Bathija A, Davis S, Trubowitz S (1978): Am J Hematol 5:315.
Bathija A, Davis S, Trubowitz S (1979): Am J Hematol 6:191.
Beard R (1950): Physiol Zool 23:47.
Beaupain D, Martin C, Dieterlen-Lievre F (1979): Blood 53:213.
Becker JE, McCulloch EA, Siminovitch L, Till JE (1965): Blood 26:296.
Becker RP, DeBruyn PPH (1976): Am J Anat 145:183.
Beeson PB, Bass DA (1977): "The Eosinophil." Philadelphia: WB Saunders.
Behnke O (1968): J Ultrastruct Res 24:412.
Behnke O (1969): J Ultrastruct Res 26:111.
Behnke O, Pedersen NT (1974): In Baldini MG, Ebbe S (eds): "Platelets, Production, Function, Transfusion and Storage." New York: Grune and Stratton, p 21.
Belman L (1967): J Ultrastruct Res 17:291.
Ben-Ishay Z, Ben-Ishay D (1970): Proc 7th Int Congr Electron Microsc, p 839.
Ben-Ishay Z, Yoffey JM (1971a): Isr J Med Sci 7:948.
Ben-Ishay Z, Yoffey JM (1971b): J Reticuloendothel Soc 10:482.
Ben-Ishay Z, Yoffey JM (1972): Lab Invest 26:637.   .
Bennett M (1973): J Immunol 110:510.
Bennett M, Cudkowicz G (1967): In Yoffey JM (ed): The Lymphocyte in Immunology and Haemopoiesis." London: Edward Arnold, p 183.
Bentley SA (1982): Br J Haematol 50:1.
Beran M, Tribukait B (1971): Acta Haematol 45:55.
Berman I (1967): J Ultrastruct Res 17:291.
Berman I, Fawcett DW (1964): Anat Rec 148:361.
Bernstein S, Russell E, Keigley G (1968): Ann NY Acad Sci 149:475.
Bessis M (1958): Rev Hematol 13:8.

Bessis M (1973): "Living Blood Cells and Their Ultrastructure." Berlin: Springer-Verlag, pp 123–126.

Beuzard Y, Vainchenker W, Testa U, Dubart A, Monplaisis N, Breton-Gorius J, Rosa J (1979): Am J Hematol 7:207.

Bhuyan RK (1965): The effect of intermittent hypoxia upon haemopoiesis in the guinea-pig. PhD dissertation, University of Bristol.

Bichat X (1802): Arch Physiol 5:169.

Bierman HR, Kelly KH, Byron RL, Marshall GJ (1961): Br J Haematol 7:51.

Bierman HR, Marshall GJ, Kelly KH, Byron R (1960): Rev Hematol 15:398.

Bizzozero G (1868): Zentralbl Med Wissensch 6:585.

Bizzozero G (1869): Zentralbl Med Wissensch 10:149.

Bizzozero G, Torre A (1884): Virchows Arch 95:1.

Blackett NM, Roylance PJ, Adams K (1964): Br J Haematol 10:453.

Bleiberg I, Feldman M (1969): Dev Biol 19:566.

Bloom W, Bloom MA, McLean FY (1941): Anat Rec 81:443.

Bloom W, Bartelmez GW (1940): Am J Anat 67:21.

Bloom W (1938): In Downey H (ed): "Handbook of Hematology." New York: Hoeber, p 865.

Boersma WJA, Daculsi R, van der Westen G (1981): Cell Tissue Kinet 14:197.

Boettcher A (1866): Virchows Arch 36:342.

Boggs DR (1967): Semin Hematol 4:359.

Boggs DR, Athes JW, Cartwright GE, Wintrobe MM (1965): Proc Soc Exp Biol Med 118:753.

Boggs DR, Boggs SS (1976): Blood 48:71.

Boggs DR, Chervenick PA, Marsh JC, Cartwright GE, Wintrobe MM (1968): J Lab Clin Med 72:177.

Boggs SS (1973): J Lab Clin Med 82:740.

Bol S, Visser J, van den Engh G (1979): Exp Hematol 7:541.

Bol S, Williams N (1980): J Cell Physiol 102:233.

Bolognari A (1949): Arch Zool Ital 34:79.

Bolognari A (1951): Arch Zool Ital 36:253.

Bond VP, Feinendegen LE, Heinze E, Cottier H (1964): Ann NY Acad Sci 113:1009.

Bond VP, Cronkite EP, Fliedner TM, Schork P (1958): Science 128:202.

Borghese E (1959): Acta Anat 36:185.

Boseila AW (1959): "The Basophil Leukocyte and Its Relation to the Tissue Mast Cell." Copenhagen: Munksgaard.

Boycott AE, Oakley CL (1933): J Path 36:205.

Bradley T, Metcalf D (1966): Aust J Exp Biol Med Sci 44:287.

Brahim F, Osmond DG (1970): Anat Rec 168:139.

Branemark PI (1959): Scand J Clin Lab Invest 11 (Suppl 38):1.

Branemark PI (1961): Bibl Anat 1:239.

Brehelin M (1973): Experientia 29:1539.

Breslow A, Kaufman RM, Lawsky AR (1968): Blood 16:1012.

Breuer M, Hirsch H (1964): Z Ges Exp Med 138:435.

Breuer M, Hirsch H, Sachveh D (1964): Pfluger's Arch Ges Physiol 278:532.

Brookes M (1965): Acta Anat 62:35.

Brookes M, Harrison RG (1957): J Anat Lond 91:61.

Brookoff D, Weiss L (1982): Blood 60:1337.

Brown JE, Adamson JW (1977): J Clin Invest 60:70.

Brown-Sequard CE, d'Arsonval A (1891): Arch Physiol 3:491.

Brown-Sequard CE, d'Arsonval A (1892): C R Acad Sci (Paris) 114:1399.

Burke WT, Harris C (1959): Blood 14:409.

Burkhardt R (1962): Blut 8:67.

Burrows PD, Kearney JF, Lawton AR, Cooper MD (1978): J Immunol 120:1526.

Burrows P, Le Jerune M, Kearney J (1979): Nature 280:838.

Caffrey RW, Everett NB, Rieke WO (1966): Anat Rec 155:41.

Calvo W (1968): Am J Anat 123:315.

Campbell FR (1972): Am J Anat 135:521.

Campbell FR (1967): J Morphol 123:405.

Campbell FR (1968): Anat Rec 160:539.

Campbell FR (1980): Anat Rec 169:101.

Campbell JA (1934): Br J Exp Pathol 16:39.

Castro F de (1929a): Trav Lab Rech Biol Univ Madrid 23:427.

Castro F de (1929b): Trav Lab Rech Biol Univ Madrid 26:215.

Castro-Malaspina H, Gay RE, Resnick G et al (1980): Blood 56:289.

Cavins JA, Scheer SC, Thomas ED, Ferrebee JW (1964): Blood 23:38.

Chajlakyan PK, Gerasinov YF, Friedenstein AJ (1978): Bull Exp Biol Med (USSR) 12:705.

Chamberlain JK, Leblond PF, Weed RI (1975): Blood Cells 1:655.

Chan B, Yoffey JM (1960): Immunology 3:237.

Chan B (1969): Acta Haematol 42:258.

Chan PC, Monette FC, LoBue J, Gordon AS (1966): Proc Soc Exp Biol Med 121:793.

Chargaff E (1968): Science 159:1448.

Charmanier M (1972): C R Acad Sci (Paris) 276D:2553.

Chen LT, Hsu YC (1979): Exp Hematol 7:231.

Chertkov JL, Gurevitch OA, Undalov GA (1982): Exp Hematol 10:90.

Chervenick PA, Boggs DR (1971a): Blood 37:131.

Chervenick PA, Boggs DR (1971b): Blood 37:568.

Cho Y, DeBruyn, PPH (1979): J Ultrastruct Res 69:13.

Clarke BJ, Nathan DG, Alter BP, Forget BG, Hillman DG, Housman D (1979): Blood 54:805.

Clementi F, Palade GE (1969): J Cell Biol 41:33.

Coggle JE, Gordon MY (1975): Exp Hematol 3:181.

Cohen JJ, Patterson CK (1975): J Immunol 114:374.

Cohen P, Gardner FH (1965): J Lab Clin Med 65:88.

Cohen SG, Kostage ST, Rizzo AP (1967): J Allergy 39:129.

Cole LJ (1963): Am J Physiol 204:265.

Cole RJ, Paul J (1966): J Embryol Exp Morphol 15:245.

Cole RJ, Hunter J, Paul J (1968): Br J Haematol 14:477.

Congdon GC, Uphoff D, Lorenz J (1952): J Natl Cancer Inst 13:73.

Cooper IA, Firkin BG (1964): Blood 24:415.

Cooper EL, Stein EA (1981): In Ratcliffe NA, Rowley AF (eds): "Invertebrate Blood Cell," Vol I. New York: Academic Press.

Cooper MD (1981): J Clin Immunol 1:81.

Cousin G (1898): C R Soc Biol Paris 5:454.

Cowden RR (1968): J Invest Pathol 14:60.

Cowden RR, Curtis SK (1981): In Ratcliffe NA, Rowley AF (eds): "Invertebrate Blood Cells," Vol I. New York: Academic Press.

Cowden RR, Curtis SK (1973): Exp Mol Pathol 19:178.

Craddock CG (1965): Acta Haematol 33:19.

Craddock CG, Perry S, Lawrence JS (1956): J Clin Invest 35:285.

Craddock CG, Adams WS, Perry S, Lawrence JS (1955): J Lab Clin Med 45:906.

Croizat H, Frindel E, Tubiana M (1976): Int J Radiat Biol 11:235.

Croizat H, Frindel E, Tubiana M (1980): Cell Tissue Kinet 13:319.

Cronkite EP (1958): Brookhaven Symp Biol 10:96.

Crosby WH (1975): Blood Cells 1:497.

Crosby WH (1976): In Seno S, Takaku F, Irino S (eds): "Topics in Hematology." Amsterdam: Excerpta Medica.

Cudennec CA, Thiery JJP, LeDuarin NM (1981): Proc Natl Acad Sci USA 78:2412.

Cudowicz G, Upton AC, Shearer GM, Hughes WL (1964a): Nature 201:165.

Cudowicz G, Upton AC, Smith LH, Gosslee DG, Hughes WL (1964b): Ann NY Acad Sci 114:571.

Cumming JD (1962): J Physiol 162:13.

Cumming JD, Nutt ME (1962): J Physiol (Lond) 162:30.

Cunningham RS, Sabin FR, Doan CA (1925): Contr Embryol Carnegie Inst 16:227.

Custer RP, Ahlfeldt FE (1932): J Lab Clin Med 17:960.

Cuthbertson EM, Gilfillan RS, Buchman RP (1964): Angiology 15:145.

Dales RP, Dixon RJ (1981): In Ratcliffe NA, Rowley AF (eds): "Invertebrate Blood Cells." New York: Academic Press.

Dalton AJ, Law LW, Maloney JB, Manaker RA (1961): J Natl Cancer Inst 27:744.

Danchakoff V (1909): Arch Mikr Anat 47:855.

Danchakoff V (1916): Anat Rec 10:397.

Daniels E (1980): Exp Hematol 8:157.

Darbre PD, Lauckner SM, Wood WG, Weatherall DJ (1981): Br J Haematol 48:133.

Darzynkiewicz A, Rogers AW, Bernard EA (1967): J Histochem Cytochem 14:915.

Davidson LSP, Davies LJ, Innes J (1943): Edinb Med J 50:226.

Debaisieux P (1953): La Cellule 55:245.

Debaisieux P (1952): La Cellule 54:253.

DeBruyn PPH, Breen PC, Thomas TB (1970): Anat Rec 168:55.

DeBruyn PPH (1964): Z Zellforsch 64:111.

DeBruyn PPH, Michelson S, Thomas TB (1971): J Morphol 133:417.

DeBruyn PPH, Becker RP, Michelson S (1977): Am J Anat 149:247.

DeBruyn PPH, Michelson S (1981): Blood 57:152.

DeBruyn PPH, Michelson S (1979): J Cell Biol 82:708.

DeBruyn PPH, Michelson S, Becker RP (1978): J Cell Biol 78:379.

DeBruyn PPH, Michelson S, Becker RP (1975): J Cell Biol 53:133.

Deckhuyzen MC (1901): Anat Anz 19:529.

De Gowin RL, Gibson DP (1976): Blood 47:315.

De Gowin RL, Hoak JC, Miller SH (1972): Blood 40:881.

DeHarven E, Friend C (1960): J Biophys Biochem Cytol 7:747.

De la Chapelle, Fantoni A, Marks PA (1969): Proc Natl Acad Sci USA 63:812.

deLeval M (1967): C R Soc Biol (Paris) 161:948.

deLeval M (1964): C R Soc Biol (Paris) 158:2198.

deLeval M (1966): C R Soc Biol (Paris) 160:2484.

deLeval M (1968a): Nouv Rev Fr Hematol 8:392.

deLeval M (1968b): Arch Biol 79:597.

Denburg JA, Davison M, Bienenstock J (1981): Acta Haematol 65:114.

Dennert G, Yogeeswaran G, Yamagata S (1981): J Exp Med 153:545.

Deur CJ, Stone MT, Frenkel EP (1981): Am J Hematol 11:309.

Dexter TM, Allen TD, Lajtha LG (1977): J Cell Physiol 91:335.

Dexter TM, Testa NG (1978): Meth Cell Biol 14:387.

Dexter TM, Moore MAS (1977): Nature 269:412.

Dicke KA, Van Noord MJ, Maat B, et al (1973): In Wolstenholme GEW, O'Connor M (eds): "Haemopoietic Stem Cells," Ciba Foundation Symposium N.S. No. 13. Amsterdam: Associated Scientific Publishers. p 47.

Dieterlen-Lievre F (1975): J Embryol Exp Morphol 33:607.

Dieterlen-Lievre F, Beaupain D, Martin C (1976): Ann Immunol (Inst Pasteur) 127C:857.

Dietz A (1944): Proc Soc Exp Biol Med 57:60.

Dineen JK, Adams DB (1970): Immunology 19:11.

Doan CA (1922): Contrib Embryol Carnegie Inst 15:27.

Donohue DM, Gabrio BW, Finch CA (1958a): J Clin Invest 37:1564.

Donohue DM, Reif RH, Hanson ML, Betson Y, Finch CA (1958b): J Clin Invest 37:1571.

Dorn A (1978): Cell Tissue Res 187:479.

Dornfest H (1970): In Gordon AS (ed): "Regulation of Hematopoiesis," Vol 1. New York: Appleton-Century-Crofts, p 237.

Downey H (1915): Folia Haematol 19:148.

Drinker CK, Drinker KR (1916): Am J Physiol 40:514.

Drinker CK, Drinker KR, Lund CC (1922): Am J Physiol 62:1.

Dubos RJ (1950: "Louis Pasteur: Freelance of Science." Boston: Little Brown.

Dukor P, Miller JFAP, House W, Allman V (1965): Transplantation 3:639.

Duplan JF (1968a): Nouv Rev Fr Hematol 8:445.

Duplan JF (1968b): C R Acad Sci Ser D 267:227.

Duplan JF, Legrand E, Castaignos C, de Calignon E (1979): Int J Rad Biol 36:595.

Dustin P (1944): Arch Biol 55:285.

Duverney M (1700): "Histoire de l'Academie Royale des Sciences," pp 202–205.

Ebbe S, Stohlman F (1965): Blood 26:20.

Ebbe S, Stohlman F, Overcash J, Donovan J, Howard D (1968): Blood 32:383.

Ecoiffier J, Prot D, Griffie R, Catach D (1957): Rev Chirurg de Orthoped 43:29.

Edmonds EH (1966): Anat Rec 154:785.

Edmonds RH (1964): J Ultrastruct Res 11:577.

Edmondson PW, Wyburn JR (1963): Br J Exp Pathol 44:72.

Efrati P, Rozenszajn L (1960): Blood 32:393.

Efrati P, Rosenszajn L, Shapira E (1961): Blood 17:497.

Ehrenstein VG, Lockner DV (1959): Acta Haematol 22:129.

Ehrlich P (1879): Arch Anat Physiol, Physiol Abt, p 571.

Ellis RE (1960): Phys in Med Biol 5:255

Elson LA, Galton DAG, Till M (1958): Br J Haematol 4:355.

Emery JL, Follett JF (1964): Br J Haematol 10:485.

Erb W (1865): Virchows Arch 34:138.

Erslev AJ (1959): Blood 14:386.

Evans HM (1915): Am J Physiol 37:243.

Evans JD, Baker JM, Oppenheimer MJ (1955): Am J Physiol 18:504.

Evatt BL, Levin J (1969): J Clin Invest 48:1615.

Everett NB, Caffrey RW (1967): In Yoffey JM (ed): "The Lymphocyte in Immunology and Haemopoiesis." London: Edward Arnold, p 108.

Everett NB, Rieke WO, Reinhardt WO, Yoffey JM (1960): "Haemopoiesis: Cell Production and Its Regulation," Ciba Found Symposium Ed. Wolstenholme GEW, O'Connor M (eds). London: Churchill, p 43.

Everett NB, Yoffey JM (1959): Proc Soc Exp Med 101:318.

Fahrenbach WH (1970): J Cell Biol 44:445.

Fairman E, Corner GW (1934): Anat Rec 60:1.

Fairman E, Whipple GH (1933): Am J Physiol 104:352.

Fand I, Gordon AS (1957): J Morphol 100:473.

Fantoni A, Bank A, Marks PA (1967): Science 157:1327.

Farr AG, DeBruyn PPH (1975): Am J Anat 143:59.

Farr AG, Cho Y, DeBruyn PPH (1980): Am J Anat 157:265.

Faulk WP, Goodman JR, Maloney MA, Fudenberg HH, Yoffey JM (1973): Cell Immunol 8:166.

Fauser AA, Lohr GW (1982): Blut 45:151.

Fauser AA, Messner HA (1978): Blood 52:1243.

Federici H (1926): Arch Biol 36:466.

Fererenko ME, Levin RF (1976): J Histochem Cytochem 24:601.

Feldman S, Rachmilewicz EA, Izak G (1966): J Lab Clin Med 67:713.

Fernbach DJ, Trentin JJ (1962): Proc VIIIth Int Cong Hematol 1:150.

Fliedner TM, Haas RJ, Stehle H, Adams A (1968): Lab Invest 18:249.

Fliedner TM, Sandkuhler S, Stodmeister R (1956): Z Zellforsch 45:328.

Florey HW (1964): J Exp Physiol 49:117.

Foot E (1965): Br J Haematol 11:439.

Ford CE, Micklem HS, Evans EP, Gray JG, Ogden DA (1966): Ann NY Acad Sci 129:283.

Frassoni F, Testa NG, Lord BI (1982): Cell Tissue Kinet 15:447.

Freedman MH, Saunders EF (1981): Am J Hematol 11:271.

French JE (1967): Br J Haematol 13:595.

Friedenstein AJ, Latzink NV, Gorskaya UF, Sidorovich SY (1981): Int J Rad Biol 39:537.

Friedenstein AJ, Chajlakhyan RK, Labykina KS (1970): Cell Tissue Kinet 3:393.

Friedenstein AJ, Petrakova KV, Kuralesova AI, Frolova GP (1968): Transplantation 6:230.

Friedenstein AJ, Kuralesova AI (1971): Transplantation 12:99.

Friedenstein AJ, Ivanov-Smolenski AA, Chajlakhayan RK, Gorskaya UF, Kuralesova AI, Latzinik NW, Gerasimow UW (1978): Exp Hematol 6:440.

Friedenstein AJ (1976): Int Rev Cytol 47:327.

Friedenstein AJ, Latzinik NW, Grosheva AG, Gosskaya UM (1982): Exp Hematol 10:217.

Friedenstein AJ, Chajlakhayan PK, Latzinik NW (1974): Transplantation 17:331.

Friedrich H (1910): Dissertation, Rostock (1890). Cited by Wetzel (1910).

Fruhman GJ (1960): Blood 16:1753.

Fruhman GJ (1964): Ann NY Acad Sci 113:968.

Fruhman GJ (1970): In Gordon AS (ed): "Regulation of Hematopoiesis," Vol 1. New York: Appleton-Century-Crofts, p 873.

Fruhman G, Fischer S (1962): Experientia 18:462.

Fruhman GJ, Gordon AS (1955a): Proc Soc Exp Biol Med 88:130.

Fruhman GJ, Gordon AS (1955b): Endocrinology 57:711.

Fukuda T (1973): Virch Arch Zellpathol B 14:197.

Fukuda T (1974): Virch Arch Zellpathol B 16:249.

Gairdner D, Marks I, Roscoe JD (1952): Arch Dis Child 27:128.

Gallien-Lartigue O (1966): Exp Cell Res 41:109.

Gallien-Lartigue O (1967): C R Acad Sci (Paris) 264:1066.

Garcia AM (1964): J Cell Biol 20:342.

Gardner FH, Nathan DG (1966): N Engl J Med 274:420.

Gathings WE, Lawton AR, Cooper MD (1977): Eur J Immunol 7:804.

Gerhartz HH, Fliedner TM (1980): Exp Hematol 8:209.

Geyer G, Schaaf P (1972): Acta Histochem 44:137.

Ghebrehiwet B, Muller-Eberhard HJ (1978): J Immunol 120:1774.

Ghisalberti AM (1960): Dizienarie Biog degli Italiani. Instituto della Enciclopedia Italiana, Rome, Vol I, Article: Biozzozero, Guilio, p 747.

Gilfillan RS, Petrakis NL, Steinbach HL (1957): Surg Forum 7:463.

Gladstone RJ, Hamilton WJ (1941): J Anat (Lond) 76:9.

Goldschneider I, Metcalf D, Battye F, Mandel T (1980): J Exp Med 152:419.

Golub ES (1972): J Exp Med 136:369.

Goodman JW (1963): Transplantation 1:334.

Goodman JW, Hodgson GS (1962): Blood 19:702.

Goodman JW, Shinpock SG (1968): Proc Soc Exp Biol Med 129:417.

Goodman JW, Shinpock SG, Basford NL (1979): Exp Hematol 7:17.

Gordon AS, Neri RO, Siegel CD, et al (1960): Acta Hematol 23:323.

Gordon AS, LoBue J, Dornfest BS, Cooper GW (1962): In Jacobson LO, Doyle M, (eds): "Erythropoiesis." New York: Grune and Stratton, p 321.

Gordon AS, Handler ES, Siegel CD, Dornfest BS, LoBue J (1964): Ann NY Acad Sci 113:766.

Goss CM (1928): J Exp Zool 52:45.

Gosselin L, Regnauld J (1849): Arch Gen Med 10:257.

Gothman L (1960): Acta Chir Scand 120:201.

Goujon E (1866): C R Soc Biol (Paris) 18:42.

Goujon E (1869): J Anat Physiol 11:399.

Gould SJ (1980): "The Panda's Thumb." New York: WW Norton.

Grasso JA, Swift H, Ackerman GA (1962): J Cell Biol 14:235.

Gregory CJ, Eaves AC (1978): Blood 51:527.

Greenberger JS (1978): Nature 255:752.

Greenberger JS (1979): In Vitro 15:823.

Greenberger JS (1980): J Supermol Struct 13:501.

Griffiths DA (1969): Blood 34:696.

Griffiths DA, Rieke WO (1969): Exp Hematol 18:36.

Griffiths DA, Rosse C, Edwards AE, Gaches CGC, Long AH, Wright JLW, Yoffey JM (1970): Acta Haematol 43:13.

Grilli F, Carbonell F, Fliedner TM (1980): Br J Haematol 44:769.

Gros M (1846): C R Acad Sci Paris 23:1106.

Grossi CW, Cadoni A, Leprini A, Ferrarini (1982): Blood 59:277.

Gurney CW, Wackman N, Filmanowicz (1961): Blood 17:531.

Haas RJ, Bohne FE, Fliedner TM (1969): Blood 34:791.

Haas RJ, Bohne F, Fliedner TM (1971): Cell Tissue Kinet 4:31.

Haas RJ, Hans-Dieter F, Fliedner TM, Fache I (1973): Blood 42:209.

Haller O, Wigzell H (1977): J Immunol 118:1503.

Halvorsen S, Finne PH (1968): Ann NY Acad Sci 149:576.

Hamazato Y (1958): J Kyu Soc 8:25.

Hammar JA (1901): Anat Anz 19:567.

Han SS, Baker BL (1964): Anat Rec 149:251.

Hanks GE (1964): Nature 203:1393.

Hansen M, Pedersen NT (1978): Scand J Haematol 20:371.

Hara H, Ogawa M (1976): Am J Hematol 1:453.

Hara H, Ogawa M (1977a): Exp Hematol 5:141.

Hara H, Ogawa M (1977b): Exp Hematol 5:161.

Hara H, Ogawa M (1978): Am J Hematol 4:23.

Harker LA (1968a): J Clin Invest 47:452.

Harker LA (1968b): J Clin Invest 47:458.

Harker LA, Finch CA (1969): J Clin Invest 48:963.

Harris, C (1961): Blood 18:691.

Harris C, Burke WT (1957): Am J Pathol 33:931.

Harris JE, Ford CE, Barnes DWH, Evans EP (1964): Nature 201:886.

Harris PF (1956): Br Med J 2:1032.

Harris PF (1960): Acta Haematol 23:293.

Harris PF, Haigh G, Kugler JH (1963): Br J Haematol 9:385.

Harris PF, Kugler JH (1963): Acta Haematol (Basel) 32:146.

Harris PF, Kugler JH (1965): Acta Haematol (Basel) 33:351.

Harris PF, Kugler JH (1971): J Anat (Lond) 108:1.

Harris PF, Menkin V, Yoffey JM (1956): Blood 11:243.

Harris RS, Herdan G, Ancill RJ, Yoffey JM (1954): Blood 9:374.

Harrison WJ (1962): J Clin Pathol 15:254.

Hashimoto M (1936): Trans Soc Pathol Jpn 26:300.

Hashimoto M (1962): Acta Hematol 27:193.

Haskill JS, McNeill TA, Moore MAS (1970): J Cell Physiol 75:167.

Haskill JS, Moore MAS (1970): Nature 226:853.

Hassan MW, Lutton GD, Levere RD, et al (1979): Br J Haematol 41:477.

Hatanaka K, Kitamura Y, Nishimune Y (1979): Blood 53:142.

Havig O, Gruner OPM (1973): Acta Pathol Microbiol Scand (A) 81:276.

Hauser JW, Ackermann GA, Knouff RA (1969): Anat Rec 124:57.

Hayem G (1889): "Dr. Duang et Ses Alterations Anatomiques." Paris: G Masson.

Heath DS, Axelrad AA, McLeod DL, Shreeve MM (1976): Blood 47:777.

Heilmeyer L (1930): Deuts Arch Clin Med 171:123.

Held D, Thron HL (1962): Arch Sci Physiol (Paris) 16:167.

Hellman S, Grate HE (1968): IAEA Symposium, Monaco. IAE Agency, Vienna, p 187.

Herberman RB (1981): Hum Lymphocyte Diff 1:63.

Herbeuval H, Duheille I, Guny G, Guerci O (1962a): C R Soc Biol 156:122.

Herbeuval H, Herbeuval R, Gany G, Duheille J, Guerci O (1962b): Nouv Rev Fr Hematol 2:619.

Herbeuval R, Herbeuval H, Duheille J (1961): C R Soc Biol 155:370.

Hesseldahl H, Larsen FJ (1971): Acta Anat 78:274.

Hibbs JB (1973): Science 180:868.

Higuchi T (1959): J Kyu Hem Soc 9:613.

Hiraki K, Sunami H, Ogawara K (1958): Acta Med Okayama 12:187.

Hodgson G (1967): Proc Soc Exp Biol Med 124:1045.

Hodgson G, Guzman E, Herrera C (1968): IAEA Symposium, Monaco. IAE Agency, Vienna, p 163.

Hoelzer E, Kurile E, Harriss EG, Fliedner TM, Haas RJ (1975): Biomedicine 22:285.

Hoffman JA (1972): Z Zellforsch Mikrosk Anat 106:451.

Hoffman JA (1973): Experientia 29:50.

Hoffman FA, Langerhans P (1869): Virch Arch Pathol Anat 48:303.

Houssaint E (1981): Cell Diff 10:243.

Howard JG (1972): J Exp Med 135:185.

Howard JG, Hunt SV, Gowans JL (1972): J Exp Med 135:200.

Howell WH, Donahue DD (1937): J Exp Med 65:117.

Hoyer H (1869): Centralbl Med Wiss 7:244.

Hoyes AD, Riches DJ, Martin BGH (1973): J Anat 115:99.

Hudson G (1958a): J Anat (Lond) 92:150.

Hudson G (1958b): Br J Haematol 4:239.

Hudson G (1959): Acta Haematol 22:380.

Hudson G (1960): Am J Physiol 198:1171.

Hudson G (1960a): J Anat (Lond) 94:274.

Hudson G (1960b): Blood 16:1199.

Hudson G (1963): Br J Haematol 9:446.

Hudson G (1964): Br J Haematol 10:122.

Hudson G (1965): Br J Haematol 11:446.

Hudson G (1966): In Yoffey JM: "Bone Marrow Reactions." London: Edward Arnold, p 86.

Hudson G (1968): Semin Hematol 5:166.

Hudson G, Osmond DG, Roylance PJ (1963): Acta Anat 53:234.

Hudson G, Smith NCW, Wilson RS, Yoffey JM (1967): Nature 213:818.

Hudson G, Yoffey JM (1963): J Anat 97:409.

Hudson G, Yoffey JM (1966): Proc R Soc Lond 165:486.

Hudson G, Yoffey JM (1968): J Anat (Lond) 103:515.

Hughes-Jones NC (1961): Clin Sci 20:315.

Hughes-Jones NC, Cheney B (1961): Clin Sci 20:323.

Huggins C (1939): Anat Rec 74:231.

Huggins C, Blocksom BH (1936): J Exp Med 64:253.

Huggins C, Noonan WJ (1936): J Exp Med 64:275.

Huggins C, Blocksom BH, Noonan WJ (1936): Am J Physiol 115:395.

Hulse EV (1964): Acta Haemat 31:50

Humble JG, Jayne WHW, Pulvertaft RJV (1956): Br J Haematol 2:283.

Hume R, West JT, Malmgren RA, Chu EA (1964): N Engl J Med 270:111.

Humphrey JH (1955): Nature 176:38.

Hunt NH, Perris AD (1973): J Endocrinol 56:47.

Hunt SV (1979): Eur J Immunol 9:853.

Hurst JM, Turner MS, Yoffey JM, Lajtha LG (1969): Blood 33:859.

Ijima H, Suda T, Miura Y (1982): Exp Hematol 10:234.

Inoue S, Ottenbreit MJ (1978): Blood 51:195.

Iscove NN, Sieber F (1974): Exp Hematol 2:278.

Iscove NN, Till JE, McCulloch EA (1970): Proc Soc Exp Biol Med 134:33.

Izak G, Nilken D, Gurevitch J (1957): Blood 12:507.

Jackson CW (1973): Blood 42:413.

Jackson JF (1962): Cancer 15:259.

Jacobsen N, Broxmeyer HE, Grossbard E, Moore MAS (1978): Blood 52:221.

Jacobson LO, Goldwasser E, Gurney CW (1960): In Wolstenholme GEW, O'Connor M (eds): "Haemopoiesis. Cell Production and its Regulation." London: J & A Churchill, p 423.

Jacobson LO, Marks EK, Gaston EO (1954): In Bacq M, Alexander P (eds): "Radiobiology Symposium." London: Butterworth's, p 122.

Jacobson LO, Marks EK, Gaston EO, Robson MJ (1949): Proc Soc Exp Biol Med 70:740.

Jacobson LO, Marks EK, Gaston EO (1959): Blood 14:644.

Johnson DR, Metcalf D (1978): Exp Hematol 6:246.

Johnson RW (1927): J Bone Joint Surg 9:153.

Jolly MJ (1905): C R Soc Biol (Paris) 58:593.

Jolly MJ (1907): Arch Anat Microsc Morphol Exp 9:133.

Jones HB, Jones JJ, Yoffey JM (1967): Br J Haematol 13:934.

Jones JC, Lin DP (1968): J Invest Physiol 14:1053.

Jones JC, Lin DP (1969): J Invest Physiol 15:1703.

Jones JC (1970): Hemocytopoiesis in Insects. In A Gordon AS (ed): "Regulation of Hematopoiesis." New York: Appleton-Century-Crofts, Vol 1.

Jones JC (1962): Current concepts concerning insect hemocytes. Am Zool 2:209.

Jordan HE (1916): Am J Anat 19:227.

Jordan HE (1926): Am J Anat 38:255.

Jordan HE, Baker JP (1927): Anat Rec 35:161.

Jordan HE, Beams HW (1930): Proc Soc Biol Med 28:181.

Jordan HE, Beams HW (1929): Proc Soc Exp Biol Med 27:67.

Jordan HE (1940): Anat Rec 77:91.

Jordan HE (1938): Comparative hematology. In Downey H (ed): "Handbook of Hematology." New York: Paul B Hoeber, p 703.

Jordan HE, Speidel CC (1923): J Exp Med 38:529.
Jordan HE, Speidel CC (1925): J Morphol Physiol 40:461.
Jordan HE, Speidel CC (1930): Am J Anat 46:55.
Jordan RK, Robinson JH (1981): In Kendall MD (ed): "The Thymus." New York: Academic Press, p 151.
Kadish J, Basch RS (1975): J Immunol 114:452.
Kalpakstoglou PK, Emery JL (1965): Br J Haematol 11:453.
Kanz L, Straub G, Bross KG, Faurer AA (1982): Blut 45:267.
Kaplan HS, Brown MB (1952): Science 116:195.
Karpatkin S (1969): J Clin Invest 48:1073.
Karrer HE (1961): J Ultrastruct Res 5:116.
Kaufman RM, Airo R, Pollack S, Crosby WH, Doberneck R (1965a): Blood 25:76.
Kaufman RM, Airo R, Pollack S, Crosby WH (1965b): Blood 26:720.
Keating A, Singer JW, Killen PD, Striker GE, Salo AC, Sanders J, Thomas ED, Thoring D, Fialkow PJ (1982): Nature 298:280.
Keiser G, Cottier H, Bryant BJ, Bond VP (1967): In Yoffey JM (ed): "The Lymphocyte in Immunology and Haemopoiesis." London: Edward Arnold, p 149.
Keiser G, Cottier H, Odartchenko N, Bond VP (1964): Blood 24:254.
Kelemen E, Janossa M, Gulya E (1982): Exp Hematol 10, Suppl 11:91.
Kempgens U, Mayer M, Schlossardt S, Muller V, Queisser W (1976): Acta Haematol 56:143.
Kerr JFR, Wyllie AH, Currie AR (1972): Br J Cancer 26:239.
Kinoti GK (1971): Parasitology 62:161.
Kincade PW (1981): Adv Immunol 31:177.
Kincade FW, Moore MAS, Schlegel RA, Pye J (1975): J Immunol 115:1217.
Kindred JE (1940): Am J Anat 67:99.
Kindred JE (1942): Am J Anat 71:207.
Kinosita R, Ohno S (1961): Bibl Anat 1:106.
Kinosita R, Ohno S (1958): Biodynamics of thrombopoiesis. In Johnson SA, Monto RW, Rebuck JW, Horn RC (eds): "Blood Platelets." Boston: Little, Brown.
Kinosita R, Ohno S, Bierman HR (1956): Proc Am Assoc Cancer Res 2:125.
Kirshner JJ, Goldberg J (1980): Exp Hematol 8:1202.
Kiyono K (1914): Die vitale Karminspeicherung. Jena: Fischer
Klemperer P (1938): In Downey H (ed): "Handbook of Hematology." New York: Paul B. Hoeber.
Kline DL, Clifton EE (1952): J Appl Physiol 5:79.
Knoll W, Pingle E (1949): Haematology 2:369.
Knospe WH, Rayudu VMS, Cardello M, Friedman AM, Fordham EW (1976): Cancer 37:1432.

Knospe WH, Blum J, Crosby WH (1968): Blood 28:398.

Knospe WH, Husseini S, Trobaugh FE (1978): Exp Hematol 6:601.

Knudtzon S (1974): Blood 43:357.

Koller PC, Davies AJS, Leuchars E, Wallis V (1967): In Yoffey JM (ed): "The Lymphocyte in Immunology and Haemopoiesis." London: Edward Arnold, p 343.

Kolliker A (1846): Z Rat Med (Zurich) 4:112.

Kolliker RA von (1953): "Manual of Human Histology," Vol 1. London: Sydenham Society.

Korbling M, Fliedner TH, Calvo W, et al (1979): Exp Hematol 7:277.

Komuro K, Boyse EA (1973): J Exp Med 138:479.

Komuro K, Goldstein G, Boyse EA (1975): J Immunol 115:195.

Koury MJ, Krantz SB (1982): Cell Tissue Kinet 15:59.

Krantz SB, Jacobson LE (1970): "Erythropoietin and the Regulation of Erythropoiesis." Chicago: University of Chicago Press.

Kretchmer AL, Conover WR (1970): Blood 36:772.

Kreutzmann H, Fliedner TM (1979): Scand J Haematol 23:360.

Kurnick JE, Robinson WL (1971): Blood 37:136.

Kuzmenko GN, Panasyak AF, Friedenstein AJ, Kulagina NN (1972): Bull Exp Biol Med (USSR) 10:94.

Lafleur L, Miller RG, Phillips RA (1972): J Exp Med 135:1363.

Lafleur L, Miller RG, Phillips RA (1973): J Exp Med 137:954.

Laing PG (1953): J Bone Joint Surg 35B:452.

LaPushin RW, Trentin JJ (1977): Exp Hematol 5:505.

Lasky LC, Ash RC, Kersey JH, Zanjani ED, McCullough J (1982): Blood 59:822.

Lau CY, Melchers F, Miller RG, Phillips RA (1979): J Immunol 122:1273.

Lautenschlager J, Borst RH, Meusers PJ (1971): Histochemistry 26:343.

Lavallard PR, Campiglia S (1975): Ann Sci Nat Zool Biol Anim 17:67.

Le Douarin NM (1978): In Clarkson B (ed): "Differentiation of Normal and Neoplastic Hematopoietic Cells." New York: Cold Spring Harbor Press, p 5.

Le Douarin N, Houssaint E, Jotereau F, Belo M (1975): Proc Natl Acad Sci USA 72:2701.

Leiter SS (1976): Folia Haematol 103:878.

Leitner SJ (1949): "Bone Marrow Biopsy. Haematology in the Light of Sternal Puncture." Translated by CJC Britton and E Neumark. London: Churchill.

Levaditi C (1902): Contribution a l'etude des mastzellen et de la mastzellen-leucocytose. These, Universite de Paris No. 183.

Levitt D, Cooper MD (1980): Cell 19:617.

Levy SB, Rubenstein CB, Tavassoli M (1976): J Natl Cancer Inst 56:1189.

Lichtman MA (1981): Exp Hematol 9:391.

Lichtman MA, Weed RI (1972): Blood 39:301.

Lichtman MA (1970): N Engl J Med 283:943.

Lichtman MA, Chamberlain JK, Simon W, Santillo PA (1978a): Am J Hematol 4:303.

Lichtman MA, Chamberlain JK, Santillo PA (1978b): In Silber R, LoBue J, Gordon AS (eds): "The Year in Hematology." New York: Plenum, pp 243–279.

Lie KJ, Heyneman D, Jeyarasasingam U, et al (1975): J Parasitol 61:59.

Lin HS (1980): Cell Tissue Kinet 13:39.

Lin HS, Stewart CC (1973): Nature New Biol 243:176.

Linke LG, Kovach AGB, et al (1965): Pfluger's Arch Physiol 283:R5.

Lipton JM, Kadisch M, Nathan DG (1981): Exp Hematol 9:1035.

Litt M (1961): J Immunol 87:522.

Litt M (1963): Am J Pathol 42:529.

Little K (1969): Gerontologia 15:155.

Liu YK, Stallard SS, Koo V, Dannaher CL (1979): Scand J Haematol 22:258.

LoBue J (1970): In Gordon AS (ed): "Regulation of Hematopoiesis," Vol 2. New York: Appleton-Century-Crofts, p 1167.

London IM, West R (1950): J Biol Chem 184:359.

Lord BI, Hendry JH (1972): Br J Radiol 45:110.

Lord BI, Testa NG, Hendry JH (1975): Blood 46:65.

Lowit M (1891): Arch Mikr Anat 38:524.

Lucarelli G, Ferrari L, Porcellini A, Carnevali C, Rizzoli V, Stohlman F (1967): Exp Hematol 14:7.

Lucy J (1970): Nature 227:815.

MacPherson GG (1971): Proc R Soc Lond (Biol) 177:256.

MacPherson GG (1972): J Ultrastruct Res 40:167.

Mahmoud AAF, Austin, KF (1980): "The Eosinophil in Health and Disease." New York: Grune & Stratton.

Malassez L (1882): Arch Physiol 9:1.

Maldonado JE, Pintado T (1974): In Baldini MG, Ebbe S (eds). "Platelets, Production, Function, Transfusion and Storage." New York: Grune & Stratton, p 105.

Malinin TI, Perry VP, Kerby CC, Dolan MF (1965): Blood 25:693.

Maloney MA, Lamela RA, Dorie MJ, Patt HM (1978): Blood 51:521.

Maloney MA, Patt HM (1978): Exp Hematol 6:227.

Maniatis AK (1969): Acta Haematol 42:330.

Maniatis A, Tavassoli M, Crosby WH (1971): Blood 37:581.

Marchesi VT, Gowan JL (1964): Proc R Soc Lond B 159:283.

Marks PA, Rifkind RA (1972): Science 175:955.

Marneffe R de (1951): Acta Chir Belg 50:469, 568, 681.

Martin C, Beaupain D, Dieterlen-Lievre F (1980): Dev Biol 75:303.

Martin K (1970): Biochim Biophys Acta 203:182.

Matter M, Hartmann JR, Krautz J, DeMarsh QB, Finch CA (1960): Blood 15:174.

Maximow A (1907): Beitr Z Pathol Anat 41:122.

Maximow A (1909): Arch Mikr Anat 73:444.

Maximow A (1927): In Von Mollendorf W (ed): "Handb d mikroskop Anat des Menschen," Bd II, Teil I. Berlin: Julius Springer, p 232.

Maximow AA (1924): Physiol Rev 4:533.

McCarthy PJ, Shmookler BM, Pierce LE (1977): Ann Intern Med 86:317.

McCluggage SG, McCuskey RS, Meineke HA (1971): Blood 38:96.

McCool D, Miller RJ, Painter RH, Bruce WR (1970): Cell Tissue Kinet 3:55.

McCuskey RS, Meinke HA, Towensend SF (1972): Blood 39:697.

McCuskey RS, McCluggage SG, Younker WJ (1971): Blood 38:87.

McDonald TP, Corttell M, Clift R (1970): Proc Soc Exp Biol Med 160:335.

McLeod DL, Shreeve MM, Axelrad AA (1976): Nature 261:492.

Mechanik N (1926): Z Anat Entwickl 79:58.

Meck RA, Haley JE, Brecher G (1973): Blood 42:661.

Medado P, Izak G, Feldman S (1967): J Lab Clin Med 69:776.

Meer JWM van der, Beelen RHJ, Fluitsma DM, van Furth R (1979): J Exp Med 149:17.

Mel HC, Schooley JC (1964): Exp Hemat 7:26.

Melamed MR, Clifton EE, Mercer C, Koss LG (1966): Am J Med Sci 252:301.

Melchers F, Abramzuk J (1980): Eur J Immunol 10:763.

Messier P, Sainte-Marie G (1972): Rev Can Biol 31:231.

Messner HA, Fauser HA (1980): Blut 41:327.

Metcalf D (1977): "Hemopoietic Colonies. In Vitro Cloning of Normal and Leukemic Cells." Berlin: Springer-Verlag.

Metcalf D, Johnson GR (1978): J Cell Physiol 96:31.

Metcalf D, Johnson GR, Mandel TE (1979): J Cell Physiol 98:401.

Metcalf D, Johnson GR, Wilson G (1977): Exp Hematol 5:299.

Metcalf D, MacDonald HR (1975): J Cell Physiol 85:643.

Metcalf D, MacDonald HR, Odartchenko N, et al (1975): Proc Natl Acad Sci USA 72:1744.

Metcalf D, Moore MAS (1971): "Haemopoietic Cells." Amsterdam: North Holland.

Metcalf D, Wakonig-Vaartaja R (1964): Proc Soc Exp Biol Med 115:731.

Metcalf D, Wilson JW (1976): J Cell Physiol 89:381.

Meyer AL, Meltzer SJ (1916): Am J Physiol 40:126.

Michaelis L, Wolff A (1902): Virch Arch Pathol Anat 167:151.

Michels NA (1931): Folia Haematol (Leipz) 45:128.

Michelsen K (1967): Acta Physiol Scand 71:16.

Michelsen K (1968): Acta Physiol Scand 73:265.

Michelsen K (1969a): Acta Physiol Scand 77:28.

Michelsen K (1969b): Acta Physiol Scand 77:52.

Micklem HS, Anderson N, Ross E (1975): Nature 256:41.

Micklem HS, Anderson N, Ure J, Jones HP (1976): Eur J Immunol 6:425.

Micklem HS, Clarke CM, Evans EP, Ford CE (1968): Transplantation 6:299.

Micklem HS, Loutit JF (1966): "Tissue Grafting & Radiation." New York: Academic Press.

Micklem HS, Ogden DA, Evans EP, Ford CE, Gray GJ (1975): Cell Tissue Kinet 8:223.

Miller AM, Gross MA, Yunis AA (1978): J Lab Clin Med 92:38.

Miller RGA, Phillips RA (1969): J Cell Physiol 73:191.

Miller SC (1982): Anat Rec 202:129A.

Miller SC, Osmond DG (1973): Cell Tissue Kinet 6:259.

Miller SC, Osmond DG (1974): Exp Hemat 2:227.

Miller SC, Osmond DG (1975): Cell Tiss Kinet 8:97

Minot CS (1901): Proc Bost Soc Nat Hist 29:185.

Minot GR (1922): J Exp Med 36:1.

Miura Y, Wilt FH (1969): Dev Biol 19:201.

Miura Y, Wilt FH (1970): Exp Cell Res 59:217.

Moffatt DJ, Rosse C, Sutherland IH, Yoffey JM (1961): Unpublished data.

Moffatt DJ, Rosse C, Sutherland IH, Yoffey JM (1964a): Acta Anat 58:26.

Moffatt DJ, Rosse C, Sutherland IH, Yoffey JM (1964b): Acta Anat 59:188.

Moffatt DJ, Rosse C, Yoffey JM (1967): Lancet 2:547.

Mollison PL (1947): Clin Sci 6:137.

Monette FC, Gilio J, Chalifoux P (1974): Cell Tissue Kinet 7:443.

Monette FC, Stockel JB (1980): Exp Hematol 8:89.

Monpeyssin M, Beaulaton J (1978): J Ultrastruct Res 64:35.

Moore DH, Ruska H (1957): J Biophys Biochem Cytol 3:457.

Moore MAS, Metcalf D (1970): Br J Haematol 18:279.

Moore MAS, Owen JJT (1967a): Lancet 2:658.

Moore MAS, Owen JJT (1967b): Nature 215:1081.

Moore MAS, Owen JJT (1965): Nature 208:956.

Moore MAS, McNeill TA, Haskill JS (1970): J Cell Physiol 75:181.

Moore MAS, Williams N, Metcalf D (1972): J Cell Physiol 79:283.

Morris RB, Nichols BA, Bainton DF (1975): Developmental Biol 44:223.

Morrison JH (1967): Brit J Haemat 13:229

Morstyn D, Nicola NA, Metcalf D (1980): Blood 56:798.

Morey ER, Baylink DJ (1978): Science 201:1138.

Morton HJ (1968): Proc Soc Exp Biol Med 128:112

Moses C, Platt M (1951): Science 113:676.

Mrlevic D et al (1970): Acta Anat 76:35.

Murphy MJ, Bertles JF, Gordon AS (1971): J Cell Sci 9:23.

Murray PDF (1932): Proc R Soc (B) Lond 111:497.

Naegeli O (1900): Deutsch Med Woch 26:287.

Naegeli O (1931): "Blutkrankheiten und Blut diagnostik," 5th Ed. Berlin: Julius Springer.

Nagahama M (1959): J Kyu Hem Soc 9:299.

Nagao K (1920): J Infect Dis 27:527.

Nagao K (1921): J Infect Dis 28:294.

Nagao K, Angrist AA (1968): Nature 217:960.

Najean Y, Ardailou N (1969): Scand J Haematol 6:395.

Nakeff A, Daniels-McQueen S (1976): Proc Soc Exp Biol Med 151:587.

Nathan DG, Chess L, Hillman DG, Clarke B, Breard G, Merler E, Housman DE (1978): J Exp Med 147:324

Necas E (1981): Cell Tissue Kinet 14:537.

Ness PM, Stengle JM (1974): In Surgenor DM (ed): "The Red Blood Cell." New York: Academic Press.

Neumann E (1868): Zentralbl Med Wissensch 6:689.

Neumann E (1869a): C R Acad Sci (Paris) 68:1112.

Neumann E (1869b): Arch Heilk 10:68.

Neumann E (1870): Arch Heilk 10:1.

Neumann E (1877): Berl Klin Wochenschr 14:865.

Neumann E (1878): Berl Klin Wochenschr 15:69.

Neumann E (1882a): Centralbl Wiss Med 6:689.

Neumann E (1882b): Zentralbl Med Wissensch 20:321.

Neumann E (1890a): Arch Pathol Anat U Physiol 119:385.

Neumann E (1890b): Virchows Arch 119:835.

Nicola NA, Metcalf D, Melchner HV, Burgess WA (1981): Blood 58:376.

Niskanen E, Olofsson T, Cline MJ (1979): Am J Hematol 7:201.

Nizet A (1946): Acta Med Scand 124:590.

Nutting WL (1951): J Morphol 89:501.

Nye RN (1931): Proc Soc Exp Biol Med 29:34.

Oberling F, Cazenove JP, Waitz R (1972): Pathol Biol 20:337.

Odell TT, Jackson CW, Gosslee DG (1965): Proc Soc Exp Biol Med 119:1194.

Odell TT, Jackson CW, Friday TJ, Charsha DE (1969): Br J Haematol 17:91.
Odell TT, Jackson CW, Reiter RS (1967): Acta Haematol 38:34.
Odell TT, McDonald TP (1964): Am J Physiol 206:580.
Odell TT Jr, McDonald TP, Assno M (1962): Acta Haematol 27:171.
Odell TT, Jackson CW (1967): Blood 30:548.
Oehlbeck LWF, Robscheit-Robbins FS, Whipple GH (1932): J Exp Med 56:425.
Ogawa M, Grush OC, O'Dell RF, et al (1977): Blood 50:1081.
Ogawa M, McEachern MD, Wilson JM et al (1976): Blood 48:980.
Ogilvie BM, Mackenzie CD, Love RJ (1977): Am J Trop Med Hygiene 26:61.
Ohuye T (1932): Sci Rep Tohoku Imp Univ 7:49.
Okos AJ, Gathings WE (1977): Fed Proc 36:1294A.
Okunewick JP, Fulton D (1970): Blood 36:239.
Okunewick JP, Hartley KM, Doreden J (1969): Radiat Res 38:540.
Orlic D, Gordon AS, Rhodin JAG (1965): J Ultrastruct Res 13:516.
Osada Y, Ogawa S (1961): Bull Inst Public Health (Tokyo) 10:205.
Osada Y, Ogawa S (1962): Bull Inst Public Health (Tokyo) 11:111.
Osada Y, Ogawa S (1964): Bull Inst Pulbic Health (Tokyo) 13:1.
Osgood EE (1954): Blood 9:1141.
Osmond DG: In Yoffey JM (ed): "The Lymphocyte in Immunology and Haemopoiesis." London: Edward Arnold, p 120.
Osmond DG (1968): Anat Rec 160:402.
Osmond DG (1975): J Reticuloendothel Soc 17:99.
Osmond DG (1980): Monogr Allergy 16:157.
Osmond DG, Everett NB (1964): Blood 23:1.
Osmond DG, Everett NB (1965): J Exp Physiol 50:1.
Osmond DG, Miller SC, Yoshida Y (1973): In Wolstenholme GEW, O'Connor M (eds): "Haemopoietic Stem Cells," Ciba Found Symposium 13 NS. Amsterdam: Associated Scientific Publishers, p 131.
Osmond DG, Nossal GJV (1974a): Cell Immunol 13:117.
Osmond DG, Nossal GJV (1974b): Cell Immunol 13:132.
Osmond DG, Roylance PJ, Lee WR, Ramsell TG, Yoffey JM (1966): Br J Haematol 12:365.
Osmond DG, Yoshida Y (1971): Proc Fourth Ann Leukocyte Culture Conference, p 97.
Osogoe B, Omura K (1950): Anat Rec 108:663.
Ottolenghi D (1902): Arch Ital Biol 37:73.
Owen JJT, Wright DE, Haba S, Raff MC, Cooper MD (1977): J Immunol 118:2067.
Padawer J, Gordon AS (1952): Proc Soc Biol Med 80:581.

Palade GE (1953): J Appl Physiol 5:1424.

Palade GE (1961): Circulation 24:368.

Papayannopoulou TH, Nute PE, Kuruchi S, Stamatoyannopoulos G (1978): Blood 51:671.

Papiernik M (1971): Biol Neonate 19:163.

Pappenheim A (1907): Folia Haematol 4:1, 142.

Pappenheim A, Ferrata A (1910): Folia Haematol I Teil (Arch) 10:78.

Parmley RT, Ogawa M, Spier SS, Bank HL, Wright NJ (1978): Exp Hematol 6:78.

Pataryas MA, Stamatoyannopoulos G (1972): Blood 39:688.

Patek BR, Bernick S (1960): Anat Rec 138:27.

Patinkin D, Grover NB, Yoffey JM (1979): Br J Haematol 41:309.

Patt HM (1957): Blood 12:777.

Patt HM, Maloney MA (1959): In Stohlman FJ (ed): "Kinetics of Cellular Proliferation." New York: Grune and Stratton, p 201.

Patt HM, Maloney MA (1964): Ann NY Acad Sci 113:515.

Patt HM, Maloney MA (1975): Exp Hematol 3:135.

Patt HM, Maloney MA, Flannery ML (1982): Exp Hematol 10:738.

Paul J, Conkie D, Freshney RI (1969): Cell Tissue Kinet 2:283.

Paulus JM (1971): "Platelet Kinetics: Radioisotopic, Cytological, Mathematical and Clinical Aspects." Amsterdam: North-Holland.

Paulus JM (1970): Blood 35:298.

Paulus JM (1967): Blood 29:407.

Paulus JM (1968a): Exp Cell Res 53:310.

Paulus JM (1968b): Nouv Rev Fr Hematol 8:394.

Paulus JM, Pennington DG, Kinet-Denol C, Jackson CW, Odell T (1971): In Paulus JM (ed): "Platelet Kinetics." Amsterdam: North-Holland, p 330.

Peabody FW (1926): Am J Pathol 2:487.

Pedersen NT (1974): Scand J Haematol 13:225.

Pedersen NT (1978): Scand J Haematol 21:396.

Pegg DR (1966): "Bone Marrow Transplantation." Chicago: Year Book Medical Publishers, p 11.

Pennington DG (1969): Br Med J 4:782.

Pennington DG, Streatfield K, Weste SM (1974): In Baldinin MG, Ebbe S (eds): "Platelets Production, Function, Transfusion and Storage." New York: Grune & Stratton, pp 115–130.

Pennington DG, Olsen TE (1970): Br J Haematol 18:447.

Perris AD, Whitfield JF, Rixon RH (1967): Rad Res 32:550.

Peschle C, Migliaccio AR, Migliaccio G, Ciccarielloo R, Lettiere F, Quatrin S, Russo G, Mastoberardino G (1981): Blood 58:565.

Peterson EA, Evans WH (1967): Nature (Lond) 214:824.

Petrakis NC (1952): J Appl Physiol 4:549.

Petrakis NL (1965): Am J Phys Anthropol 25:119.

Petrakis NL, Davis M, Lucia SP (1961): Blood 17:109.

Petrakis NL (1966): Am J Phys Anthropol 25:119.

Petrakis NL, Pons S, Lee RE (1969): In Vitro 4:3.

Piersima AH, Ploemacher RE, Brochbank KGM (1982): Exp Hematol 10 (Suppl 11):82.

Piney A (1922): Br Med J 2:792.

Pisciotta AV, Santos AS, Keller C (1964): J Lab Clin Med 63:445.

Pisciotta AV, Stefanni M, Dameshek W (1953): Blood 8:703.

Playfair JHL, Wolfendale MR, Kay HEM (1963): Br J Haematol 9:336.

Ploemacher RE, Van Soest PL, Wagemacher G, Van Thull E (1979): Cell Tissue Kinet 12:539.

Pluznik DH, Sachs L (1965): J Cell Comp Physiol 66:319.

Ponfick E (1869): Virch Arch Pathol Anat 48:1.

Ponzio NM, Speirs RS (1975): Immunology 28:243.

Popp RA (1960): Proc Soc Exp Biol NY 104:722.

Post M, Shoemaker WC (1964): J Bone Joint Surg 46A:111.

Pouchet G (1878): C R Soc Biol (Paris) 30:37.

Prchal JF, Axelrad AA (1974): N Engl J Med 290:1382.

Press O, Rosse C (1977): Cell Immunol 28:218.

Press O, Rosse C, Clagett J (1977): J Exp Med 146:735.

Prindull G, Prindull B, Palti Z, Yoffey JM (1975): Biol Neonate 27:318.

Prindull G, Prindull B, Meulen NVD (1978): Acta Paediatr Scand 67:413.

Prindull G, Gabriel M, Prindull B (1981): Blut 43:109.

Prothero JW, Starling M, Rosse C (1978): Cell Tissue Kinet 11:301.

Quesenberry P, Levitt L (1979): N Engl J Med 301:755, 819, 868.

Rabellino EM, Nachman RL, Williams N, Winchester RJ, Ross GD (1979): J Exp Med 149:1273.

Radley JM, Scurfield G (1980): Blood 56:996.

Radley JM, Haller CJ (1982): Blood 60:213.

Radley JM, Haller CL (1983): Br J Haematol 53:277.

Raff MC, Megson M, Owen JJT, Cooper MD (1976): Nature 259:224.

Ramsell TG, Yoffey JM (1961): Acta Anat 47:55.

Ranvier LA (1899): "Traite Technique d'Histologie." Paris: F Savy.

Ranvier LA (1874): Arch Physiol 11 (Ser 2):429.

Rappaport H, Braum M, Horrell JB (1951): Am J Pathol 27:407.

Ravindranth MH (1977): Cytologia 42:743.

Rebuck JW, Crowley JH (1955): Ann NY Acad Sci 59:757.

Reid CDL, Baptista LC, Chanarin I (1981): Brit J Haemat 48:155.

Rencricca NJ, Howard D, Kubanek B, Stohlman F (1976): Scand J Haematol 16:189.

Rencricca NJ, Rizzoli V, Howard D, Duffy P, Stohlman F (1970): Blood 36:764.

Rhoads CP, Miller DK (1938): Arch Pathol 26:648.

Rice FAH (1966): Proc Soc Exp Biol Med 123:189.

Rich IN, Kubranek B (1976): Blut 33:171.

Rich IN, Kubranek B (1980): J Embryol Exp Morphol 58:143.

Riches CK, Sharp JG, Littlewood V, Briscoe CV, Thomas DB (1976a): J Anat 172:717.

Riches AC, Thomas DB, Briscoe CV, Littlewood V, Sharp JG (1976b): Wadsley Med Bull 6:35.

Richman CM, Chess L, Yankee RA (1978): Blood 51:1.

Rickard KA, Rencricca NJ, Shadduck RK, Monette FC, Howard DE, Garrity M, Stohlman F (1971): Br J Haematol 21:537.

Rifkind RA, Chui D, Epler H (1969): J Cell Biol 40:343.

Riley JF (1959): "The Mast Cells." London: Livingstone.

Rind H (1967): Handb Kinderheilkunde 6:740.

Rindfleisch GE (1880): Arch Mikr Anat 17:21.

Robertson OH (1917): J Exp Med 26:221.

Robin C (1849): C R Sci Biol (Paris) 1:149.

Robin C (1875): "Dictionnaire Encyclopedique des Sciences Medicales," pp 1–33.

Robinson WA, Mangalik A (1975): Sem Hematol 12:7.

Robinson WA, Pike BL (1970): In Stohlman F (ed): "Haemopoietic Cellular Proliferation." New York: Grune & Stratton, p 249.

Rohlich K (1941): Z Mikr Anat Forsch 49:425.

Rolovic Z, Baldini M, Dameshek W (1970): Blood 35:173.

Rollet A (1870): Untersuch Inst Physiol Histol Graz Leipz 1:1.

Ropke C, Everett NB (1974a): Cell Tissue Kinet 7:137.

Ropke C, Everett NB (1974b): Cell Tissue Kinet 6:499.

Ropke K, Hougen HP, Everett NB (1975): Cell Immunol 15:82.

Rosenberg M (1969): Blood 33:66.

Rosenquist GC (1966): Contrib Embryol 38:71.

Rosse C (1969): Blood 34:72.

Rosse C (1970a): Nature 227:73.

Rosse C (1970b): Zeiss Inform 73:90.

Rosse C (1971): Blood 38:372.

Rosse C (1972a): Blood 40:90.

Rosse C (1973): In Wolstenholme GEW, O'Connor M (eds): "Haemopoietic Stem Cells." Ciba Found Symposium No. 13. Amsterdam: Associated Scientific Publishers, p 105.

Rosse C (1976): Int Rev Cytol 45:155.

Rosse C, Beaufait DW (1978): Anat Rec 191:135.

Rosse C, Cole SB, Appleton C, Press OW, Clagett J (1978): Cell Immunol 37:254.

Rosse C, Griffiths DA, Edwards AE, Gaches CGC, Long ALH, Wright JLW, Yoffey JM (1970): Acta Haematol (Basel) 43:80.

Rosse C, Kraemer MJ, Dillon TL, McFarland JG, Smith MJ (1977): J Lab Clin Med 89:1225.

Rosse C, Press OW (1978): Blood Cells 4:65.

Rosse C, Trotter JA (1974a): Blood 43:885.

Rosse C, Trotter JA (1974b): Am J Anat 141:41.

Rosse C, Yoffey JM (1967): J Anat 102:113.

Rothermel JE (1930): Anat Rec 47:251.

Rous P (1923): Physiol Rev 3:75.

Rozing J, Brons NHC, Benner R (1978): Immunology 34:909.

Rubinstein AS, Trobaugh FE (1973): Blood 42:61.

Rudnick D (1938): Anat Rec 70:395.

Russell ES, Bernstein SE (1966): Blood and blood formation. In Green EL (ed): "Biology of the Laboratory Mouse." New York: McGraw-Hill, p 351.

Ryfkind RA, Terada M, Marks PA (1971): Ser Haematol 4:7.

Ryser J, Vassalli P (1974): J Immunol 113:719.

Rytomaa T (1960): Acta Pathol Microbiol Scand (Suppl) 140:1.

Sahebekhtiari HA, Tavassoli M (1976): Scand J Haematol 16:13.

Sahebekhtiari HA, Tavassoli M (1978): Cell Tissue Res 192:437.

Sabin FR (1928): Physiol Rev 8:191.

Sakakeeny MA, Greenberger JS (1982): J Natl Cancer Inst 68:305.

Sawada U, Adler SS (1981): Blut 42:1.

Scharrer E (1944): Anat Rec 88:291.

Scheinin TM, Korvuniemi AP (1962): Cancer 15:972.

Scheinin TM, Korvuneimi AP (1963): Blood 22:82.

Schlecht H (1910): Deutsch Arch Klin Med 98:308.

Schlecht H, Schwenker G (1912): Deutsch Arch Klin Med 108:405.

Schleicher EM (1946): Anat Rec 95:379.

Schleiden MJ (1838): Muller's Arch Anat Physiol Wissensch Med 5:137.

Schlesinger M, Hurvitz D (1968): J Exp Med 127:1127.

Schofield R (1970): Cell Tissue Kinet 3:119.

Schooley JC, Giger K (1962); Semiannual Report, Donner Laboratory, Lawrence Radiation Laboratory Report UCRL 10683, p 176.

Schooley JC, Garcia JF, Cantor LN, Havens VW (1968): Ann NY Acad Sci 149:266.

Schridde H (1907): Zbl Allg Path 18:823.

Schotton D (1978): Nature 272:16.

Schulz H (1968): "Thrombocyten and Thrombose in electronmikroskipischen Bild." Berlin: Springer-Verlag.

Scuderi P, Rosse C, Everett NB (1977): Anat Rec 189:141.

Schwann T (1847): "Microscopical Researches Into the Accordance in the Structure and Growth of Animals and Plants." Smith H (Trans). London: Sydenham Society.

Seip M (1953): Acta Med Scand 146, Suppl 282:1.

Seki M (1973): Transplantation 16:544.

Settle GW (1954): Contrib Embryol 241:223.

Shaklai M, Tavassoli M (1977): Lancet 2:305.

Shaklai M, Tavassoli M (1978a): J Ultrastruct Res 62:270.

Shaklai M, Tavassoli M (1978b): Am J Anat 151:139.

Shaklai M, Tavassoli M (1979): J Ultrastruct Res 69:343.

Shapiro M (1968): J Insect Physiol 43:999.

Sharp JG, Thomas DB, Briscoe CV, Littlewood V, Riches AC (1976): Wadsley Med Bull 6:23.

Shaw NE (1964): Ann R Coll Surg Engl 35:214.

Sheard A (1924): "Pernicious Anaemia and Aplastic Anaemia." New York: Williams Wood.

Shinpock SG, Goodman JW (1978): Cell Tissue Kinet 11:111.

Shortman K (1972): Ann Rev Biophys Bioeng 1:93.

Shotton D (1978): Nature 272:16.

Siegel CD (1970): In Gordon AS (ed): "Regulation of Hematopoiesis." New York: Appleton-Century-Crofts, p 67.

Silini G, Pozzi LV, Pons S (1967): J Embryol Exp Morphol 17:303.

Silini G, Andreozzi U, Pozzi L (1976): Cell Tissue Kinet 9:341.

Silini G, Pons S, Pozzi CV (1968): Br J Haematol 14:489.

Simar IJ, Haot J, Betz EH (1968): Eur J Cancer 4:529.

Siminia T (1974): Cell Tissue Res 150:443.

Siminia T (1972): Z Zellforsch Microsk Anat 130:497.

Simionescu M, Simionescu N, Palade GE (1981a): J Cell Biol 90:605.

Simionescu M, Simionescu N, Silbert JE, Palade GE (1981b): J Cell Biol 90:614.

Simionescu M, Simionescu N, Palade GE (1982a): J Cell Biol 94:406.

Simionescu M, Simionescu N, Palade GE (1982b): J Cell Biol 95:425.

Siminovitch L (1965): Radiat Res 24:482.

Simpson CE, Kling JM (1967): J Cell Biol 35:237.

Skutelsky E, Danon D (1969): J Cell Biol 43:8.

Skutelsky E, Danon D (1972): Anat Rec 173:123.

Slavin BG (1972): Int Rev Cytol 33:297.

Slavin BG, Yoffey JM, Yaffe P (1981): Prog Clin Biol Res 59B:231.

Smith EB, Butcher J (1952): Blood 7:214.

Smith H (1962): J Clin Pathol 15:260.

Sokol J, Wales J, Norris PD, Hudson G (1982): J Anat 135:615.

Sorensen GD (1961): Ann NY Acad Sci 111:45.

Spicer S, Greene WB, Hardin JH (1969): J Histochem Cytochem 17:781.

Spiers RS (1958): Ann NY Acad Sci 73:283.

Spiers RS, Dreisbach ME (1956): Blood 11:44.

Spry CJF (1971): Cell Tissue Kinet 4:351.

Stamatoyannopoulos G, Nienhuis AW (1978): "Cellular and Molecular Regulation of Hemoglobin Switching." New York: Grune & Stratton.

Stamatoyannopoulos G, Nienhuis AW (1981): "Hemoglobins in Development and Differentiation." New York: Alan R. Liss.

Starling MR, Rosse C (1976): Cell Tissue Kinet 9:191.

Steinberg B, Martin RA (1950): Am J Physiol 161:14.

Stephensen JR, Axelrad A, McLeod DL, Shreeve MM (1971): Proc Natl Acad Sci USA 68:1542.

Stites DP, Wybran J, Carr MC, Fudenberg HH (1972): In Wolstenholme GEW, O'Connor M (eds): Ciba Found Symposium "Development of Cellular Immunocompetence in Man." London: Ciba Foundation, p 113.

Stohlman F (1961): Proc Soc Exp Biol Med 107:751.

Storer JB, Lushbaugh CC, Furchner JE (1952): J Lab Clin Med 40:355.

Stricker S (1868): Arch Ges Physiol 1:590.

Sugijama S (1926): Embryology 97:121.

Suit HD (1957): J Clin Pathol 10:267.

Suit HD, Lajtha LG, Oliver R, Ellis F (1957): Br J Haematol 3:165.

Sutherland DJA, Till JE, McCulloch EA (1971): Cell Tissue Kinet 4:479.

Symann M, Anckaert MA, Cordier A, Rodhain J, Sokal G (1978): Exp Hematol 6:749.

Symann M, Fontebruonie A, Ansesnberry PL, Howard F, Stohlman F (1976): Cell Tissue Kinet 9:41.

Tateno K (1957): J Kyu Hem Soc 7:150.

Tavassoli M (1974a): Acta Anat 90:608.

Tavassoli M (1974b): Experientia 30:424.

Tavassoli M (1974c): Arch Pathol Lab Med 98:189.

Tavassoli M (1974d): J Reticuloendothel Soc 15:163.

Tavassoli M (1975a): Exp Hematol 3:213.

Tavassoli M (1975b): West J Med 122:194.

Tavassoli M (1976a): Arch Pathol Lab Med 100:16.

Tavassoli M (1976b): Acta Anat 94:65.

Tavassoli M (1977a): Br J Haematol 35:25.

Tavassoli M (1977b): Br J Haematol 36:323.

Tavassoli M (1978a): In Hibino S, Takakn F, Shahich NT (eds): "Aplastic Anemia." Tokyo: University of Tokyo Press.

Tavassoli M (1978b): Scand J Haematol 20:330.

Tavassoli M (1978c): Exp Hematol 6:257.

Tavassoli M (1979a): Blood Cell 5:89.

Tavassoli M (1979b): Br J Haematol 41:297.

Tavassoli M (1980a): Blood 55:537.

Tavassoli M (1980b): Exp Hematol 10:435.

Tavassoli M (1981a): Br J Haematol 49:660.

Tavassoli M (1981b): In Acosta-Virido E, Salvia MA (eds): "Advances in the Morphology of Cells and Tissue." New York: Alan R. Liss, pp 249–256.

Tavassoli M (1982a): Blood 60:1059.

Tavassoli M (1982b): Scanning Electron Microscopy 1:349.

Tavassoli M (1982c): Exp Hematol 10:435.

Tavassoli M, Aoki M (1981): Br J Haematol 48:25.

Tavassoli M, Aoki M, Shaklai M (1980): Exp Hematol 8:568.

Tavassoli M, Crosby WH (1968): Science 161:54.

Tavassoli M, Crosby WH (1973): Science 173:912.

Tavassoli M, Crosby WH (1970): Science 169:291.

Tavassoli M, Eastlund DT, Yam OT, Neiman RS, Finkel HE (1976): Scand J Haematol 16:311.

Tavassoli M, Friedenstein AJ: Am J Hematol (in press).

Tavassoli M, Houchin DN, Jacob P (1977): Scand J Haematol 18:47.

Tavassoli M, Khademi R (1980): Experientia 36:1126.

Tavassoli M, Maniatis A, Crosby WH (1972): Br J Haematol 23:707.

Tavassoli M, Maniatis A, Crosby WH (1974): Blood 43:33.

Tavassoli M, Ratzan RJ, Maniatis A, Crosby WH (1973a): J Reticuloendothel Soc 13:518.

Tavassoli M, Ratzan RJ, Crosby WH (1973b): Blood 41:701.

Tavassoli M, Shaklai M (1979): Br J Haematol 41:303.

Tavassoli M, Takahashi K (1982): Am J Anat 164:91.

Tavassoli M, Watson LR, Khademi MR (1979): Cell Tissue Res 200:215.

Tavassoli M, Weiss L (1971): Anat Rec 171:477.

Tavassoli M, Weiss L (1973): Blood 42:267.

Terry RW, Bainton DF, Farquhar MG (1969): Lab Invest 21:65.

Thiele J, Ballard AC, Georgii A (1977): Virchow's Arch B Cell Pathol 23:33.

Thiery JB, Bessis M (1956a): C R Acad Sci (Paris) 242:290.

Thiery JB, Bessis M (1956b): Rev Hematol 2:162.

Thomas DB (1971): J Anat 110:297.

Thomas DB (1973): In Wolstenholme GEW, O'Connor M (eds): "Haemopoietic Stem Cells," Ciba Found Symposium. Amsterdan: Associated
Scientific Publishers, p 71.

Thomas DB, Yoffey JM (1962): Br J Haematol 8:290.

Thomas DB, Yoffey JM (1964): Br J Haematol 10:193.

Thomas DB, Sharp JG, Briscoe V (1977): J Anat (Lond) 124:21.

Thomas DB, Yoffey JM (1962): Br J Haematol 8:290.

Thomas DB, Yoffey JM (1964): Br J Haematol 10:193.

Thomas ED, Fliedner TM, Thomas D, Cronkite EP (1965): J Lab Clin Med
65:794.

Till JE, McCulloch EA (1961): Radiat Res 14:213.

Tillmann W, Prindull G, Schroter W (1976): Eur J Pediatr 123:51.

Timonen T, Ortaldo JR, Herberman RB (1981): J Exp Med 153:569.

Timonen T, Saskela E, Ranki A, Hayry P (1979): Cell Immunol 48:133.

Tinggaard Pedersen N, Cohen J (1981): Scand J Haematol 27:51.

Tocantins LM, O'Neill JF (1941): Surg Gynecol Obstet 73:281.

Toldt C, Zuckerkandel E (1875): SB Akad Wiss Wein Math Nat Kl 72:241.

Trachtenberg F (1932): Folia Haematol 46:1.

Trentin JJ (1970): In Gordon AS (ed): "Regulation of Hematopoiesis." New
York: Appleton-Century-Crofts, p 161.

Trentin JJ (1971): Am J Pathol 65:621.

Tribukait B, Forssberg A (1964): Naturwissenschaften 51:12.

Trobaugh FE, Lewis JP (1964): J Clin Invest 43:1306.

Trubowitz S, Bathija A (1977): Blood 49:599.

Tsien RY, Pozzan T, Rink TJ (1982): Nature 295:68.

Turner MS, Hurst JM, Yoffey JM (1967): Br J Haematol 13:942.

Turner AR, Pfrimmer WJ, Torok-Storb BJ, Boggs DR (1978): Am J Hematol
4:105.

Turpen JB, Knudson CM (1982): Dev Biol 89:138.

Turpen JB, Knudson CM, Hoefen PS (1981): Dev Biol 85:99.

Tyan ML (1968): J Immunol 100:535.

Tyan ML, Herzenberg LA (1968): Proc Soc Exp Biol Med 128:952.

Tyan ML, Herzenberg LA, Gibbs PR (1969): J Immunol 103:1238.

Tyler RWC, Everett NB (1966): Blood 28:873.

Tyler RW, Everett NB (1972): Blood 39:249.

Tyler RW, Rosse C, Everett NB (1972): J Reticuloendothel Soc 11:617.

Uchida M (1958): J Kyu Hem Soc 8:905.

Ueno Y, Korizume S, Yamagami M, Miara M, Taniguchi N (1981): Exp Hematol 9:716.

Unanue ER, Grey HM, Rabellino E, Campbell P, Schmidtke J (1971): J Exp Med 133:1188.

Vainchenker W, Guichard J, Breton-Gorius J (1979): Blood Cells 5:25.

Van den Berghe L, Blitstein I (1945): C R Soc Biol (Paris) 139:325.

Van der Stricht O (1892): Arch Biol 12:199.

Van Dyke D (1967): Clin Orthop 52:37.

Van Dyke DC, Huff RL (1951): Am J Physiol 165:341.

Variot P, Remy CH (1880): J Anat Physiol 6:73.

Vazquez JJ, Lewis JH (1960): Blood 16:968.

Volkman A (1966): J Exp Med 124:241.

Volkman A, Gowans JL (1966): Br J Exp Pathol 46:62.

Vos O, Luiten F, Erkens-Versluis ME (1981): Blut 43:33.

Warren A (1965): "Comparative Hematology." New York: Grune & Stratton.

Watanabe Y (1966): Tohoku J Exp Med 89:167.

Weber EH (1846): Z Rat Med (Zurich) 4:160.

Weber TH, Stantesson B, Skoog VT (1973): Scand J Haematol 11:177.

Weinrel EL (1958): Zoologica 43:145.

Weinrel EL (1963): Anat Rec 147:219.

Weiskotten HG (1930): Am J Pathol 6:183.

Weiss L (1965): J Morphol 117:467.

Weiss L (1970): Blood 36:189.

Weiss L (1976): Anat Rec 186:161.

Weiss LP, Wislocki GB (1956): Anat Rec 126:143.

Weitz-Hamburger A, LoBue J, Sharkis SH, Gordon AS, Alexander P (1971): J Anat 109:549.

Wertheim G, Silverman H, Yoffey JM (1982): In preparation.

Westen H, Bainton DF (1979): J Exp Med 150:919.

Wetzel C (1910): Arch Entw Mech Org 30:507.

Wharton-Jones T (1846): Phil Trans R Soc Lond (Biol) 136:63.

Whitby L (1948): Blood 3:934.

Whitby LEH, Britton CJC (1963): "Disorders of the Blood," 9th Ed. London: Churchill.

Wigglesworth VB (1959): Ann Rev Ent 4:1.

Williams N, Moore M (1973): J Cell Physiol 82:81.

Willie AH (1980): Nature 284:555.

Wilson FD, Tavassoli M, Greenberg BR, Hinds D, Klein AK (1981): Stem Cells 1:15.

Wilt FH (1965): Science 147:1588.

Winquist G (1960): Exp Cell Res 19:7.

Winter GCB, Byles AB, Yoffey JM (1965): Lancet 11:932.

Wintrobe MM (1961): "Clinical Hematology," 5th Ed. London: Hery Kimpton.

Wislocki GB (1921): Johns Hopkins Hosp Bull 32:132.

Wislocki GB (1924): Am J Anat 32:423.

Wolf NS (1979): Clin Haematol 8:469.

Wolf N, Rosse C (1982): Am J Anat 163:131.

Woodard HQ, Holodny E (1960): Phys Med Biol 5:57.

Worton RG, McCulloch EA, Till JE (1969): J Cell Physiol 74:171.

Wright JH (1906): Boston Med Surg J 154:643.

Wright JH (1910): J Morphol 21:263.

Wright RK (1981): In Ratcliffe WA, Rowley AF (eds): "Invertebrate Blood Cells," Vol I. New York: Academic Press.

Wyllie AH, Kerr JFR, Currie AF (1980): Int Rev Cytol 68:251.

Yamada E (1957): Acta Anat 29:267.

Yaffe P, Yoffey JM (1982): J Anat 134:739.

Yoffey JM (1929): J Anat 63:314.

Yoffey JM (1954): Bone Marrow. Br Med J 11:193.

Yoffey JM (1957): Brookhaven Symp Biol 10:1.

Yoffey JM (1962): J Anat (Lond) 96:425.

Yoffey JM (1965): Bibl Anat 7:298.

Yoffey JM (1966): Bone Marrow Reactions. London: Edward Arnold.

Yoffey JM (1968): J Anat (Lond) 102:583.

Yoffey JM (1971): Israel J Med Sci 7:825.

Yoffey JM (1974): "Bone Marrow in Hypoxia and Rebound." Springfield, IL: Chas C. Thomas Co.

Yoffey JM (1977): Advances in Microcirculation 7:49.

Yoffey JM (1980): Int Rev Cytol 62:311.

Yoffey JM (1981): In Kendall MD (ed): "The Thymus Gland." New York: Academic Press, p 185.

Yoffey JM, Ancill RJ, Holt JAG, Owen-Smith B, Herdan G (1954): J Anat 88:115.

Yoffey JM, Brynmor TD (1964): J Anat 95:613.

Yoffey JM, Courtice FC (1970): "Lymphatics, Lymph and the Lymphmyeloid Complex." New York: Academic Press.

Yoffey JM, Everett MB, Reinhardt WO (1959): In Stohlman FJ (ed): "Kinetics of Cellular Proliferation." New York: Grune & Stratton, Inc., p 69.

Yoffey JM, Hudson G, Osmond DG (1965): J Anat 99:841.

Yoffey JM, Jeffreys RV, Osmond DG, Turner MS, Tahsin SC, Niven P (1968): Ann NY Acad Sci 149:179.

Yoffey JM, Makin GS, Yates AK, Davis CJF, Griffiths DA, Waring IS (1964): Ann NY Acad Sci 113:790.

Yoffey JM, Patinkin D, Grover NB (1978): Israel J Med Sci 14:1247.

Yoffey JM, Rich WJCC, Tidman MK, Cummins BH, Roy RR (1964): Ann NY Acad Sci 113:1053.

Yoffey JM, Ron A, Prindull G, Yaffe P (1978): Clin Immunol Immunopathol 9:491.

Yoffey JM, Rosse ZC, Moffatt DJ, Sutherland IH (1965): Acta Anat 62:476.

Yoffey JM, Smith NCW, Wilson RS (1966): Scand J Haematol 3:186.

Yoffey JM, Smith NCW, Wilson RS (1967): Scand J Haematol 4:145.

Yoffey JM, Thomas DB (1964): J Anat 65:913.

Yoffey JM, Thomas DB, Moffatt DE, Sutherland IH, Rosse C (1961): "Biological Activity of Leukocytes," Ciba Foundation Study Group #10. London: J. & A. Churchill, pp 45–54.

Yoffey JM, Weinberg A (1976): Proc 6th Europ Congress Electron Microscopy, p 590.

Yoffey JM, Yaffe P (1980a): J Reticuloendothel Soc 28:37.

Yoffey JM, Yaffe P (1980b): J Anat 130:333.

Yoffey JM, Yaffe P (1982): Unpublished Observations.

Yoshida Y, Osmond DG (1971): Blood 37:73.

Zach E, Shafrir E (1974): Israel J Med Sci 10:1541.

Zachary D, Hoffman JA (1973): Z Zellforsch Mikrosk Anat 141:55.

Zajicek J (1957): Acta Physiol Scand (Suppl) 40:138.

Zakaria E, Shafrir E (1967): Proc Soc Exp Biol Med 124:1265.

Zamboni J, Pease DC (1961): J Ultrastruct Res 5:65.

Zanjani ED, Hjamm LJ, Burlington H, Gordon AS, Wasserman LR (1974a): Blood 44:285.

Zanjani ED, Peterson EN, Gordon AS, Wasserman LR (1974b): J Lab Clin Med 83:281.

Zanjani ED, Poster J, Burlington H, Mann LI, Wassermann LR (1977): 89:640.

Zinkernagel RM, Callahan GN, Althage A, Cooper NS (1978): J Exp Med 147:882.

Zucali JR, Van Zant G, Rakowitz P, Gordon AS (1974): Exp Hematol 2:250.

Zucker-Franklin D (1969): Sem Hematol 6:4.

Zucker-Franklin D (1974): Adv Int Med 19:1.

Zucker-Franklin D (1980): Blood 56:534.

Zucker-Franklin D (1970): In Gordon AS (ed): "Regulation of Hematopoiesis." New York: Appleton-Century-Crofts, p 1553.

Zucker-Franklin (1981): Blood 58:545.

Zuckerman KS, Wicha MS (1983): Blood 61:540.

Zweig SE, Tokuyasu KT, Singer JS (1981): J Supramol Struct Cell Biochem
17:163.

Index

Transitional (stem) cell compartment,
cont'd
labeling index, 223, 224, 228
leptochromatic, 220, 221, 226
"lymphoid cells," 218, 226, 228, 233
morphology, 218–225
nuclear structure, 221–222
proliferation gradient, 223–225
schema, 229
self-replication and differentiation
equilibrium, 228–229, 232, 234
size spectrum, 219–221
terminology, 218, 232–234
velocity sedimentation test, 224
see also Stem cells
Transplantation, marrow
early, abdominal grafts, 14–15
fetal, 231
stem cells after, 250–251
stroma in, 62
Trichinella spiralis, 156
Trout, hemopoiesis, 24, 25
Tubular bones, 62
Tubules, transfer, marrow, 96
Twins, 58
Typhoid (TAB) vaccine, neutrophil
effects, 147–151
blood, 147, 149, 150, 151
marrow, 148

Urine, paroxysmal nocturnal
hemoglobinuria, 255
Urodeles, hemopoiesis, 26

Vaccine, typhoid (TAB), neutrophil
effects, 147–151
blood, 147, 149, 150, 151
marrow, 148
Valéry, Paul, 8
Veins, marrow, 66–68; see also
Circulation, marrow
Vertebrae, caudal, and red and yellow
marrow distribution, 111
Vesicle transfer between cells, 53, 61

Weight, body, and marrow volume, 108
White bodies, 21
White cells precede red cells in
phylogeny, 19
Worms, 19–21
Wright-Giemsa satin, 201

X cells, 233

Yolk sac in ontogeny of hemopoeisis,
32–39
blood islands, 32–34
CFU-GM, 36–38
CFU-S, 36, 37
dependence on endoderm, 33, 34
fetal hemopoiesis, 235, 236
migration to liver, 40
primitive cf. definitive, 34–39
stem cell precursor, 35–36
see also Stem cells